W9-CQM-254

A Massage Therapist's Guide to Business

Laura Allen, NCTMB

Wolters Kluwer | Lippincott Williams & Wilkins
Health

Philadelphia • Baltimore • New York • London
Buenos Aires • Hong Kong • Sydney • Tokyo

Acquisitions Editor: Kelley Squazzo
Product Manager: Linda G. Francis
Development Editor: Betsy Dilernia
Marketing Manager: Shauna Kelley
Design Coordinator: Teresa Mallon
Compositor: SPi Global

Copyright © 2012 Lippincott Williams & Wilkins
351 West Camden Street
Baltimore, MD 21201
530 Walnut Street
Philadelphia, PA 19106

All rights reserved. This book is protected by copyright. No part of this book may be reproduced in any form or by any means, including photocopying, or utilized by any information storage and retrieval system without written permission from the copyright owner.

Library of Congress Cataloging-in-Publication Data

Allen, Laura, NCTMB.
    A massage therapist's guide to business / Laura Allen.
        p. ; cm.
    Includes bibliographical references.
    ISBN 978-1-58255-827-1
  1. Massage therapy—Practice. I. Title.
    [DNLM: 1. Massage. 2. Entrepreneurship—organization & administration. 3. Practice Management—organization & administration. WB 537]

    RM722.A415—2010
    615.8'22068—dc22

                                                                        2010034964

The publisher is not responsible (as a matter of product liability, negligence, or otherwise) for any injury resulting from any material contained herein. This publication contains information relating to general principles of medical care that should not be construed as specific instructions for individual patients. Manufacturers' product information and package inserts should be reviewed for current information, including contraindications, dosages, and precautions.

RRS1011

Dedicated to my parents,
Margaret Lawson and Jim Rich

Laura Allen is a nationally certified massage therapist and bodyworker and an approved provider of continuing education under the NCBTMB. She is on the visiting faculty of The Obus School of Healing Therapies in Leixlip, Ireland, as an instructor of Advanced Massage Techniques and travels all over the United States teaching continuing education classes in Professional Ethics and Marketing for Massage Therapists.

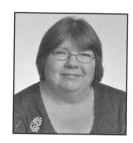

Laura acts as a consultant to massage schools seeking initial licensure, educators seeking approval from the National Board, and therapists who desire to increase their communication and marketing skills in order to effect positive change in their businesses.

Laura is a member of AMTA and ABMP and is a frequent contributor to trade journals. She is also a blogger with three popular blogs currently on the Internet, mainly about the politics and legislation of massage. She is a founding member of the Alliance for Massage Therapy Education, a recent delegate to the Federation of State Massage Therapy Boards, and is currently in the last year of a 5-year term on the North Carolina Board of Massage & Bodywork Therapy.

Born in Savannah, Georgia, to a military family, Laura attended 15 different schools during her family's travels to different military bases. She attended Isothermal Community College to study social work, dropping out just short of graduation to enter a career in the restaurant business. Laura owned four restaurants over the next 20 years and worked as a chef in some of North Carolina's most prestigious dining establishments. In 1998, she sold her business and returned to school to earn a B.A. in psychology from Shaw University in Asheville, North Carolina. She distinguished herself there by winning the Bronze Award and the Pinnacle Award for academic excellence and was elected to Psi Chi, the National Honor Society in Psychology.

She graduated from The Whole You School of Massage & Bodywork in Rutherfordton, North Carolina, in 2000, while simultaneously pursuing a graduate degree in psychology through online classes. She has completed an additional 120 hours of specialized training in techniques for releasing emotional stress and also completed a counseling internship under the direction of a licensed psychologist, a licensed clinical social worker, and a certified family therapist.

Laura remained at The Whole You as an instructor and administrator for 5 years, before leaving to open a private practice that has grown to include six licensed massage therapists, a chiropractor, an acupuncturist, a professional clinical herbalist, and an RN certified in natural health and microdermabrasion. She is frequently called upon to speak about the clinical use of therapeutic touch in hospitals, nursing homes, and schools.

Laura is regionally well-known as a musician and songwriter in Western North Carolina and has made numerous public appearances, including being featured on public radio and public television, as well as being a contributor on five CDs. She has been a member of the band Hogwild for over two decades and enjoys playing guitar, piano, and harmonica professionally as well as for stress relief. Laura resides with her husband Champ, a builder, in Rutherfordton, North Carolina.

PREFACE

A Massage Therapist's Guide to Business is written for massage therapists and bodyworkers. It will be useful as well for the extended family of people working in the different areas of complementary and alternative health care. The ideas and resources can be easily adapted to suit all holistic professions.

People in the holistic healing arts share a philosophy that the natural way is the best way. We concern ourselves with the body, the mind, and the spirit of those we serve, in the belief that you can't affect one without affecting the other. We are caregivers; we are caretakers. We have chosen a path of trying to help others live in wellness and in balance. We sometimes feel that instead of choosing the path, the path has chosen us. For those of you who have decided that this path is your livelihood, this book is for you.

Along with the desire to help others, we all have the desire to make a comfortable and prosperous living, to be able to provide for ourselves and our families while doing a job that we love. Many people in the holistic healing arts are lacking in business education; they may be self-educated or schooled in ways other than through a traditional education, such as by attending workshops or participating in apprenticeships. Even those who may have attended school in an institutional setting, or are still attending one now, are sometimes taught a lot about the theoretical side of business, while receiving too little information about the practicalities of opening and maintaining a business that not only survives but also thrives. *A Massage Therapist's Guide to Business* is meant to fill that void.

STRUCTURAL ORGANIZATION

This book is divided into five distinct parts. Part I, *Mapping Your Route*, is full of guidelines for preparing you to become an entrepreneur. Chapter 1 discusses inventorying your strengths and weaknesses, setting concrete goals, and using resources and the help of professional experts before taking the big leap into the business world. It also describes the importance of keeping a positive attitude. Chapter 2 describes constructing and adapting a viable business plan. Chapter 3 discusses the importance of conducting business and therapeutic relationships in an ethical manner.

Part II, *Setting Out*, covers the preliminary details to think through and take care of before opening a business. Chapter 4 is a discussion of the legal, logistical, and financial issues involved in a massage therapy business. Chapter 5 discusses how to manage obstacles any business owner might face and addresses successfully growing your business.

Part III, *Staying on Course*, helps you stay on track and avoid missteps. Chapter 6 discusses managing technology, record keeping, and documentation. Chapter 7 explains budgeting, taxes, managing inventory, bartering, reimbursement, planning for retirement, and valuing a business in preparation for selling. Chapter 8 discusses working alone, assembling and managing a staff, the differences between employees and independent contractors, and interviewing and hiring. Chapter 9 is a discussion of the necessity of written business policies and enforcing them.

Part IV, *Traffic Signals*, addresses everyday business communications. Chapter 10 discusses cultivating self-confidence and client confidence by projecting professionalism. Chapter 11 discusses effectively communicating in a clear and professional way with clients, staff members, mutual referral practitioners, and others in the business setting.

Part V, *Highway Visibility*, discusses marketing your business. Chapter 12 explains three of the four essential "P's" of marketing—Product, Place, and Price—and how they can enhance the success of any massage therapy business. Chapter 13 provides an in-depth discussion of the fourth "P," Promotion of your business in the community. Chapter 14 explores the many different kinds of advertising venues available in today's marketplace and how to get the most benefit for your advertising dollars.

At the end of the book is an appendix: Business Forms for Every Need. A glossary of the boldfaced terms that occur in the book is provided as well.

SPECIAL FEATURES

Throughout the book, reader-friendly features follow the theme of a personal and professional journey.

The features reinforce the cultivation of a positive attitude and the performance of proactive exercises along the route to success.

- An inspirational quotation sets the tone for each chapter.
- *Key Concepts* introduce the main ideas covered in the narrative.
- *Roadside Assistance* captures my personal tips and observations from years of experience in business.
- *Postcards from the Highway* is a feature that presents success stories and timely advice from some of the most successful people in the field of massage therapy and bodywork.
- *Words of Wisdom* are positive affirmations or motivational sayings included in each chapter.
- *Going with the Flow* examines current trends in massage therapy and other forms of holistic health care and business in general.
- Traffic signs and cartoons lend humor to offset the challenges of learning something new.
- *Explorations* are activities for the reader to perform, such as visiting the local office of the Small Business Administration or researching a particular topic.
- *My Personal Journey* is a journaling feature that requires the reader to take positive steps on the way to success.

ANCILLARIES

The website at http://thePoint.lww.com/Allen-Business1e provides access to a variety of resources to supplement this textbook, for students/practitioners and instructors. (Use the access code on the inside cover.)

For instructors, the website contains

- Lesson plans
- Test bank

- PowerPoint presentations for each chapter, including "Points to Ponder" at the end of each, with questions for discussion and reflection

In addition, there is a supply of sample forms that students can use for practice assignments and practitioners can adapt for their own business.

CONTINUING THE JOURNEY

This book continues the personal journey to success that began with my book, *One Year to a Successful Massage Therapy Practice* (Lippincott Williams & Wilkins, 2008). Both books share the practical presentation of ideas, the road signs to help readers along the way, and the journaling feature that spurs the readers into taking action and documenting responsibility for their own success. The information in *A Massage Therapist's Guide to Business*, and the no-cost and low-cost marketing strategies in *One Year to a Successful Massage Therapy Practice*, can be very easily applied to other holistic health care businesses, such as chiropractic, acupuncture, or naturopathy.

HAPPY TRAVELS

I believe that we're all meant to prosper; prosperity lets us share with others and perform good works that we can't necessarily do when we're worried about our next rent or mortgage payment. Please let me know if this book is a help to you, and send me your practical business advice and your success stories for inclusion in the next edition. I wish you the best of luck on your personal journey and pray that you have half the fun that I've had in mine. We're all blessed to be in this business; there isn't a better job in the world than that of helping people feel good—and being able to cultivate prosperity at the same time.

Laura Allen, NCTMB

ACKNOWLEDGMENTS

Thank you so much to my editors, Betsy Dilernia and Linda Francis, all the rest of the great folks at LWW, and the reviewers who took the time to help make this book as good as possible. Thanks to Imagineering for realizing my vision on the artwork. I am grateful to my family of origin and my family of selection. Thanks to my staff members, who have made my business what it is and who keep my business rocking whether I'm here or not. A great big thanks to Champ Allen, my husband, who good-naturedly claims my back is the only thing he sees of me for weeks at a time while I'm typing. Special gratitude goes out to the therapists and educators who contributed to the book: Thomas Myers, Ruthie Piper Hardee, Ralph Stephens, Joel Tull, Linda Roisum, Felicia Brown, Ruth Werner, Ann Catlin, James Waslaski, John Barnes, Tamsin Stewart, and Angela Palmier. I cannot say thank you enough to Christine Courtney, not only for contributing to the book but also for feeding my addiction for Ireland and giving me a place to land. Nina McIntosh passed away while I was writing this book, and I am grateful for her contribution and everything else she has done for me. Thanks to the Sunday Night Music gang for keeping me sane. Finally, thank you so much to the whole family of hands, my colleagues in the massage profession, for cheering me on and supporting me. I appreciate all of you.

REVIEWERS

Dianne Bunn, AS, CMT
Newton, North Carolina

Kelly Carpenter, LMT
All that Matters
Wakefield, Rhode Island

Heidi Homerding, LMT
New Lenox, Illinois

Stephanie Meyers-Roche, BS
South Shore Massage Therapy
Weymouth, Massachusetts

Eric Munn, BSID, CMT
Berdan Institute
Wayne, New Jersey

Sharlene Philip, MT, NCTMB
National Holistic Institute
Emeryville, California

Lori Robertson, CMT, LMT
The Healing Arts Center
Winchester, Virginia

Eddy Van Hunnik, PhD
The Career Institute of American International College
Braintree, Massachusetts

CONTENTS

Mapping Your Route

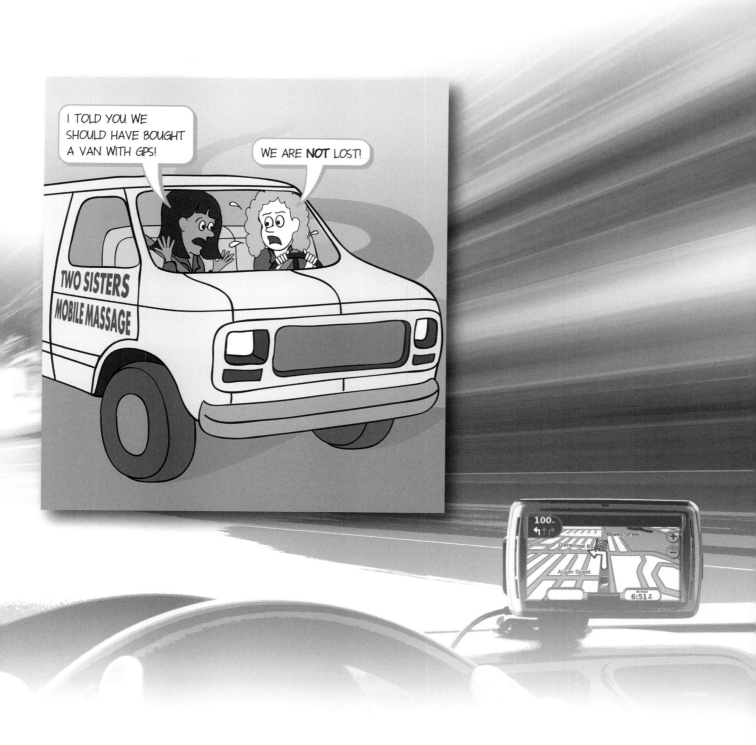

Preparing for Your Career

The victory of success is half won when one gains the habit of setting goals and achieving them. Even the most tedious chore will become endurable as you parade through each day convinced that every task, no matter how menial or boring, brings you closer to fulfilling your dreams.

OG MANDINO

KEY CONCEPTS

- Taking a self-inventory is crucial to capitalizing on strengths and minimizing weaknesses and can help you decide whether to be self-employed or work for someone else.
- Many options are available to those seeking a career in massage therapy.
- Therapists who want to work for an employer instead of being self-employed must prepare for employment with a professional resume and interviewing skills.
- Learning the discipline of setting goals and following through on them is the most direct route to success.
- Utilizing all the available resources at your disposal is smart strategy.
- Cultivating a positive attitude and the willingness to persevere will serve you well when you encounter bumps in the road.
- Banishing as much negativity as possible from your personal and professional life helps you keep a positive attitude and builds confidence.

Whether your discipline is massage therapy or another holistic practice, chances are you have spent a lot of money and invested a lot of time preparing. Many people are drawn to a career in massage therapy or other holistic health practices because of a personal health crisis, when conventional medical approaches might not have been completely satisfying or successful. Becoming a practitioner in the healing arts can be a second career for adult learners who return to school after the kids are grown and out of the house, or even following retirement from a first career. Others may be fresh out of high school when they embark on an education in massage therapy or other branches of holistic health.

Many disciplines of natural healing exist—literally dozens of modalities of massage and bodywork, plus naturopathy, energy work, chiropractic, homeopathy, aromatherapy, acupuncture, and so much more—and different curricula, philosophies, and types of education are available. The majority of schools focus on the theory and practice of the art, and the business end of being in practice, along with basic job-seeking skills, is often given short shrift. Many holistic practitioners are intuitive or self-taught, or have taken a learning path outside a traditional school, such as learning through online study, attending workshops, or serving apprenticeships. Even the National Certification Board for Therapeutic Massage & Bodywork (NCBTMB) revised their policy in 2007, to allow up to 300 hours of their 500-hour educational requirement to be completed through distance learning, leaving only the hands-on practical part of the education to actually be done in the presence of an instructor.

Just as a degree in international finance does not prepare you to be a massage therapist, neither does a degree in massage prepare you for the realities of the daily running of a business. In states where there are still no legal requirements, or in the case of certain disciplines that aren't regulated, such as energy work, the practitioner who is self-educated or who learned in workshops may have had no business training at all. Many who have never been self-employed, as well as those who may have previously tried going into business by themselves, have attended the school of hard knocks—jumping in and finding out as they go along what works and what doesn't. Being prepared is the better way, and certainly a lot less stressful.

The Associated Bodywork & Massage Professionals (ABMP) sponsors a public education website, www.massagetherapy.com. According to the latest statistics in an article entitled *Explosive Growth Rate for Massage Training Begins to Flatten*, 1500+ massage schools in the United States are training around 63,000 new massage therapists every year, but that is offset by the estimated 50,000 who leave the profession annually. While some of those leaving are retiring, many more leave because they are suffering from career burnout, have sustained a career-ending injury, or have proved to be unable to run a profitable business. You don't want to be a statistic in any of those categories.

HELP JUST AHEAD

It's easy to become overwhelmed when you're in a new practice, to the point that instead of running your business, you may find it's running you. If that applies to you, don't give up. If you haven't yet gotten your business off the ground, don't be discouraged. Being a successful businessperson is largely a function of the Boy Scout motto: "Be Prepared." If you feel your business education was nonexistent or wasn't thorough enough, you can and must educate yourself—starting here. There are lots of resources available to the entrepreneur, many of them low-cost or free, and they will be discussed throughout this book. Read other business books, attend classes, do Internet research, and talk to other therapists and business owners. The more prepared you are, the better off you'll be.

Not everyone is cut out to be self-employed, and some practitioners prefer to focus on massage and let someone else deal with the responsibilities associated with running a business. Some therapists initially seek a job when they're new graduates, with the intent of being entrepreneurs at some point in the future. If you haven't yet decided which route you want to take, a self-inventory is a good way to start.

THE SELF-INVENTORY

For anyone considering going into business or entering the job market, taking a thorough inventory of your motivations, your hopes, your dreams, and your goals is a necessity. For those who want to *succeed* in business, a "searching and fearless" self-inventory must go beyond. There are numerous psychological profiles you can complete to find out where your talents do or don't lie, to identify your traits and qualities. Many are available at no charge on the Internet.

The bottom line is that you must be brutally honest with yourself about your strengths and weaknesses, if you want to maximize your chances for success. Figure 1-1 provides a basic format to get your self-inventory started; you can build on it as you see fit. The point is to help you recognize your talents as well as areas that need improvement and not to become discouraged by your less-than-perfect qualities. Your self-inventory can be a good indicator of whether to take the plunge into self-employment, or whether you might be more suited to working for someone else.

Practical Considerations

Before starting out in business, recognize what you can and can't do well, and think about ways you can handle any potential issues. Here are a few examples to consider. Are you on time for appointments? If you're someone who likes to sleep until 10:00 and don't really feel motivated until noon, it would be silly to set your office hours to begin at 8:00 a.m. There are plenty of clients who work during the day and would welcome the opportunity to get a massage in the evenings.

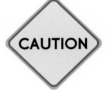

Can you balance your own checkbook, and do you do it every single month? Do you know where your tax records for the past 3 years are located? Can you put your hands on your insurance policies without having to dig around for them? Those things are just a few of the responsibilities that come with owning your own business. The idea of being your own boss is often romanticized, and the realities don't appear until you're knee deep in a situation you aren't prepared for. There are many practicalities to consider before committing to becoming an entrepreneur.

Attention to Detail

Running a successful business requires attention to detail—particularly keeping good records and a close watch on financial information. If you're constantly overdrawing on your bank account, that's not a good sign. It doesn't mean you can't open a business—but it does mean you'd be better off to have someone more conscientious taking care of the books and organizing your finances (see Chapter 4). The cost of paying someone to do your bookkeeping will be worth the assurance you'll have that your business checks are not bouncing. If you're just starting out and think you can't afford an accountant, perhaps you can trade services with someone (see Chapter 7).

If you become an independent contractor and work in someone else's office, you will still be considered self-employed and will be responsible for paying your own taxes—and for keeping up with your own deductions. If you're an employee, the employer will deduct the tax you owe from your paycheck. You may still be entitled to tax deductions for certain expenses, but you'll have a lot less paperwork to keep up with than a self-employed therapist (see Chapter 8).

The Compassionate Communicator

Are you ready to spend your day with people who are stressed or in pain and want to tell you all about it? This can be the case for any therapist, whether self-employed or not. Can you listen to that every day with compassion, without feeling as if you're taking on the problems of the world? Will you be stressed or depressed by it? Do you possess good listening skills? Are you a good communicator? You'll have to conduct intake interviews, give clients after-care instructions, and the like. Do people feel comfortable talking with you? Can you make them feel as if you're listening to every word they have to say and that you are genuinely interested? The elements of the therapeutic relationship are covered in Chapter 3, while Chapter 11 discusses how to have effective communications.

The self-inventory is intended to give you an idea of your strengths and weaknesses. Choose the statement that best suits you, and be brutally honest. Ask your friends and family, and vow not to get mad when they tell you the truth!

Practical Considerations

I am a punctual person who believes it's important to be on time.

All of the time	Most of the time	Some of the time	Rarely	Never
☐	☐	☐	☐	☐

I'm able to balance my work and personal life.

All of the time	Most of the time	Some of the time	Rarely	Never
☐	☐	☐	☐	☐

I'd prefer to be working with others instead of by myself.

All of the time	Most of the time	Some of the time	Rarely	Never
☐	☐	☐	☐	☐

Attention to Detail

I pay attention to detail.

All of the time	Most of the time	Some of the time	Rarely	Never
☐	☐	☐	☐	☐

I think it's important to plan ahead and be well-organized.

All of the time	Most of the time	Some of the time	Rarely	Never
☐	☐	☐	☐	☐

I believe in keeping my workspace clean and dressing neatly in order to present a professional image.

All of the time	Most of the time	Some of the time	Rarely	Never
☐	☐	☐	☐	☐

The Compassionate Communicator

I'm a good listener.

All of the time	Most of the time	Some of the time	Rarely	Never
☐	☐	☐	☐	☐

I'm very clear in my professional conversations, and people feel comfortable talking with me.

All of the time	Most of the time	Some of the time	Rarely	Never
☐	☐	☐	☐	☐

I'm sympathetic, but I don't get caught up in other people's problems.

All of the time	Most of the time	Some of the time	Rarely	Never
☐	☐	☐	☐	☐

FIGURE 1-1 A sample self-inventory.

Management Material

I enjoy being in charge, but I'm diplomatic when I need to be.

All of the time	Most of the time	Some of the time	Rarely	Never
☐	☐	☐	☐	☐

I'm comfortable taking on responsibility and confident in my abilities.

All of the time	Most of the time	Some of the time	Rarely	Never
☐	☐	☐	☐	☐

I'm calm and rational when it comes to handling problems.

All of the time	Most of the time	Some of the time	Rarely	Never
☐	☐	☐	☐	☐

Financial Realities

I'm disciplined when it comes to finances; I balance my bank statements and pay my bills on time.

All of the time	Most of the time	Some of the time	Rarely	Never
☐	☐	☐	☐	☐

I could go for a year without a salary and still meet my obligations.

All of the time	Most of the time	Some of the time	Rarely	Never
☐	☐	☐	☐	☐

I think it's important to keep good records and I'm meticulous about doing so.

All of the time	Most of the time	Some of the time	Rarely	Never
☐	☐	☐	☐	☐

Key:

All the time = 5 points

Most of the time = 4 points

Some of the time = 3 points

Rarely = 2 points

Never = 1 point

Add your points together to get your final score.

60-75 points: You're a good candidate to be an entrepreneur!

45-59 points: You may want to work for someone else for a couple of years before deciding whether or not to take the next step into self-employment.

Less than 45 points: You'd probably be happier without the responsibilities of management, and would be more satisfied working for someone else.

FIGURE 1-1 *(Continued).*

Management Material

If you plan to have associates or employees working for you, you have to strike a balance between being an authority figure and being too lenient. Everyone enjoys working for a boss who is a good communicator and a genuinely nice person. No one enjoys working for someone who shouts orders and acts like a commando. Can you show appreciation for the work people do for you? Are you capable of being a courteous supervisor for whom people will want to work? If you're thinking of being a member of a group practice, are you someone your co-workers will enjoy being around, or someone they'll try to avoid? Those who can't work well with others do better in a solo practice.

As an employee or an independent contractor, you would hope to work for a manager who is fair and courteous to the staff. The number of long-term employees who are working in a business is often a good indication of whether or not there are management problems; people don't want to stay where they're unhappy. A business that has a high turnover usually has management issues.

Financial Realities

Are you financially secure enough to open your own business? (This issue will be reiterated many times throughout this book.) Can you last for a year without a paycheck and still meet your obligations? Many new businesses open and don't last beyond a few months. Inexperienced and unprepared new business owners often have unrealistic expectations of drawing a big salary in just a few short months—and that rarely happens. According to the Bureau of Labor Statistics (BLS), as of May 2008, the median pay for massage therapists was slightly less than $17 per hour, with those in the highest 10% earning more than $33 per hour. The ABMP website lists the average yearly income for a massage therapist at $17,750, as of 2007, the last year for which the figure was available. That's not most people's idea of wealth. However, the potential is there for much more, and preparing yourself with knowledge of effective business practices is the key if you want to be above the norm.

If you have advanced training and certification in a specialty modality of massage or bodywork, such as Rolfing or orthopedic massage, you are in a position to charge more than the average therapist for your services. However, you will still have the same opening expenses as any other practitioner considering going into business.

If you're seeking a job, chances are you have the same issue as an entrepreneur: You need a certain amount of money in order to support yourself and meet your financial obligations. While taking any job that comes along is tempting when you're unemployed, it's often a mistake; the job you truly want might be just around the corner. Try to plan ahead and save enough money to live on for a few months after you graduate from massage school, and/or have your license or whatever credential is required in your state. That will allow you the time to find your ideal job without feeling the pressure to accept something you don't want in order to survive.

REALITY CHECKPOINT

ROADSIDE ASSISTANCE

Sometimes, we just plain fool ourselves; we're human. We have strengths and weaknesses. There's no shame in admitting weaknesses, especially when it comes to business. If there's a quality or skill you don't have, try to cultivate it. Reward yourself for learning positive new habits!

CAREER OPTIONS IN MASSAGE AND BODYWORK

While many take the plunge into self-employment, it's not for everyone. Some practitioners will choose to work for someone else, either permanently or as a valuable way to gain experience until the day comes to take the next step into business ownership.

There are many possibilities for a career in massage and bodywork, in terms of settings, and each has its own merits to consider when you're deciding which situation best suits you and your goals. Table 1-1 summarizes career options, special training that may be needed, and pros and cons of each. You can maximize your chances of success by choosing a workplace that's the right "fit" for you.

Deciding Where to Work

Massage therapists can practice on the beach, or in the park. They can do chair massage in a coffeehouse or on the street corner, in tents at races and festivals, backstage at concerts, and many other places outside traditional massage settings. One airline is even putting massage therapists in their first-class cabins for the convenience of their wealthy clientele. It must be a lot of fun to be doing massage as you watch the clouds float by!

There are many things to consider when deciding on a work venue you like. Different opportunities, as well as drawbacks, often depend on the work environment. Here are some of the issues when you're choosing a place to work:

- Whether you want to work alone or with others.
- Whether you want to work as an employee, independent contractor, or employer.
- Whether you want to work in a clinical setting or a more relaxed setting.
- What type of massage you want to provide.
- What days and hours you want to work.
- How many massages you are comfortable performing daily or per shift.
- What type of benefits you want, such as health insurance or a retirement plan.

A home office may be practical for some therapists for a variety of reasons, such as wanting to be home with their children, preferring to work alone, or simply because they have the space and can save on the rent and other **overhead** costs that go with having a commercial location. Many home practitioners are (wisely) selective about their clientele and work strictly by word-of-mouth referrals out of concern for letting strangers into their homes.

Cultivating doctor referrals and insurance clients may be more challenging for home practitioners. Part of the process for joining an insurance network may include submitting photographs of your facility as proof that it is in compliance with the ADA (Americans with Disabilities Act), such as providing a wheelchair ramp and a therapy room and restroom with handicap accessibility. For practicing medical massage, a hospital, chiropractic clinic, medical office, or holistic wellness clinic may be more appropriate.

A practice in a commercial location means more visibility to the public and more income opportunities than a home practice, and, as mentioned above, more overheads.

Athletic venues and gyms, both commercial and those affiliated with colleges, are good places to set up shop for those who have an interest in sports and/or rehabilitative massage.

Salons and spas offer opportunities for practitioners who prefer doing relaxation massage or spa treatments. There are different categories of spas: cruise ship spas, day spas, destination spas, medical spas, and resort spas.

TABLE 1-1	Career Options in Massage and Bodywork
Athletic Venue Such as Stadium or Track	
Worker status	Self-employed and renting space, independent contractor, or employed by venue or sports team
Specialty training required	Sports massage, techniques for assisting injury recovery, such as orthopedic massage
Pros	Variety of sports and training seasons means year-round steady employment; may include travel opportunities if employed by a team
Cons	Involves transporting table and other supplies if you travel
Chiropractic Office	
Worker status	Independent contractor or employee
Specialty training required	Medical massage, stretching techniques, joint mobilizations (not manipulations; that's chiropractic)
Pros	Working with medical professionals offers valuable experience and lends credibility; office personnel handle booking and advertising
Cons	May be fast-paced with short sessions, as little as 15 min
Client's Home or Accommodation	
Worker status	Usually self-employed; some business may offer outcalls and expect employees to perform them
Specialty training required	None
Pros	Staying on the go suits some therapists; hardly any overhead
Cons	Safety issues in working with people you don't know in their own environment; involves transporting equipment and supplies
Corporate Office	
Worker status	Employee, self-employed renting space from the corporation, or independent contractor
Specialty training required	None
Pros	Clients are on the premises; no need to spend money advertising
Cons	Clientele is usually limited to employees of the corporation, leaving little room for growth

(continued)

TABLE 1-1	*(continued)*
Cruise Ship	
Worker status	Employee; work on commission basis plus gratuities and commissions on product sales
Specialty training required	150 hours of training in Swedish massage is the only requirement for most cruise lines
Pros	Opportunity to travel and see the world
Cons	Tiny living quarters; expected to perform as many as 10–14 massages daily; pressure to sell retail products
Day Spa	
Worker status	Self-employed owner, employee, or independent contractor
Specialty training required	Spa techniques such as hot stone massage, body wraps, mud, and exfoliations
Pros	Supplies and linens are usually provided; venue does advertising and handles booking
Cons	May be pressure to sell retail products and upsell other services to client
Destination Spa	
Worker status	Usually employee; can be independent contractor
Specialty training required	Spa techniques such as hot stone massage, body wraps, mud, and exfoliations
Pros	Supplies and linens are usually provided; spa does advertising and handles booking
Cons	Depending on location, business may be seasonal; clients are tourists, not potential regulars
Franchise Massage Business	
Worker status	Usually employees; some may use independent contractors
Specialty training required	None
Pros	Management handles booking and advertising and provides linens and supplies; some opportunities for advancement
Cons	Lower pay than normal for self-employed therapists; if scheduled, you are required to be on the premises whether you have appointments or not

(continued)

TABLE 1-1   *(continued)*

Gym or Health Club

Worker status	Independent contractor renting space (usually)
Specialty training required	Sports massage
Pros	Clients are on the premises; no need to spend money advertising
Cons	Clientele is limited to membership, leaving little room for growth

Holistic Wellness Clinic

Worker status	Self-employed owner, employee, or independent contractor
Specialty training required	None
Pros	Opportunity to work with and cross-refer to holistic health care practitioners, such as naturopaths or acupuncturists
Cons	May be required to provide own linens and supplies, handle advertising, and book clients

Home Office

Worker status	Self-employed
Specialty training required	None
Pros	Low overhead; home office tax deduction; convenience
Cons	Isolation; may be limited to word-of-mouth advertising; takes effort to keep business and personal life separate

Hospice

Worker status	Employee or independent contractor
Specialty training required	Geriatric and/or oncology massage helpful, but probably not a job requirement
Pros	Rewarding to assist clients during their transition; possibility of appointments with family and staff members as well
Cons	Emotionally challenging to work with terminally ill clients

Hospital

Worker status	Employee or independent contractor
Specialty training required	Geriatric massage, pregnancy massage, oncology massage, or other modalities for working with people who are ill

(continued)

TABLE 1-1 (continued)	
Pros	Clients are on the premises; practicing in medical setting enhances credibility
Cons	May be required to provide own equipment and supplies; working with people who are ill can be emotionally challenging
Mobile Chair Massage	
Worker status	Self-employed
Specialty training required	None
Pros	Ability to work wherever there is room for a chair; minimal overhead
Cons	Involves transporting equipment
Physician's Office	
Worker status	Employee or independent contractor
Specialty training required	May depend on physician's specialty (e.g., pregnancy massage if working in an OB/GYN office)
Pros	Booking and advertising provided by physician or staff; practicing in medical setting enhances credibility
Cons	May be required to provide own equipment and supplies; may be fast-paced, with shorter sessions
Private Practice in a Commercial Location	
Worker status	Self-employed; employee or independent contractor if working in someone else's practice or renting space from another therapist
Specialty training required	None
Pros	Self-employed and independent contractors will be in control of their own schedule
Cons	Self-employed have total responsibility for all business aspects; independent contractors responsibility for own equipment and supplies and possibly bookings and advertising
Resort	
Worker status	Employee, independent contractor, or self-employed person renting space
Specialty training required	Management may desire specific skills, such as hot stone massage or spa treatments
Pros	Tend to be located in tourist areas, with opulent surroundings
Cons	Work may be seasonal depending on location

(continued)

TABLE 1-1	(continued)
	Salon
Worker status	Independent contractor rending space or employee on a commission basis
Specialty training required	Management may desire specific skills, such as hot stone massage or spa treatments
Pros	Clientele is on the premises, usually referred by hairdressers and nail technicians
Cons	May be subjected to chemical odors common in salons; may have difficulty getting outside clients unless the salon promotes your services

"Specialty training" refers to any training beyond basic massage skills. Note that this table is a general sample of the possibilities; specific practices may vary.

Day spas are sometimes attached to salons. In addition to bodywork and spa treatments, they usually offer hair and nail services and may also have fitness classes, pools, light meals, and many of the same amenities offered at destination and resort spas, minus the lodging.

Destination spas are usually all-inclusive, meaning visitors pay a package fee that includes their lodging, meals, classes, and a certain number of massage and spa treatments for the duration of their stay. Some are located in tourist areas; others may be well off the beaten path.

Medical spas are becoming increasingly popular as places where people go to address health problems, while combining their medical care with relaxation and pampering. Many medical spas specialize in weight loss or quitting smoking, some cater to clients who are in recovery from anything from addiction to plastic surgery, and there are even dental spas.

Resort spas and cruise ships offer massage and spa treatments à la carte, although some may offer spa credit or a package deal as a booking incentive. Therapists may also be expected to sell retail products as part of the job, especially on cruise ships. The pace on cruise ships is much more intense than what most practitioners are used to, with12-hour shifts being the norm and therapists expected to perform 10 to 12 massages per shift.

In 2008, I interviewed over a dozen massage therapists who have worked on cruise ships for an article I was writing and heard the same comments from all of them: It is a great way to see the world. However, in addition to the fast pace, you are expected to meet sales quotas of retail products, you must be comfortable sharing a tiny room with three or four people, and there are numerous rules relating to dress, behavior, and time off.

Steiner Leisure, based in London, has been recruiting and training therapists and other service professionals to work on cruise ships since 1947 and currently provides service staff to 116 cruise ships. The training period may vary according to the needs of the cruise lines at any time and the experience of the applicant. Among the therapists I interviewed, the time range averaged from a few weeks to as long as 6 months; one therapist stated she was in training for only 2 days before she was on board the ship because of emergency staffing needs. Others reported that the training was heavy on product education; you can't sell products if you don't know anything about them. It's not for everyone, but for the energetic and outgoing, it can be an adventure.

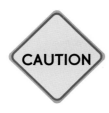

Be sure to thoroughly investigate the requirements and costs associated with training and employment before you sign any agreements.

Providing massage in a hospice setting requires special dedication and the emotional stamina to work with clients who are dying. Sometimes therapists in hospice settings make massage available to staff or family members, in addition to giving a comforting touch to the dying. The situation is similar in a hospital, working with those who are ill or injured, and may include making massage available to others as well.

Some therapists choose not to have a permanent location at all, and instead do outcalls for a living, performing massage in the client's home, office, or accommodations. A therapist who has a mobile chair massage practice may be in the park 1 day and in the offices of a major corporation the next.

Clients expect to pay more for massage by a therapist who comes to them. Operating expenses are usually less for an outcall business than the expense of maintaining an office, although there are transportation and advertising costs to consider. Due to travel and set-up time, outcall therapists may do fewer appointments a day than a therapist who has a set location.

There's also the hassle of hauling equipment; you may sometimes find yourself lugging a massage table and your supplies up several flights of stairs. There are also safety precautions to consider, if going to the home or accommodations of people you don't know. Still, providing mobile massage is appealing to practitioners who enjoy a constant change of scenery and venue.

Related to the choice of where to work is the question of whether to work alone or with others. Some prefer working as an employee, while others prefer being independent contractors or employers. Some therapists may choose to go into business with others and form a partnership. These topics will be discussed in detail in Chapter 8.

Seeking a Job

The job market is a competitive place, and you want to be well prepared. The self-inventory in Figure 1-1 and the work settings listed in Table 1-1 can give you some idea of the kind of career situation you want to pursue. If you're seeking employment, there are several ways to maximize your chances of getting the position you want, and you should use all the resources at your disposal. If you're looking for your first job as a professional massage therapist, what you lack in experience can be made up for with enthusiasm and the willingness to learn and grow through continuing education and on-the-job training.

The Professional Resume

A professional **resume** is essential for any job candidate. You won't make a good impression by walking into a nice spa or medical office and leaving them your name and number on a sticky note. You must have a resume that documents your qualifications.

There are three basic types of resumes: chronological, functional, and combination.

- A chronological resume lists your employment experience in reverse chronological order (from the present backwards), showing that you have experienced steady growth in your field and your career accomplishments. An example of a chronological resume appears in Figure 1-2.
- A functional resume focuses on what you have done, rather than timeframes or settings. An example of a functional resume appears in Figure 1-3.
- A combination resume uses a functional style listing of *relevant* skills and accomplishments, and then describes employment and education histories

---

Priscilla Evans, A.A., NCMTB
145 Wysteria Lane
Cold Mountain NC 28043
828-288-3727
pevans@coldmtn.net

Skills:

- Nationally Certified in Massage Therapy and Bodywork since 2000.
- Licensed as an Emergency Medical Technician since 1995.
- Computer literate with abilities in word processing, database management, and spreadsheet functions.
- Bilingual in Spanish and English.
- Excellent customer service and communication skills.

Experience:

2005-present
Lead Massage Therapist at the Cold Mountain Spa and Resort.
- Responsible for training all new employees in spa techniques.
- Prepare work schedule for a staff of 15 massage therapists.
- Handle daily tasks such as ordering linens and spa supplies.
- Greet clients, bridge communications between clients and therapists.

2000-2005
Massage Therapist for Carolina Mobile Massage.
- Provided chair massage to corporate accounts.
- Successfully solicited over 20 new corporate accounts in a 5-year period.

1995-2000
Emergency Medical Technician (EMT) employed by Cold County Emergency Services, North Carolina.
- Acted as a first responder to accidents and medical emergencies.
- Volunteered EMT services one night per week to the local county search and rescue squad for 5 years.

Education:

Associate of Arts in Therapeutic Massage,
Cold Mountain School of Holistic Arts, 1999.

Emergency Medical Technician Certification,
Cold Mountain Community College, 1994.

FIGURE 1-2 **A chronological resume.**

in reverse chronological order. The experience section directly supports the functional section. An example of a combination resume appears in Figure 1-4.

A cover letter should accompany your resume. A **cover letter** is a brief introduction to prospective employers that clearly states the job you wish to apply for

Priscilla Evans, A.A., NCMTB
145 Wysteria Lane
Cold Mountain NC 28043
828-288-3727
pevans@coldmtn.net

Summary of Qualifications

- Nationally Certified in Therapeutic Massage & Bodywork.
- Licensed as an Emergency Medical Technician.
- Additional 25 hours continuing education in hot stone massage.
- 5 years of experience in supervising, scheduling, and ordering supplies for a spa employing 15 massage therapists.
- Additional 5 years of experience in dealing with corporate clients as provider of chair massage for a mobile massage company.
- Successfully solicited over 20 new corporate accounts in a 5-year period.

Additional Skills

- Computer literate with abilities in word processing, database management, and spreadsheet functions.
- Bilingual in Spanish and English.

Education

- **Associate of Arts in Therapeutic Massage,** Cold Mountain School of Holistic Arts, 1999.
- **Emergency Medical Technician Certification,** Cold Mountain Community College, 1994.

Activities and Interests

- Volunteer as instructor for English as a Second Language (ESL) for Spanish-speaking immigrants through Community Outreach Center.
- Volunteer chair massage to local Hospice staff one day per month.
- Volunteered services as a first responder to the county search and rescue squad for five years.
- Member of Toastmasters and the Sertoma Club.

FIGURE 1-3   **A functional resume.**

and highlights the key points of your resume. An example of a cover letter appears in Figure 1-5.

Whichever type of resume you choose to use, follow a few basic rules:

- Represent your qualifications honestly, and in the best possible light.
- Submit your resume to places you think you'd like to work in. Call first and ask the name of the person to send it to.

Priscilla Evans, A.A., NCMTB
145 Wysteria Lane
Cold Mountain NC 28043
828-288-3727
pevans@coldmtn.net

Objective

Position in massage therapy/spa setting with opportunity for advancement into management.

Career Profile

- Since earning certification in therapeutic massage and bodywork in 1999, I have completed additional certification in hot stone therapy, spa treatments, and reflexology.
- Recognized as Employee of the Year two years in a row at Cold Mountain Spa and Resort based on guests voting.
- Was actively employed as an Emergency Medical Technician for 5 years and still maintain licensure.
- Active as a volunteer in my community since 1995, working for Hospice and teaching English as a Second Language (ESL) to immigrants.
- Proven skills in computer operations including word processing, database management, and spreadsheet use.

Experience

Lead Massage Therapist: Cold Mountain Resort , Cold Mountain, NC (2005-present).
- Training massage therapists in spa techniques.
- Responsible for scheduling for 15 staff members.
- Handle ordering of spa supplies.

Chair Massage Therapist: Carolina Mobile Massage, Cold Mountain, NC (2000-2005).
- Provided chair massage to corporate clients.
- Successfully solicited over 20 new corporate accounts in a 5-year period.

Emergency Medical Technician
- Licensed as an Emergency Medical Technician since 1995, employed by Cold County NC (1995-2000).

Education

- **Associate of Arts in Therapeutic Massage,** Cold Mountain School of Holistic Arts, 1999.
- **Emergency Medical Technician Certification,** Cold Mountain Community College, 1994.

Other Facts

- **Volunteer service:** Volunteer monthly massage to staff members at Hospice. Previously volunteered for 5 years as a first responder for the county search and rescue squad. I am an active member of Sertoma, and teach English as a Second Language (ESL) classes to immigrants in my community
- **Civic Activities:** Member of Toastmasters, enjoy improving my skills in public speaking.

FIGURE 1-4   A combination resume.

Priscilla Evans, A.A., NCMTB
145 Wysteria Lane
Cold Mountain NC 28043
828-288-3727
pevans@coldmtn.net

Mr. Andrew Huffy
The Spa at Oakbrook
1000 Ocean Drive
Oakbrook, South Carolina, 27777

August 27, 2009

Dear Mr. Huffy,

I am responding to the ad in the August 27 Mountain Express for a management trainee at The Spa at Oakbrook. My resume is enclosed. I am nationally certified in massage therapy and bodywork. I have excellent communication skills, computer skills, and supervisory experience. I am also a licensed Emergency Medical Technician.

I am currently employed in a similar position at the Cold Mountain Resort and Spa in western North Carolina. I have been very happy here, but my parents are in a retirement community in the Oakbrook area and I feel that I should move to be closer to them.

You may feel free to contact my present employer, and I will be happy to provide you with other references on request. I believe I have the experience and enthusiasm you are looking for in a management candidate.

May I schedule an interview with you at a mutually agreeable time to further discuss my qualifications? I look forward to hearing from you at your convenience.

Thank you for your consideration,

Priscilla Evans

FIGURE 1-5 A sample cover letter.

- Call within a week or two to follow up on your submission, and to ask for an appointment for an interview. Speak professionally on the telephone and during your job interview, avoiding the use of slang, profanity, "ums," and other conversation fillers.
- References other than past employers should be listed on a separate sheet of paper instead of on the resume itself. Be sure your contact information is on the heading.

The Job Interview

The job interview is your all-important chance to shine. You probably won't be the only person applying for the job, and you want the odds to be in your favor so that you'll be the one who gets hired. Managers are usually busy people. If you are greeted by a receptionist or assistant when you arrive for your interview, be as nice as possible to that person. A word from the receptionist to the boss about your polite (or impolite) demeanor could make or break the interview before it gets started.

When you go to the interview, conduct yourself accordingly:

- Arrive on time.
- Dress professionally.
- Exude professionalism and a positive attitude.
- Answer all questions honestly.
- If you require a certain salary or benefit, state that honestly.
- If you have a scheduling preference, such as having to be home with your children by a certain time, see if the manager would be willing to negotiate.
- Don't complain about your present or past employers, or about anything else.
- Ask intelligent questions, such as how long the company has been in business and how many staff members are employed; ask about employee benefits, opportunities for advancement, and anything else that is important to you. Keep your questions brief and neutral.
- Conclude by thanking the interviewer for seeing you.
- Follow up a few days later by sending a thank-you note to the interviewer, regardless of whether you know the hiring decision.

If a question makes you uncomfortable, consider it from the interviewer's point of view, instead of resisting or becoming defensive. For example, a potential employer may ask if you have a criminal record, and anyone can understand the need to keep people who have been convicted of certain crimes out of our profession. If there's anything negative in your past, it's better to be upfront about it than have it discovered later that you covered it up. You could say, "Yes, I was arrested for disturbing the peace during a nuclear power plant protest when I was in college, but that was 10 years ago and I haven't been in trouble since." Honesty is the best policy.

If a potential employer asks a discriminatory question, such as your religion or sexual orientation, you don't have to answer. Not only is that against the law, but it's also probably a good sign that you wouldn't want to work there.

ALTERNATE ROUTES: PREPARING FOR YOUR CAREER

Employees

If you intend to work for someone else as a stepping-stone on the way to owning your own business, it's never too early to network and start making connections with people with whom you'll want to do business in the future. If you plan to spend your massage career as an employee, seek a quality employer who is established, and who doesn't have a lot of turnover. That's usually a good sign that employees are treated fairly. You might schedule a massage or two there before applying, chat a little with the therapists, and just soak in the atmosphere. Does it seem like there's a serene ambience, or does the staff seem rushed and overworked?

Independent contractors

If you work as an independent contractor in someone else's business, you may be responsible for bringing in your own clients. Network with other practitioners by becoming a member of a professional association and cultivating mutual referrals.

Business partners

If you're considering a partnership with one or more people, all of you should take the same self-inventory and compare answers. An advantage of being partners is that one person may possess qualities or skills the other doesn't have, and that knowledge can be used to decide how to divide the tasks needed for running the business.

INFORMATION AHEAD

You might be fortunate enough that your first job turns out to be your last—you immediately find your niche and stay put until retirement. However, many therapists take a job after getting licensed as a means to an end; perhaps they plan to work for someone else for a year or two to gain experience, or to give them time to save the money to go into business for themselves.

SETTING GOALS

Even if you're still getting your education and graduation is a year away, set a goal for yourself for Opening Day or for Get-a-Job-Day. Write it down: *Launch Day, January 2, 2012*, or whatever you decide. Procrastination is your vital enemy. Don't wait until a week before your goal date to write your business plan or to start a list of possible places for job hunting. There are many details for you to address. Don't get in your own way by lack of action.

CAUTION

Wherever you are today—working, in school, at home, or playing somewhere—do you think it's where you'll want to be a year from now, 5 years, or even 20 years from now? When you're setting goals, think about not only your actual physical place in the world, but your *circumstances*—your employment, your finances, your personal relationships, your life situation. If you want *more*—more money, more job security, more enjoyment from your work, more time to play, and enjoy your family and friends—learning how to be a smart businessperson is an important step toward achieving those goals.

Your Wish List

An important first step in goal setting is to define your personal vision—your wish list—of what you will require in order to consider yourself to be conducting your business successfully. To some people, success might mean seeing six clients a day, 6 days a week. Some might want six clients a week and plenty of time to spend with the family. Things become clearer when you have to write them down (Fig. 1-6). Making lists is not a prerequisite to being successful, but it is a tool many successful people use. Be specific.

Building a business takes time, and having a timeline set for yourself can keep you motivated as you move along the path to achievement. For instance, in the one-year plan below, the therapist is focused on finishing school and finding a job that will pay the bills, but looking ahead by scouting locations for her future business. By year 2, she's planning to rent space and share the premises with other practitioners, and by year 5, she's realizing her long-range plan of buying a building to house her business.

To maximize your chances for a successful business, focus on setting goals to help you: Go Out And Live Successfully (GOALS). After you've defined what you want, start defining the actions you can take to make it happen by writing down a plan. We'll get to the actual **business plan** in Chapter 2. This is a general list of actions you'll need to take in order to start meeting your goals.

The One-Year Plan

1. Join a professional association. (Note: all massage associations admit student members.)
2. Finish massage school.
3. Scout for good locations to open my office.
4. Take the necessary exam for licensure (exams for licensure and certification are discussed in Chapter 4).

Wish List

- Be self-employed (or employed at a spa, clinic, etc.)
- Have an office close to home
- Get home each night by 6 p.m.
- Have thirty clients a week
- Be off every weekend
- Be able to afford health insurance
- Have two weeks off every year
- Fund college for kids
- Pay off mortgage early
- Be able to retire at 50
- Be able to give to charity

FIGURE 1-6   Setting goals; getting started. You can adapt this wish list to your own desires and strengths, whether you are considering owning your own business or being a business partner, an employee, or an independent contractor.

5. Work at a resort spa for a year to gain experience and save money for opening my own office.
6. Visit the local office of the Small Business Administration (SBA) and Chamber of Commerce to find what resources are available.

The Two-Year Plan

1. Rent an office with at least two treatment rooms on the west side of town.
2. Line up a couple of other practitioners to share the office.
3. Open for business.
4. Enter esthetician school so that I can offer other services.

The Five-Year Plan

1. Buy a building of my own that can be retrofitted with a wet room.
2. Have a dozen practitioners of different disciplines together in one clinic.
3. Be able to hire a permanent receptionist, and laundry and cleaning services.

These plans are simple, just to give you the idea. Writing down your goals will help you have them clearly in mind when you start writing your business plan.

> ### ROADSIDE ASSISTANCE
>
> My goal: every day I spend at work is to make money and to have fun while I'm doing it. My own wish list is ever-evolving, and I always keep it on a sticky note on the corner of my computer screen. It's my way of "keeping my eyes on the prize," and it's fun to check those goals off as they're met.

The Balancing Act

Working hard is usually a prerequisite to meeting goals, but it can be both an asset and a liability when you own your own business. You have to be *willing* to work hard. As the owner, you're the one with the ultimate responsibility, even if you have many staff members. However, you can't enjoy your work nearly as much if you're resentful of the amount of time you have to spend at the workplace. You don't want to look back years from now and regret that you didn't spend enough time with your children or your spouse, or that you never went on that trip you wanted to take, or learned how to crochet or bungee-jump because you were too busy working. There has to be a balance, and it's up to you to find it. All of us need time to play, no matter how much we enjoy our work.

RECREATION AREA AHEAD

Here are some guidelines for entrepreneurs:

- Decide on your opening hours, and adhere to them.
- Plan for emergencies. Another therapist in your office may become ill and you'll have to step in and take over some clients.
- Don't keep your business open 7 days a week. Then, even if an emergency occurs, you will still have 1 day off. Think carefully about that if you are considering buying into a franchise massage business that may require staying open 7 days a week.
- Schedule your time off work, giving it the same importance as work time. Take time to do the things you enjoy outside of work, things that leave you feeling refreshed and restored.

If you're working for someone else, your schedule may be at their whim, but you still have to make time for self-care and other obligations you may have. Prioritize, and don't put getting your own massage at the bottom of your list!

Words of Wisdom
I take care of myself, so I can take care of my business.

RESOURCES TO HELP YOU GET STARTED

Some of the best resources for people who own and operate small businesses are free or are available at a reasonable price. They include the SBA, the Chamber of Commerce, and the various professional associations that serve massage therapists and others in the healing arts. Remember to check the IRS website for tax requirements and instructions.

The Small Business Administration

The SBA was created in 1953 as an independent agency of the federal government to aid, counsel, assist, and protect the interest of small business concerns, thereby helping to maintain and strengthen the overall economy of our nation. Can you imagine our country without small businesses? You can't get your clothes cleaned at IBM, your car serviced at AT&T, or your health care from General Motors. Small businesses are the backbone of the U.S. economy, and the SBA has numerous programs to facilitate the success of small business owners. There are programs specifically to help women business owners, minority business owners, disabled business owners, and even teenage entrepreneurs.

The SBA website has pages that provide instructions and helpful templates on such myriad topics as writing a business plan, naming your business, obtaining financing, leasing equipment, finding a **mentor**, getting licenses and permits, and many more items of interest. There are free video courses you can view on the website, including starting a small business on a shoestring, from none other than Donald Trump. The SBA does not actually lend money, but they do guarantee loans if you obtain a small business loan from your local bank in order to start or expand your business.

Most small towns have an SBA office, where you can get all kinds of literature and free advice. SBA offices in your town may be located in a government building. Sometimes they are located in the business department at local community colleges. SBA staff members will provide you with a free folder containing invaluable information about the local permits and licenses you may need to obtain, tax information for small businesses, and a checklist of things to take care of in preparing for opening day.

The Chamber of Commerce

The U.S. Chamber of Commerce is the world's largest federation of businesses, representing more than 3 million businesses of every size and description. As with the SBA, there is a Chamber office in most towns and cities. The Chamber differs from the SBA in that local Chambers are not necessarily affiliated with the national Chamber; many are independent organizations. You must pay annual dues to join, but the fee is reasonable. In small towns, dues for individual business owners start at about $100 per year and go up based on the number of employees you have. There are many benefits to membership listed in Box 1-1.

BOX 1-1   Benefits of Chamber of Commerce Membership

- Free publicity and promotional opportunities for your business.
- Networking opportunities with the public and other business owners at Chamber functions.
- Free listing on the Chamber's website.
- Free listing in the Chamber's membership directory.
- Opportunities to receive discounts from other Chamber merchants.
- Discounted advertising opportunities.
- Free space to place your business literature and cards in the Chamber office.
- Combining your voice with other small business owners in local politics concerning economic development.
- Business referrals from the Chamber office.
- Exposure to newcomers who often visit a Chamber website before vacationing or moving to the area.
- Inexpensive access to the Chamber's mailing list.
- Educational programs offered by the Chamber to enhance the skills and knowledge of small business people.
- Free access to members of SCORE (Service Corps of Retired Executives) to help advise and mentor you.
- Displaying the Chamber seal in your business lends credibility and indicates your involvement in the local business community.

Market Research

Your local Chamber of Commerce is a goldmine of information free for the asking. Chambers traditionally maintain statistics on population and **demographics**. This information will be very useful to you when you conduct your **market study** (see Chapter 2).

Education

The Chamber sponsors inexpensive or free classes on such topics as tax help for small businesses, and **marketing** your business on the Internet. Members have free access to SCORE, the Service Corps of Retired Executives, who are available for consulting and mentoring. The business advice alone is worth the cost of Chamber membership. More about the various opportunities associated with the Chamber of Commerce and Internet marketing appears in Chapters 13 and 14.

Networking

Members have the opportunity of **networking** with other members. The Chamber also has a member-to-member discount program, in which members discount their goods and services to each other. You can participate in the frequent Chamber functions to help to get your name out to the public. A popular Chamber function in many towns is known as Business After Hours, or in some places, a breakfast or lunch meeting. The Chamber advertises it by fax and e-mail to all the members, and in the "local events" section in the newspaper. Local business owners provide refreshments, and some also supply entertainment. These events give others a chance to come in and see what the business is all about. They are attended by other merchants and businesspeople who really appreciate the value of networking.

When you network with other business owners, it can be a marketing bonanza for your business and for theirs. You may establish mutual referral relationships, with everyone from a physician to a local florist. Trade business cards with as many people as possible at Chamber functions. Talk to others about who you are and what you do, and listen to others so that you can find out about their business. Other people are eager to make beneficial connections, too. It's a win-win situation.

Benefits for All

The Chamber bends over backward to help small businesses, especially those just starting out. They *want* you to succeed. It's in the interest of the local economy for your business to succeed, and that filters all the way up to the national economy.

Your service-oriented business will be promoted by the Chamber of Commerce to tourists and to newcomers. As a member, you can display your business cards or literature in the Chamber office, which in many towns or cities is in a high-visibility location. You can have a listing on their website at no additional charge other than your annual membership fee.

Getting Off to a Good Start

One function of the Chamber of Commerce is to welcome new businesses to the area. They will arrange a ribbon-cutting ceremony, with invited local dignitaries like the mayor, the members of the town council, and neighboring merchants. They usually have a photographer from the local newspaper. Many newspapers will run "new business opens" announcements for free. Any time a new member joins the Chamber, it is announced to other members by way of fax, e-mail, and in Chamber publications.

EXPLORATIONS

Even if you're not ready to join yet, call or visit your local Chamber of Commerce and ask for a membership packet. The staff there will be happy to answer any questions you may have, and to talk to you about what the Chamber does to help promote small businesses.

Professional Associations

As a holistic health care practitioner, you have access to at least one professional association for business tips and marketing materials, online support, free website listings, networking opportunities: the American Holistic Health Association. Massage therapists have the American Massage Therapy Association (AMTA) and ABMP, both of which are open to students; you don't have to wait until graduation to join. Reiki practitioners have the International Reiki Professionals Association. In addition, there are the American Naturopathic Medical Association, the North American Society of Homeopaths, the American Association of Acupuncture and Oriental Medicine, and dozens more. Canada has many such associations, and so does most of Europe. The Internet has made the world a smaller place. Even if you live in a remote area with no local chapters of your professional association, you can still participate online.

Professional associations often sponsor continuing education classes, have lending libraries, and maintain a list of business coaches and mentors. Many practitioners belong to more than one organization, so they can avail themselves of different services and opportunities.

Attending conventions is one of the great joys of belonging to a professional association. The annual AMTA convention has been held in some great cities like Denver, Albuquerque, Atlanta, Phoenix, and Cincinnati, just to name a few. There is something awesome about being with a thousand or so people who do what you do, and who understand the joys and the challenges that we face as massage therapists. It's like a big family reunion every year, lots of social events are planned, and the speakers and continuing education opportunities are the cream of the crop. Sign up for a great experience—you'll be glad you did.

THE POWER OF A POSITIVE ATTITUDE

A positive attitude is one of the most important components of success. Believing in yourself and your capabilities is the key, and so is recognizing your shortcomings and taking steps to rectify them or asking for help when necessary. It's hard to have a positive attitude if you're worried about your rent check bouncing, or when you're overwhelmed and can't seem to keep up with your clients, keep the office clean, and stay on top of your bookkeeping. A positive attitude is something you often have to work at, and not everyone is wired to be upbeat and happy all the time.

When you work in a job that involves serving the public, your attitude can make or break your business. Even on those days when your child is being a monster, your tire went flat on the way to work, and your washing machine is on the fritz, it's important to "keep the faith" and at least maintain the appearance of a positive attitude. You can go to pieces if you want to after all the clients have gone for the day, but realize that during business hours, people want to be greeted by someone with a smiling face and a cheerful disposition.

Keeping a positive attitude will make your business and your life in general go more smoothly; otherwise, you'll find that little things that are just temporary bumps in the road seem like a train wreck. When things go wrong, and they will, a negative attitude isn't going to help the situation. You might feel a little better if you kick the flat tire; then again, you might break your foot! Everyone has an occasional setback.

ROADSIDE ASSISTANCE

My rule of thumb for whether to have a meltdown when something bad happens is to ask myself: Is what happened going to make any difference a year from now? If the consequences are so serious that I'll still be feeling the effects a year from now, then I go ahead and get mad, have a pity party, or whatever I need to do in order to diffuse the upset and make myself feel better. Then, I can get to work figuring out what to do about the problem. In the long run, it isn't worth it to waste energy on something minor like a jam in the copy machine. In situations like these, I take a deep breath—and let it go—instead of letting it ruin my day.

Banishing Negativity

There's no room for negativity in a successful business—particularly a service-based business where you are constantly dealing with the public. *Practice* having a positive attitude. Seek out positive people to be around.

Sometimes people with good intentions will disparage your plans. *The economy's bad right now. It isn't the time. Wait until your kids graduate from college. How many people get massage anyway? That office isn't very fancy. People might not want to drive five miles out of town to see you.* Consider the source. Is it someone who is already a successful businessperson giving you advice? If it's your brother-in-law who sits on the couch watching sit-coms all day and doesn't have enough ambition to fill up a thimble, tune him out.

Words of Wisdom
If you can't avoid negative people, surround yourself with a cloak of optimism before you go near them.

People sometimes sabotage themselves in ways they aren't even aware of. Procrastination, looking at the glass as half-empty instead of half-full, being around others who have that view—all of these are obstacles to succeeding. Gradually break those habits, and you'll be better off. Don't get in your own way by succumbing to self-sabotage.

When someone close to you, such as a spouse, significant other, or best friend, constantly disapproves of your desire to follow your dreams, one of two things will happen once you decide to proceed with your plan. Ideally, he will see how happy you are for coming into your own and doing what you want to do, and he will be happy *for* you. If that doesn't happen, it might become a losing battle. Sometimes, deciding to follow your own heart means distancing yourself from relationships that are no longer serving you.

Showing Confidence

If you're a new therapist looking for a job, employers want people who have a confident, positive attitude. In fact, many potential employers value positivity more than skill. If you're applying for a job, apply with a smile on your face. Even if you get turned down at that moment, you want to be remembered in a positive way later on when they might be looking to hire someone. Represent your talents honestly, and be upbeat about the opportunity to learn things you don't know. Put on a happy face! Be confident! Psychological studies have shown that *acting* happy can actually make you a happier person.

Clients want to see practitioners with a positive attitude because some of that rubs off on them. People seek holistic practitioners because they are looking for a more natural approach to health care, and nothing's more natural and welcoming than a smile. Go to work every day wearing one, and you'll be that much closer to success.

Debra Benton, an executive development coach and author, reminds us that cultivating self-confidence and keeping a positive attitude are all about choosing perspective. When you don't succeed, you can say you're a failure, think about all the things you should have done, and tell yourself you might as well give up because you don't have what it takes to make it. Conversely, you can say you've learned something new, think about how you'll use that information in the future, and tell yourself that—now that you know what *not* to do the next time—you're closer than ever to achieving your goal.

SUCCESS NEXT EXIT

If you think you need help keeping a positive attitude, *The Power of Positive Thinking* by Dr. Norman Vincent Peale is a great motivator. Although Dr. Peale's book is written from a Christian perspective, the premises have been adopted by many authors and self-help groups—because they work. First published in 1952, the book has sold millions of copies and been translated into 15 languages. Dr. Peale offers simple suggestions for letting go of stress, resentment, and worry; he describes ways of visualizing happiness and success, and removing self-doubt and fear. It's powerful!

Going with the Flow

To keep up with the latest trends in the massage and bodywork business, subscribe to the trade journals. *Massage Magazine*, *Massage Therapy Journal*, *Massage & Bodywork*, and *Massage Today* are all good resources for the latest in massage research, the latest products, tips for practice, and timely business advice from experts in the field.

POSTCARDS from the HIGHWAY

Tom Myers

I've been in this trade for over 30 years now, through many ups and downs.

There are two measures of your practice skill—the soaring, intuitive session you give on your best day, and the plodding, distracted session you give on your worst day. Keep a close watch on the latter; the sessions you give when you are having a bad day are a better measure of your basic skill and professionalism.

How to be successful in manual therapy: We are born into three instincts: the instinct to preserve ourselves, the instinct to relate to others, and the instinct to orient to what's happening in the world. The way to success is to follow your instincts. If you forget yourself and get lost in others, you will suffer in your own practice. Make sure your practice is feeding your spirit and making you inside-happy. If you are not getting up each morning happy to go to work, you are not in this instinct. Each client is a relationship—listen! There is nothing as interesting as people, so if you're losing your interest in them, take a break. So much new is happening in this field; don't be satisfied with your same old routine. Take your commitment to keep yourself educated and fresh seriously, by making the time for classes, mentoring, or getting work yourself.

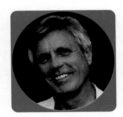

Thomas Myers is the author of *Anatomy Trains* (Churchill Livingstone; 2nd ed., 2008). An internationally known speaker and instructor, he received direct training from Drs. Ida Rolf, Moshe Feldenkrais, and Buckminster Fuller, and he has been practicing and teaching integrative manual therapy all over the world for more than three decades. Visit his website at www.anatomytrains.com.

SUGGESTED READINGS

American Association of Acupuncture and Oriental Medicine. Membership. http://www.aaaomonline.com/index.php?act=viewCat&catId=4. Accessed 07/24/2009.

American Holistic Health Association. Join/Donate. http://ahha.org/joindonate.asp. Accessed 07/24/2009.

American Massage Therapy Association. Join AMTA. http://www.amtamassage.org/membership-intro.html. Accessed 07/27/2009.

American Naturopathic Medical Association. Application for membership. http://www.anma.org/pdf/application.pdf. Accessed 07/24/2009.

Anatomy Trains. http://www.anatomytrains.com/at/people/tom-myers. Tom Myers. Accessed 07/24/2009.

Benton D. *Lions Don't Need to Roar: Using the Leadership Power of Personal Presence to Stand Out, Fit in, and Move Ahead.* New York, NY: Grand Central Publishing, 1993.

Bureau of Labor Statistics. Massage therapists. http://www.bls.gov/oco/pdf/ocos295.pdf. Accessed 07/24/2009.

Explosive Growth Rate for Massage Therapy Training Begins to Flatten. http://www.massagetherapy.com/media/metricsgrowth.php. Accessed 07/24/2009.

Internal Revenue Service. Tax Information for Businesses. http://www.irs.gov/businesses/index.html?navmenu=menu1. Accessed 08/28/2009.

International Association of Reiki Professionals. Join IARP-Register. http://iarp.org/registration.php. Accessed 07/24/2009.

Massage & Bodywork Magazine. http://www.massageandbodywork.com. Accessed 07/24/2009.

Massage Magazine. http://www.massagemag.com. Accessed 07/24/2009.

Massage Therapy Journal. http://www.amtamassage.org/journal. Accessed 07/24/2009.

Massage Today. http://www.massagetoday.com. Accessed 07/24/2009.

National Certification Board for Therapeutic Massage & Bodywork. New Distance Education Component. http://www.ncbtmb.org/pdf/infoline/vol_2007_no3.pdf. Accessed 5:52 pm EDT, 07/24/2009.

North American Society of Homeopaths. Join. http://www.homeopathy.org/join.html. Accessed 07/24/2009.

Peale, Dr. Norman Vincent. *The Power of Positive Thinking*. Fireside, 2007.

Resume Goals. http://www.careerowlresources.ca/Resumes/Res_Frame.htm?res_overview.html.right. Accessed 08/27/2009.

Service Corps of Retired Executives. Ask Score for Business Advice. http://www.score.org/index.html. Accessed 07/24/2009.

Small Business Administration. Programs and Services to Help You Start, Grow, and Succeed. http://www.sba.gov. Accessed 07/24/2009.

Steiner Leisure. www.str.co.uk. Accessed 07/24/2009.

United States Chamber of Commerce. http://www.uschamber.com. Accessed 07/24/2009.

My Personal Journey

In this chapter, we've discussed the importance of setting concrete goals as a prerequisite to creating a business plan or beginning a job search. Make a list of your goals for the future in three different categories: (1) short-term goals that you want to meet immediately, within the next few weeks or months; (2) longer-term goals that you want to meet within 1 year; and (3) five-year goals, things you want to accomplish within the next few years, whether you are self-employed or working for others. Consider carefully the most important priorities on your lists, with the intent to accomplish them first.

My goals _____

_____

_____

What's in my way? _____

_____

_____

What action can I take to remedy the situation? _____

_____

_____

One-year progress update _____

_____

_____

CHAPTER 2

The Business Plan

Create a definite plan for yourself and begin at once, whether you are ready or not, to put this plan into action.

NAPOLEON HILL

KEY CONCEPTS

- Writing a formal business plan should be the first step in preparing to open a business, and it is a necessity for those who are seeking a business loan.

- Examining your desires and needs for the future before writing your plan can help identify the strategies to help you meet those objectives.

- A certified financial planner will help determine whether or not your plan is financially feasible.

- Resources are available from the Small Business Administration, the Chamber of Commerce, and professional associations; many Internet companies and software programs provide business plan services and templates.

- The components of a well-thought-out business plan are pulled together by the executive summary into a cohesive statement.

- The key parts of the business plan are the objectives, the mission statement, a description of the keys to success as visualized by the entrepreneur, the company highlights, biographies of the owners, start-up budget projections, details of the services and products that will be offered, a market study and survey analysis, and a plan for marketing strategies.

Starting a business without a business plan would be like driving across the country with no map to guide you. You may eventually get where you want to go, but it will be a long and winding journey with many wrong turns along the way. Your sweat equity, determination, and enthusiasm will be invested in your business, and they're vital parts of it. Taking those parts and combining them with a carefully thought-out business plan is like having a great set of directions. You'll reach your destination faster with a good plan.

EXPRESS LANE AHEAD

THE IMPORTANCE OF PLANNING

You may think you don't need a written business plan if you're a lone practitioner, if you intend to only do outcalls, or if you aren't borrowing money to start your business, but you should prepare one just the same. The act of preparing a business plan will have a far more positive effect than just kicking around vague ideas in your head; it will help you meet your personal and financial goals. James L. Silvester, president of Business Experts, Inc., and a motivational coach and speaker, says no operation is too small for planning, even home-based business, and he points out that a lack of planning leads to missed opportunities for income and growth. "Today's challenging economic environment demands extra diligence in that even a few mistakes may prove to be unforgiving no matter the size of your business," Silvester says. "Even the smallest operation needs a plan of action, a road map so to speak, that will assist the owner down the highway to ultimate business success. To quote the great French Chemist Louis Pasteur, 'chance favors the prepared mind.'" (Silvester, personal communication.)

A **business plan** is a written summary of the purpose, goals, and strategies for starting a business. It includes details about how the objectives of the business will be accomplished, and the reasons *why* the owner believes his or her goals for the business are obtainable. A business plan may be written with the intent of gaining a bank loan or attracting investors, or it can simply be for the owner's use as a tool for getting started, maintaining momentum, and growing a business.

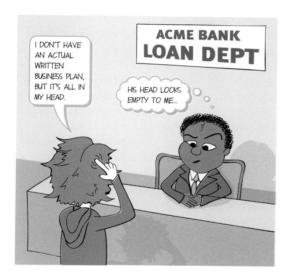

Different Strokes for Different Folks

If everybody wanted the same thing, one plan would work for everybody, but your business plan should be as individual as you are. A person who doesn't have children may need a business plan that varies greatly from that of a parent with four young kids. A 40-year-old massage therapist who is switching careers will probably have a plan that's a lot different from that of a therapist who is 20 and just starting her working life. People have different priorities, different financial needs and desires, different ideas about the amount of time they want to spend working, and their own unique ideas about what constitutes success. These are all issues to consider before writing your business plan.

Resources for Planning

There is plenty of footwork to do to get ready to open your business. If you plan to borrow start-up funds from a bank or other source, you *must* prepare a professional business plan; showing up at a bank to borrow money without a business plan would be just as irresponsible as showing up without any proof of identification. Even if you're borrowing money from your mother, she should have the expectation that you have a concrete plan for your business, including a plan to repay the loan. Don't feel overwhelmed; there are many resources available to help you create your plan.

The Small Business Administration, the Chamber of Commerce, and the professional associations mentioned in Chapter 1 are good sources for sample business plans and financial forms. There are hundreds of businesses on the Internet devoted to writing business plans for potential entrepreneurs, costing anywhere from $299 for a basic plan to thousands of dollars for a plan that's guaranteed to impress the bank or potential investors. You could go that route, but writing a business plan is really not as difficult as you might think. An example of an actual business plan is shown in Box 2-1 later in the chapter.

BOX 2-1   Business Plan for THERA-SSAGE, LLC

Executive Summary

THERA-SSAGE is a holistic health clinic and educational facility located in Rutherfordton, North Carolina. We offer nine comfortable and tastefully decorated treatment rooms and a classroom for community education classes as well as continuing education classes for massage therapists and others in the holistic healing arts. Our team of health care practitioners includes massage therapists, acupuncturists, an R.N. trained as an aesthetician, a chiropractor who is also a naturopath, and energy workers. Our organization is already an approved provider of continuing education under the NCBTMB (National Certification Board for Therapeutic Massage and Bodywork) for several disciplines. Our focus is on being a venue for natural health and wellness, and although some spa-type treatments, such as therapeutic mud and exfoliations, are offered, we have no plans to add other spa services, such as nail or hair services, because we do not want any chemicals in our setting. Our services are wellness based, and future expansion will focus strictly on wellness treatments and educational offerings.

This business plan has been developed to track our progress from opening through our five-year expansion plan; the projected growth during these 5 years is illustrated in the accompanying bar graph. Although we are using money from our savings as start-up funds, we may seek additional financing from outside sources in the future as the need to expand our facilities becomes necessary as projected.

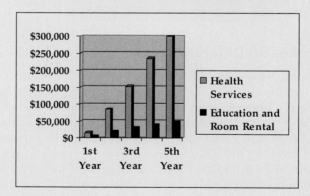

Objectives

1. To establish ourselves as a one-stop destination for holistic health and wellness services.
2. To expand our visibility and reputation as a provider of high-quality wellness-based education for the community at large, as well as the practitioner community seeking continuing education.

(continued)

BOX 2-1 Business Plan for THERA-SSAGE, LLC

3. To increase our income every year by gaining one new client every day, 365 days a year.
4. To have a word-of-mouth referral rate of 95%.
5. To have a client retention rate of 65%, allowing for the fact that we are located just on the outskirts of a popular tourist destination and that some of our clients will just be passing through.
6. To perform 20 treatments per day by the end of the first year, increasing to 50 or more treatments per day by the end of the fifth year.
7. To increase attendance at our educational offerings by 50% every year, and increase the number of classes that are offered.

Mission Statement

We seek to serve our community and beyond by honoring the human body, mind, and spirit of every person who comes through our door.

The Keys to Our Success

1. *Experience:* The owner has been a massage therapist, as well as an instructor and administrator, for more than a decade. Prior to that, she had a 20+ year career as the owner of four successful restaurants and catering operations. She has vast experience in marketing, daily business operations, and being a team leader. In addition, the practitioners who are joining the business have a combined strength and track record of many years both in practice and as educators.
2. *Professional credentials:* The team of practitioners we have assembled are all professional and dedicated and will be bringing many of their own existing clients into the business. Our massage therapists are all graduates of massage schools requiring at least 500 hours of education, nationally certified and licensed by the North Carolina Board of Massage and Bodywork Therapy. Our acupuncturists are Masters of Oriental Medicine, Fellows of the National Certifying Commission of Acupuncture and Oriental Medicine (NCCAOM), and licensed by the state Board of Acupuncture. Our chiropractor is licensed and has been practicing for more than 20 years. Our registered nurse has been licensed for more than 30 years and is certified in aesthetic procedures as well as nutritional counseling. Licensure is not required of energy workers in our state, but they are educated and qualified to perform their modalities.
3. *Availability of services:* Our services will accommodate those who seek massage and bodywork, acupuncture, chiropractic, and other forms of holistic health in one location, as well as outcalls. We also serve massage therapists who need to maintain licensure by offering a number of continuing education classes at our facility. While there are massage therapists, chiropractors, and an acupuncturist operating elsewhere in our county, we are the only business to provide all these services in one location.
4. *Mutual referrals:* Our practitioners will refer their clients to the other practitioners in the group; for example, the massage therapist will send someone to the chiropractor, who will refer someone to the acupuncturist, and so forth. We also expect to receive referrals from physicians, dentists, and other health care professionals.
5. *Location:* Rutherfordton, North Carolina, is just 15 minutes away from the popular tourist destinations of Chimney Rock and Lake Lure. It is along the busy main route for popular skiing and other winter sports destinations. Our attractive new and modern office is conveniently located in a complex housing other service businesses just south of the Historic District of town. The building is highly visible at 431 S. Main Street. Both parking and the facility are handicapped-accessible. The setting is professional without being too clinical, and we are striving for an aesthetic of uncluttered, serene simplicity.

(continued)

BOX 2-1 Business Plan for THERA-SSAGE, LLC

Company Highlights

We will provide services to appeal to both men and women of all ages, at a price that is affordable to the general public. We will also have a retail section where we will sell organic oils, skin products, and nutritional products. Our organization has already been successful in offering continuing education classes, which we formerly held in rented hotel conference facilities; our new location will allow us to teach classes on-site in a highly visible location that is convenient to transportation, other professionals, businesses offering many goods and services, and restaurants and lodging. The convenience of offering such a variety of wellness services and practitioners of different disciplines, as well as education, in one location makes us unique in our area.

Company Ownership

THERA-SSAGE is owned by Champ and Laura Allen. Laura Allen has been a massage therapist and educator for more than a decade. She is the author of three books related to the field of massage and bodywork, and a frequent contributor to trade journals. Champ Allen has been self-employed for many years in the construction business and has experience working with the public. He is also a graduate of massage school and an energy worker. Although he will not be involved in daily business operations, he will perform energy work on a part-time basis, and his support of Laura's management and presence in the business are assets. As the owner of his own contracting business, he will also handle all maintenance and repairs not covered under our lease, thereby saving money that would be spent paying someone else.

Start-Up Budget Projections

The start-up expenses for the business, such as rent, utility deposits, office equipment and other necessities, will be invested solely by the owners. The practitioners in the business are independent contractors who will provide their own equipment other than basic furnishings, thus lowering the start-up costs. The accompanying tables detail the company's assets, start-up/first year expenses, liabilities, and owner's equity.

Assets

Décor and office furnishings	$15,000
Computer equipment and software	$2000
Laundry equipment	$2000
Linens	$2000
Spa treatment supplies	$1000
Products to retail	$2000
Signage	$1000
Total value of assets	$25,000

Start-Up/First Year Expenses

Legal expenses	$1000
1 year lease on building	$17,400
Utility and phone deposits	$600
Printing brochures, cards, and misc. business literature	$3000

(continued)

BOX 2-1   Business Plan for THERA-SSAGE, LLC

Website development	$1000
Advertising	$7500
Accounting	$1200
Office supplies	$500
Janitorial supplies	$500
Total start-up expenses	$32,700
Total funding needed	$57,700

Liabilities and Equity

Money used from owner's savings	$20,000
Owner's equity at start-up	$37,700

Services and Products

All services are provided by independent contractors, who are paid a commission for the services they provide, meaning there is compensation only when the business brings in money; no sales, no cost. The products we will be retailing are high-end organic products and items recommended by our staff chiropractor, such as custom orthotics and orthopedic pillows, with a 40% to 60% profit margin. We project an additional gross income of $50,000 per year by our fifth year from the use of our classroom facility, which can accommodate between 14 and 40 participants, depending on whether the class is a lecture class or a hands-on massage class.

Market Study and Survey Analysis

Our services are directed at everyone and priced so that everyone can afford them. Our primary market is composed of residents all over Rutherford County, who we believe will visit our business because of the uniqueness of having so many holistic services under one roof. We are also in close proximity to tourist areas that are popular year-round. On four consecutive Sundays in January, we asked skiers stopping at the Rutherford County Hospitality Center if they would be inclined to use massage and spa services en route to and/or from the ski area and received a positive response.

Other solo massage therapists are located a minimum of 5 miles away from our location. The only other licensed acupuncturist in the county is located 15 miles away. There is only one other chiropractor in town; although there are several more located in other communities throughout the county, there are none in a group practice such as ours.

We expect our clientele to be equally distributed among people who are seeking stress relief through massage and others who need help in pain management or are recovering from trauma or injury. We will be set up to accept health insurance as the presence of the chiropractor in our office means that many plans will cover that service, as well as the massage therapy he will prescribe.

We hesitate to name a specific target market because we intend to target everyone who has an income above poverty level. Our pricing is in line with what others in the area charge. Our services will be in the range of $30 to $120 per session, depending on the procedure and the time involved (sessions as short as 30 minutes are available). The individual contractors have the right to discount or "comp" their services for clients who genuinely need services and can't afford them at full price. We think this practice will serve the community at large and our business in the long run by creating good will.

(continued)

> ### BOX 2-1   Business Plan for THERA-SSAGE, LLC
>
> #### Marketing Strategies
>
> We will initially do a media blitz announcing our opening through advertising in the county newspaper and on local cable channels and radio, and by staff members handing out cards and brochures to the public. We will advertise in the Yellow Pages and have a website that will be listed on all our printed business materials. Our color brochures will be placed in as many of the guesthouses, motels, and hotels in the local area and the adjoining resort/tourist area as possible.
>
> We will have booth space at all the main festivals in our town, such as the Octoberfest and the Spring Fling. Our staff members will be going out to many venues such as the Fire Department, Police Department, and other locations of public service, hospice houses, health food stores, the Hospitality Center, and other appropriate places that will allow us to come in and do chair massage as a way of publicizing our business while performing community service.
>
> Prior to opening, Laura Allen has done a personal mailing on business letterhead to all physicians and many other health care professionals in the area, detailing our services and the fact that we accept health insurance, along with the assurance that we will be diligent in following through with referrals and will reciprocate when warranted. We have already gotten a positive response. We believe that as with most successful service businesses, once the word gets out, the majority of our clients will come from word-of-mouth referrals from other clients. We are well prepared to open our business and look forward to seeing it grow.

THE COMPONENTS OF A BUSINESS PLAN

A well-thought-out business plan is composed of several important components:

- An executive summary.
- A list of business objectives.
- The mission statement of the business.
- The keys to success: strengths that give your business the potential to thrive, including the experience and professionalism of the staff, availability of services, plans for mutual referrals, and location.
- Company highlights: specifics about your business that will make it stand out from other similar businesses in your area. Using a bulleted list is one way of emphasizing these features and calling more attention to the unique details of your plan.
- Company ownership: biographical information about the owner(s) of the business.
- A start-up budget: projected income and expenses for at least the first year. A five-year plan is ideal because it shows you intend to have growth and staying power.
- Information about the services and products your business will offer.
- A market study and market survey analysis.
- A statement about the marketing strategies you intend to implement.

Executive Summary

A business plan actually begins with an **executive summary**; however, it's best not to write it until you've written the rest of your plan. When you are satisfied with the rest of the plan, write the executive summary to pull all the key points together, and use it as the introduction to your plan.

Objectives

Objectives are the concrete goals of the business; for example, gaining one new customer every day, hiring two additional therapists within a year, or selling $1000 worth of gift certificates every month. If you're seeking financing for your business, the objectives—and any other sections of your business plan that quote numbers—are enhanced by including a visual aid such as a chart, table, or graph, like the one in Box 2-1.

People who choose the healing arts as a profession usually have an objective other than financial success—such as the desire to help people—but we all want to make a comfortable living in exchange for the work we do. Referring to the wish list in Chapter 1 (Figs. 1-1 to 1-6), let's refine those goals and treat them as concrete objectives for your business plan. Instead of a wish list, it will become an *action* list. If an office close to home is your first wish, start by taking positive action toward making that happen, such as scouting available locations and inquiring about the cost of properties for rent and for sale in the area, and weighing the options of renting versus owning.

Buying property is a much bigger commitment than being a renter, but on the other hand, it will be *your* property, and ownership builds **equity**. Keep in mind that one of the main purposes of the business plan is to *identify the strategies that will enable you to meet the objectives*, so do your research. Given the facts, you can make a more informed decision about whether to rent or own. Here are the main differences:

Owning

- A substantial down payment is usually required.
- The mortgage can be any length, up to as much as 30 years.
- Property taxes are your responsibility.
- Maintenance is your responsibility.
- You build equity in the property as you pay off the mortgage.
- Property is a tangible investment that you can sell if you decide to move or leave the business.

Renting

- No cash investment is required except a deposit and commitment to monthly rent.
- The owner, or landlord, may require a lease of any duration, or rent month-to month.
- Property taxes are the owner's responsibility.
- Maintenance is the owner's responsibility, possibly with some stipulations.
- You have no equity and no real property.

The second wish shown in Figures 1-1 to 6, 30 clients a week, sounds like a great goal to aspire to. It looks even better when you plug in the figures. According to Associated Bodywork & Professionals, the median price for a massage is currently $60 per hour; that may be more or less in your location. Body workers who perform Rolfing or other specialties may charge $100 or more per hour. Based on the median, 30 clients per week at $60 per hourly session, 50 weeks a year (remember, another goal is 2 weeks off every year!) yields the tidy sum of $90,000 before taxes and expenses; this is known as **gross income**. (A full discussion about pricing your services appears in Chapter 12.)

If you take weekends off (another one of the goals listed in Figs. 1.1–1.6), that means six clients a day, 5 days a week, which is possible for some and not for others. That could be a tough pace to maintain. Paying careful attention to your body mechanics and your health in general will prolong your career, and only you can decide how many sessions a day you can perform without overdoing it.

Use your own wish list to refine the goals for your business as a preliminary step to creating the plan that will help you meet your objectives.

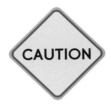

The Mission Statement

Your motivations for going into business will help shape your **mission statement**, a concise statement (usually up to three sentences) of the goals and purposes of a business. Here is an example:

> The mission of Sunset On-Site Massage is to provide massage therapy to older adults with respect and compassion, at their location, at an affordable price.

Keys to Success

This section of your business plan should detail the reasons you are convinced—the ones that will convince an investor or lender—that your business will be a success. It's important to strike a balance between enthusiasm and realism. If you're seeking financing, a loan officer doesn't want to see grandiose projections of profit in the first year; in fact, any potential lender would probably expect most businesses to operate at a loss the first year and might immediately turn down your plan if you're making wild claims of instant profitability. The keys to success should highlight the strengths that will ultimately lead your business to profitability, with a realistic perspective.

Experience

Experience can be presented in a positive light, regardless of what kind of background you have. If you've ever been self-employed, had a job, done volunteer work, been involved in extracurricular activities at school, or run a household prior to coming to massage as a career—name the responsibilities you've had and the talents and skills you possess. Examples are experience in time management and scheduling, analytical and problem solving skills, and written and verbal communication skills.

Professional Credentials

Mention the credentials you and any other staff members are bringing to the business. If you have licensure, certification, registration, or whatever authorization is required in your state, mention it. Particularly if you are practicing in a state that has no licensure or registration requirements, stating your professional training and certification(s) can set you apart from others.

Availability of Services

Define the services you intend to offer. Highlight anything that's unique about your services, such as a modality that isn't available anywhere else nearby. Include something that makes your business different from your competitor's business, such as "Each person who receives a massage is encouraged to use our far-infrared sauna afterward at no additional cost."

Mutual Referrals

If you plan to cultivate mutual referrals (and you definitely should), note that in your business plan. It is helpful to state the professionals with whom you intend to collaborate: "I have mutual referral relationships with a chiropractor and an acupuncturist who are located in my community, and also intend to cultivate relationships with the nearby physicians and dentists." Attach letters of reference or testimonials from physicians or other health care providers that have referred to you.

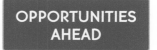

Location

Describe your location in the best possible light, including parking availability, handicap access, and proximity to other goods and services. Don't fail to mention anything that would make the location stand out, such as "Our business is located in the Historic District in the former Halifax Hotel that dates from 1849," or "Our business is located in the new, modern medical building at 101 Main Street in Burton."

Company Highlights

This section should highlight anything that makes your business accessible, market-friendly, competitive, relevant, and timely. Examples:

- My business is connected to a busy gym that's open 24/7 and has over 3000 members. The gym owner has agreed to refer people to my business in exchange for a free afternoon of chair massage once a month for his employees. (Again, it's a good idea to attach a letter from the gym owner or other referral source to reinforce your claim.)
- Our close proximity to the university and the sliding scale fees we plan to offer to students will help our business succeed.
- The upscale salon next door has agreed to do collaborative advertising on several strategically located billboards.
- My business is the only place in town that offers massage therapy, acupuncture, and yoga classes in the same place.
- Our staff members are trained in over 30 modalities of massage and bodywork.
- We offer discounts to students and senior citizens.
- Every Friday, members of the Police Department, Fire Department, and other public servants will receive massage for half price as our way of contributing back to the community.

Company Ownership

This section introduces the owner(s) of the business. You may opt to include a resume (see Chapter 1), or write a summary of your qualifications, talents, experience, and education. This component is basically a short biography, but leave out your childhood details unless they're relevant, such as "I grew up working every weekend and summer vacation in my mother's spa, which was a successful operation for more than 25 years until her retirement."

Start-up Budget Projections

A preliminary **budget** is a part of your business plan. (The operating budget is discussed in Chapter 7.) You'll have one-time expenses related to furnishing and equipping the office space that have to be factored in; those costs are subject to **depreciation** over a period of years on your tax returns. Make a list of the things you need, set a budget for how much you can afford to spend, and shop around for the best price. Use the classified ads, "swap & shop" papers, second-hand stores, freight-damaged furniture stores, and even garage sales as possible sources for furnishings.

Any tangible items, such as equipment or furnishings that you purchase for your business, are **assets**; in the event that you decide to buy property instead of renting, property is also an asset. The money that you owe for a mortgage or other debt that you incur related to your business is a **liability**. You may want to use tables like those in Box 2-1 to list assets, start-up expenses, liabilities, and owner's equity.

HELP JUST AHEAD

ROADSIDE ASSISTANCE

Even though I didn't borrow money from a bank to start my business, I still wrote a business plan worthy of taking to the bank, and so should you. Writing my plan and referring to it has often helped keep me on track as I refine my vision of how I want my business to evolve and grow.

Getting advice from a tax planner or financial advisor at the outset is a wise idea. Even if your business loses money for the first year or two, you may still be obligated to pay **self-employment tax**, and you should be prepared for that. Construct your start-up budget and then let an expert pick it apart for you. He might notice an expense or a tax advantage that you overlooked. He can also tell you the most beneficial way for you to set your business up, either as a **sole proprietorship**, **partnership**, or one of the variants of a **corporation**, depending on your individual circumstances. (The various types of business structures are discussed in Chapter 4, and taxes are discussed in Chapter 7.)

If you're moving into an existing office, you can find out by calling the utility companies how much the power, gas, and water have historically cost. Most utility companies offer the option of paying a predetermined equal amount every month, and once a year will bill you or credit you according to your actual usage. It's always wise to err on the side of caution by estimating high for an expense, rather than low. If you overestimate an expense, that becomes extra money in your pocket.

REALITY CHECKPOINT

Words of Wisdom
A penny saved is a penny earned.

For most business owners, the rent or mortgage payment is usually the biggest monthly expense. When you're just starting out, you have to be prepared to meet that and other obligations, such as the utilities, even when your business doesn't bring in enough money to cover those costs at the outset. Planning ahead is a necessity.

ROADSIDE ASSISTANCE

In the start-up budget for my business, I inserted the amount of the first year's rent in one lump sum as opposed to having it broken down month-by-month. That's because I wanted to know if I could pay the rent on the building for 1 year regardless of whether I got enough clients to do so. I wanted to be able to last for a year without worrying about paying the rent, so I planned for that. If possible, it's wise for you to do the same.

Services and Products

Name the specific services and products you are going to offer, such as treatments or services in addition to massage. List them, along with any other sources of customer revenue, such as selling products, giving community education classes, or renting space to others for classes or meetings. If you have classroom space, mention the particulars in the interest of projecting revenue. Here are some ideas:

- Our meeting space accommodates up to 40 people for lecture classes, 20 for movement classes, and 14 for table (hands-on massage) classes.
- We project holding classes in yoga 50 weeks of the year, which will account for approximately $1000 per month in additional revenue.

- We will be providing continuing education classes to other massage therapists by holding monthly classes. Based on our past history of attendance, we expect an additional $30,000 per year in gross revenue from these classes.
- Our meeting space will also be available to the public for a reasonable hourly fee of $25. Tables and chairs are provided, and there is a small kitchenette available. We are projecting revenue of $5000 per year from rental fees.

MARKET STUDY AND SURVEY ANALYSIS

A **market survey analysis** is simply a compilation of the results from your investigation of the market in your area. If you are going to the bank to ask for a start-up loan, the loan officer will want to know that you have researched the competition in the area and the probable demand for your services. A **market study** doesn't have to be complicated; it can be as simple as looking in the phone directory, searching the Internet, and driving around town to see how many businesses of your type are already up and running, taking note of their location, their prices, and their customers. Office location can tell you a lot about the customer base—yours and that of the competition. A fancy spa in a galleria filled with high-end luxury stores will have a different clientele than a day spa in a strip mall, or compared to a home practice.

A market study can include a survey of area residents to ask what services they would be interested in supporting, but unless you personally conduct face-to-face interviews, this can be an expensive task. Even with bulk mailing prices, sending a survey to every resident in your immediate area would be cost-prohibitive for most people, and a survey that yields a 2% to 3% return is considered successful. That's not much return for your effort. As mentioned in Chapter 1, the Chamber of Commerce is a good source of demographic information for your market study.

EXPLORATIONS

Conduct your market study by doing the following:

- Look in the phone book or online for massage therapy listings.
- Drive around within a 10 to 15 mile radius of the location you're considering, and note the concentration of similar businesses in surrounding neighborhoods.
- Note the kind of places they are; for example, an upscale day spa, a stand-alone office, or a practice in a medical complex.
- Notice the overall appearance of prosperity in the area you're considering; for instance, too many empty or run-down storefronts, or going-out-of-business signs, can indicate that the general economic atmosphere in the area is depressed.
- Visit the Chamber of Commerce to pick up literature (cards and brochures) about similar businesses that are Chamber members.
- Best of all, book an appointment; it's a surefire way to find out about the customer experience at other places.

Marketing Strategies

This section of the business plan discusses the ways you intend to market and promote your business. Your goal should be to get as much value for your advertising dollars as possible. Performing community service, for instance, is a no-cost way to get your name out there, as is cultivating mutual referrals and attending networking events. In addition to naming the advertising sources from which you plan to purchase space, be sure to mention the things you'll do to spread the word without spending money. Obtain pricing from the advertising sources you intend to use before writing this part of the plan, so you have a realistic idea of what ad space costs before deciding how much money to budget for it. (Chapters 12–14 discuss marketing your business.)

ROADSIDE ASSISTANCE

If there is a lack of specialty massage available in your area, a good strategy is to host a practitioner in your office on a regular or semiregular basis and announce it to your established clients. I've been keeping a Rolfer busy 2 days a month in my office for the past 5 years, and I get a percentage of what he earns.

Going with the Flow

Consumers expect businesses to have an Internet presence these days. Your website serves the purpose of informing the public about your business, and you can also use it to sell gift certificates and even make it possible for people to book appointments online.

A SAMPLE BUSINESS PLAN

The sample plan in Box 2-1 is a relatively short business plan. Yours may be even shorter, or it might be longer and more detailed. If you need to borrow money to start your business, make sure your plan is thorough because a lender will want to see that you have carefully thought everything through.

ROADSIDE ASSISTANCE

The example is adapted from my own business plan; feel free to use it to suit your own purpose. Note that my plan strikes a balance between professionalism and speaking in a personal way about my dreams and desires for my business. A banker or investor reading my plan will know that I put a lot of thought into personalizing my plan and did not just copy a generic plan from a business book.

ALTERNATE ROUTES

Employees and Independent Contractors

Even though you're not writing a business plan, there are components you'll want to keep in mind as you're seeking a job: experience and professionalism. Volunteer experience is no less valuable because you weren't paid for it. Making the most of your professionalism is important, and as stated previously, it can make you stand out from the crowd when you're in a locale that doesn't require it; you'll appear all the more credible because you went to the trouble to obtain professional credentials.

(continued)

Business Partners

The most important part of a business plan for partners is to be absolutely certain that all partners are in agreement with the terms of the plan, and any legal dealings associated with it, such as lease or rental agreements and other contracts. Taking the time at the outset to craft a plan and business agreements that satisfy all concerned parties is much better than trying to settle a disagreement or even a lawsuit later.

REVISITING AND ADAPTING YOUR PLAN

For the first year you are in business, you will need to revisit your business plan regularly to see what's working out and what isn't. You may need to adjust your budget, or change marketing strategies, or make other adaptations. Make adjustments as soon as you become aware of the need.

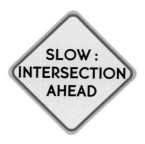

Bear in mind as you're trying to adhere to your start-up budget that you must pay for your necessities first before you spend a lot on advertising (see Chapter 14). Marketing your business won't help you if the power gets cut off because you didn't pay the bill. Keep your operating expenses as low as you can while you're getting established, and pay your bills on time. Avoid using credit cards to pay for advertising or anything else that can't be classified as an asset.

A useful way to see if you need to adjust your business plan is to survey your clients to find out what they like and don't like about your business. This can be done in the form of a written questionnaire, or it can be more informal by asking them what they'd like to see happen with your business. Responses might be different operating hours, or accepting credit cards if you don't do so already, or offering more or different services. A lot of people, for instance, think working 9 to 5 is the ideal for operating hours and that sounds good to you—you don't have to get up too early, and you're home in time for the 6:00 news. However, most of corporate America works 9 to 5, so by choosing that timeframe for your operating hours, you're cutting many people out of your potential client list. You obviously can't work around the clock and accommodate everyone's schedule, so you have to figure out what works best for you.

You may have to adapt your plan because you haven't quite gotten the number of clients you had planned to have—or you might have to adapt it because you got a lot more! If you're in a small town where there isn't much competition, you might find yourself being overwhelmed with more clients than you can handle. Wouldn't that be great? If you're lucky enough to be in that situation, don't tell people you can't take any new clients. Ask them for their phone numbers and tell them you'll be happy to put them on your waiting list. Alternatively, you can refer them to another therapist whose abilities are well established.

Massage, like any service business, is subject to the whims of the public. You'll lose clients because people will feel they no longer need massage and stop coming. Clients will move away, find a therapist more convenient to home, or have to reduce their expenses. Don't take any of it personally. If you maintain a waiting list, you'll have some backup for replacing lost clients. Moreover, telling people you have a waiting list gives the impression that you must be someone really special and talented if you have people waiting to get an appointment—and you are, aren't you?

Revisit your business plan often, and by the end of the first year, you'll have a clear picture of whether or not you met your goals and projections. Staying on top of it will serve you well as you plan for the future.

Ruthie Piper Hardee

I knew the first week I was in massage school back in 1990 that I would never make it in this field if I had to bend at the waist to deliver deep tissue effleurage with my hands. I was born with lumbar scoliosis, which has developed into ankylosing spondylitis with moderate stenosis. I loved the thought of becoming a massage practitioner but my back condition didn't agree, so I developed a Swedish effleurage modality that I could give to my clients standing up, holding a bar, using my feet, and letting gravity do the work.

When my clients started spreading the news around town of their pain-free results, local therapists started calling me to ask how it was done and whether I could teach them.

Putting my creation in curriculum form with case studies with exact methodologies for teaching it to others was the challenge. At the time the Florida Department of Health, the AMTA, and the NCBTMB were reluctant to approve such a course. Many doors were slammed in my face. "It will never fly," they said. "Massage is supposed to be done with the hands, not the feet!" Well, perseverance proved "them" wrong, and what a passionate ride it has been for 13 years.

I taught the first Ashiatsu Oriental Bar Therapy seminar in November 1998 in Denver, Colorado. The mission was to change therapists' lives—to give body workers, who were willing, a chance to have a healthy (deep tissue) practice for years to come, to teach them how to use their feet like their hands, and keep them from bending at the waist and suffering from hand problems. I was filled with passion for the modality and the prospect of teaching it to others. I am living proof that the mission was sound then and is still on track today. With more than 3000 graduates, 11 training facilities throughout the United States, and a core team of instructors who fully embrace my vision, we have countless inspiring stories of change and renewal from hundreds of therapists.

You can often tell the difference between a continuing education provider who is only teaching for money and a provider who is *passionate* about what she is delivering, and the same applies to massage therapists. If you are merely in business to make money, you will never be as successful as you could be. *Passion* fuels us, motivates us, and inspires us.

Having your own business is not for the weak and faint of heart. It takes time to build, it takes time to see monetary returns, and it takes such a degree of dedication that if you do not have *passion* in the mix, your efforts will be in vain. I attribute my success to honesty, with truthful innovation, following my heart, and believing in what I do.

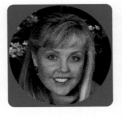

Ruthie Piper Hardee is the founder of Ashiatsu Oriental Bar Therapy. She created the first nationally approved course of study for a Western barefoot technique using bars on the ceiling and invented the Hardee-Ashiatsu Portable Bar apparatus, which is currently used worldwide. The trademarked therapy was named one of the top 25 life-changing treatments by *Spa Magazine* 2006 World Wide Guide, and in 2007, *Spa Finders Magazine*. Hardee has been a guest speaker and presenter at numerous AMTA chapter meetings across the United States and workshops in Canada, Mexico, and the Dominican Republic. Visit her website at www.deepfeet.com.

SUGGESTED READINGS

American Massage Therapy Association. A Guide to Starting Your Own Business. http://www.amtamassage.org/journal/spring05_journal/GuideToStartYourOwnBusiness.pdf. Accessed 06/07/2008.

Krass P, ed. *The Little Book of Business Wisdom: Rules of Success from More Than 50 Business Legends.* New York, NY: John Wiley & Sons, Inc., 2001.

Silvester JL. *401 Questions Every Entrepreneur Should Ask.* Franklin Lakes, NJ: Career Press, 2006.

Small Business Administration. Write a Business Plan. http://www.sba.gov/smallbusinessplanner/plan/writeabusinessplan/index.html. Accessed 06/08/2008.

United States Chamber of Commerce. Writing Your Business Plan. http://business.uschamber.com/P02/P02_5001.asp. Accessed 06/08/2008.

Weltman B, Silberman J. *Small Business Survival Book.: 12 Surefire Ways for Your Business to Survive and Thrive.* New York, NY: John Wiley & Sons, 2006.

My Personal Journey

In this chapter, we've discussed the importance of creating a business plan, defined the components of an effective business plan, and provided an example of a completed plan.

Compile the information you gathered during your market study into a market survey analysis, and begin writing down the key points of your business plan. If you are interested in pursuing employment or being an independent contractor rather than starting a business, see if you can construct a "business plan" that details what *you* have in mind.

My goals _____

_____

_____

What's in my way? _____

_____

_____

What action can I take to remedy the situation? _____

_____

_____

One-year progress update _____

_____

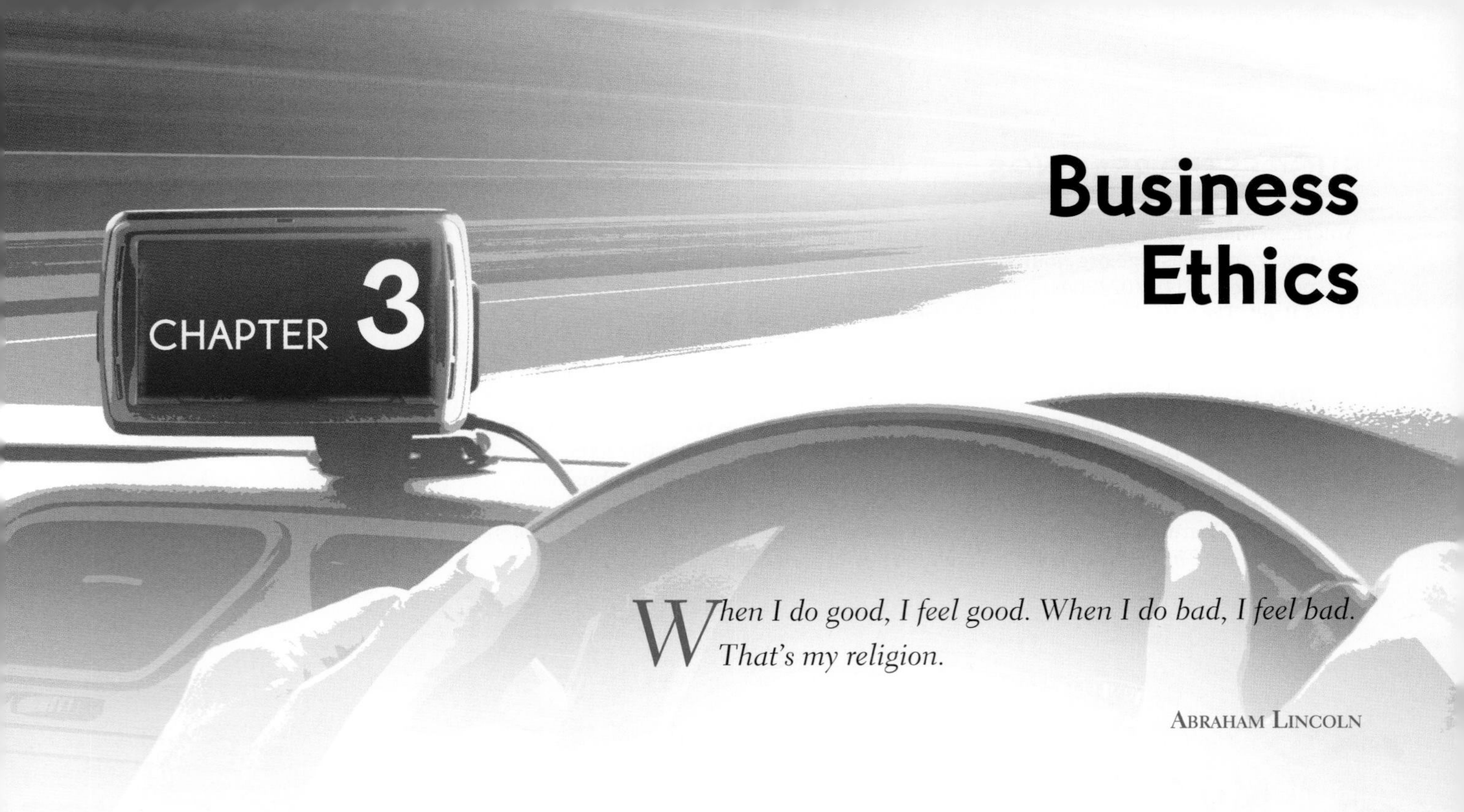

CHAPTER 3

Business Ethics

When I do good, I feel good. When I do bad, I feel bad. That's my religion.

Abraham Lincoln

KEY CONCEPTS

- Professional organizations and boards governing massage and bodywork have a code of ethics that members, certificate holders, and licensees are obligated to observe.
- HIPAA requirements serve to protect client confidentiality.
- The Standards of Practice of the NCBTMB are good guidelines that can be used by any practitioners to ensure they are conducting business ethically.
- You may adopt your own code of ethics from professional sources.
- Caring for yourself is essential when your profession is about taking care of others.
- Business relationships should be governed by recognizing the roles and boundaries of each individual; respecting client boundaries is a professional ethical obligation, and maintaining your own boundaries will help you handle the challenges of running a business.
- The massage and bodywork business is based on the therapeutic relationship between therapist and client.
- Educating clients about practicing self-care is an important part of ensuring the continued benefits of therapy and gives the client a positive reinforcement of your role as a knowledgeable professional therapist.
- Dealing with business associates in an ethical manner and expecting the same from them are the keys to prosperity.
- Learning to handle difficult clients in a professional manner is a necessity for maintaining business roles and boundaries.
- A mentor can be invaluable in helping you respond to business and ethical dilemmas.

The nature of what we do, placing our hands on people who may be partially or fully unclothed and in a vulnerable position, dictates that a grounding in ethical behavior is an essential part of preparing to go into the massage therapy business. As practitioners who are involved in the care of the human body, mind, and spirit, we are obligated to *first do no harm.* Massage therapists and other holistic health care professionals have a **code of ethics**, a set of rules governing professional moral behavior that practitioners agree to observe while performing their duties. A code of ethics is meant to safeguard the safety, modesty, and privacy of clients, and to define the roles and boundaries practitioners should observe. Adhering to the code is the only acceptable route.

CODES OF ETHICS

Hippocrates is regarded as the father of medicine, and the Hippocratic Oath for physicians is the foundation of the codes of ethics in use today governing those who work in the health care professions. It is one of the oldest binding documents in history, written in the fourth century by Hippocrates, or perhaps one of his pupils (historians are not sure). Here is a modern adaptation of the Hippocratic Oath:

I swear to fulfill, to the best of my ability and judgment, this covenant:

- I will respect the hard-won scientific gains of those physicians in whose steps I walk, and gladly share such knowledge as is mine with those who are to follow.
- I will apply, for the benefit of the sick, all measures [that] are required, avoiding those twin traps of over-treatment and therapeutic nihilism.
- I will remember that there is art to medicine as well as science, and that warmth, sympathy, and understanding may outweigh the surgeon's knife or the chemist's drug.
- I will not be ashamed to say "I know not," nor will I fail to call in my colleagues when the skills of another are needed for a patient's recovery.
- I will respect the privacy of my patients, for their problems are not disclosed to me that the world may know. Most especially must I tread with care in matters of life and death.
- If it is given me to save a life, all thanks. But it may also be within my power to take a life; this awesome responsibility must be faced with great humbleness and awareness of my own frailty. Above all, I must not play at God.
- I will remember that I do not treat a fever chart, or a cancerous growth, but a sick human being, whose illness may affect the person's family and economic stability. My responsibility includes these related problems, if I am to care adequately for the sick.
- I will prevent disease whenever I can, for prevention is preferable to cure.
- I will remember that I remain a member of society, with special obligations to all my fellow human beings, those sound of mind and body as well as the infirm.
- If I do not violate this oath, may I enjoy life and art, respected while I live and remembered with affection thereafter. May I always act so as to preserve the finest traditions of my calling and may I long experience the joy of healing those who seek my help.

It's easy to see how the Hippocratic Oath has been modified to create the ethical codes that apply to massage therapy and other health care modalities. The ethics codes of various organizations and disciplines all have common threads: utmost respect for the client; protection of the client's modesty and privacy; the expectation that we will observe confidentiality; the expectation that we will work only within our scope of practice and will initiate referrals to other health care professionals as needed; the expectation that we will not accept gifts intended to influence treatment or referral; and that we will perform work only when it is for the good of the client.

Know your code, and follow it to the letter. The phrase "respected while I live" is a key phrase in the Hippocratic Oath; an unethical practitioner will eventually be found out. If you don't respect your clients, you can't expect them to respect you.

Let's look at a code of ethics specifically for our profession. This one is from the American Massage Therapy Association. Massage therapists shall

1. Demonstrate commitment to provide the highest quality massage therapy/bodywork to those who seek their professional service.
2. Acknowledge the inherent worth and individuality of each person by not discriminating or behaving in any prejudicial manner with clients and/or colleagues.
3. Demonstrate professional excellence through regular self-assessment of strengths, limitations, and effectiveness by continued education and training.
4. Acknowledge the confidential nature of the professional relationship with clients, and respect each client's right to privacy.
5. Conduct all business and professional activities within their scope of practice, the law of the land, and project a professional image.
6. Refrain from engaging in any sexual conduct or sexual activities involving their clients.
7. Accept responsibility to do no harm to the physical, mental, and emotional well-being of self, clients, and associates.

That's pretty thorough, although some codes are much longer and spell out a lot of details. Let's explore the meaning of the above points a little further:

1. *Demonstrate commitment to provide the highest quality massage therapy/bodywork to those who seek their professional service.* Naturally, you want to provide the highest quality of care you can to everyone who seeks your services. You want the last client of the day to have the same high-quality experience as the first client of the day. If you chronically run late on appointments, or are overworked and don't schedule yourself for adequate days off or even adequate downtime between clients, your quality of care will suffer. There's more to follow about self-care for the therapist; this part of the code of ethics illustrates that self-care is an obligation—not just a good idea.
2. *Acknowledge the inherent worth and individuality of each person by not discriminating or behaving in any prejudicial manner with clients and/or colleagues.* Recognizing the inherent worth of all individuals and not discriminating against anyone obviously means that the people who seek our help should all be treated the same, regardless of their color, race or ethnicity, gender, religion, sexual orientation, or any other characteristic that makes them the unique people they all are. Prejudice and bigotry have no place in a health care business.
3. *Demonstrate professional excellence through regular self-assessment of strengths, limitations, and effectiveness by continued education and training.* For practitioners who want to maintain National Certification, professional membership in the AMTA, and/or licensure in their state, continuing education (CE) is a requirement that must be met, including regular CE pertaining specifically to observing professional ethics. If you plan to practice professionally in a state with no licensure as of yet, and no education requirements, that's all the more reason to continue your education; it can set you apart from

the "recreational" therapists. Why wouldn't you jump at the tax-deductible chance to expand your education and learn new things that will benefit you and your clients, not to mention the opportunity to enhance your menu of services? Be sure to educate yourself about the requirements that apply to you.

Words of Wisdom
Don't view CE as a burden; think of it as an opportunity!

4. *Acknowledge the confidential nature of the professional relationship with clients, and respect each client's right to privacy.* **Confidentiality** and respecting a client's right to privacy are two of the most important tenets in the ethics code of any health care discipline. People who seek our care should be able to rely on the fact that they can tell us anything and that it will remain between client and practitioner. You can't go home and share details around the dinner table, or even discuss them with another practitioner, physician, or insurance company, unless the client has given specific permission for you to do so by signing an **authorization** to release information form.

5. *Conduct all business and professional activities within their scope of practice, the law of the land, and project a professional image.* Working within your **scope of practice** is essential. If you are a massage therapist, it would be irresponsible, for example, to present yourself as an herbalist, unless you are qualified. Taking a weekend class doesn't count. Be honest about your qualifications and training. Maintaining a professional image, whatever and wherever your practice, will earn you respect in the eyes of clients and the community at large. If you work at your home, you have to be especially mindful of this. Just because your office is at home is no excuse for greeting clients in your bathrobe and slippers.

6. *Refrain from engaging in any sexual conduct or sexual activities involving their clients.* It goes without saying—and yet it must be said—that no sexual behavior of any kind should enter into the therapeutic relationship. We all want to believe that everyone who comes into our profession is going to behave in an ethical manner, but unfortunately, that isn't so. Read the newsletter of the NCBTMB or your state licensure board, and you will be shocked and saddened at the number of therapists who are accused of sexual impropriety and other ethics offenses. It's a problem everywhere. Sexualizing a relationship with a client can do just as much, if not more, harm to the practitioner as well when the professional relationship falls apart. Losing your license to practice can be compounded by a ruined reputation and a ruined career. Both the NCBTMB and the Federation of State Massage Therapy Boards (FSMTB) are working to create national disciplinary databases so that a therapist who has committed an offense in one state cannot practice in another state.

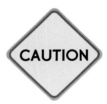

7. *Accept responsibility to do no harm to the physical, mental, and emotional well-being of self, clients, and associates.* Agreeing to "do no harm" includes, of course, observing sexual boundaries, and although that is very important, doing no harm also means not performing treatments of any kind when there is a contraindication. People have the right to choose the health care they want, as well as the right to refuse treatment. You are obligated not to promise a cure for any condition, even if it's just a taut muscle, and not to cause a client further harm by any techniques you use. We must remember that people who seek massage are sometimes suffering from mental or emotional issues as well as pain or tension in their body, and we're obligated to treat every client with the utmost caution, care, and compassion.

ROADSIDE ASSISTANCE

I've actually experienced a home practitioner coming to the door wrapped in a bath towel with another one on her head. I was on time for the appointment—not so early that I might have caught her (un)dressed like that. She quickly threw on a pair of sweats and gave me the massage with the towel still on her head. While her appearance had no negative effect on her technique, it did affect my perception of both her and my experience of the massage. It felt like she wasn't prepared for the appointment and didn't care about presenting a professional image. The client *perceives* more benefit out of the session when the therapist is presentable and prepared for the session.

Words of Wisdom
You only get one time to make a first impression.

Avoiding Unintended Offenses

There is always the possibility of committing an ethics offense inadvertently. For instance, a therapist might have a temporary lack of good judgment, or he might be careless in his choice of words or techniques. We all have days when we're tired, or distracted by a personal problem. If you're in the middle of a session and the drape accidentally falls off and exposes a private part of the client's body, apologize right away and place the drape back on.

If you find yourself attracted to a client, take that energy and apply it toward giving a massage like the professional you are. The slightest flirtation on your part is a pathway to disaster.

If a client asks you for a date, and you happen to be attracted to the person, take a step back from the table and explain to him that your workspace is sacred, and that if you are going to enter into another type of relationship, you will have to excuse yourself from having a therapeutic relationship with him. If you're not inclined to pursue a social relationship, address it immediately by stating your position. A simple "Thanks, but I have a strict policy of not dating clients" will suffice.

If a client makes a blatantly sexual comment or gesture, say right away that such behavior is unacceptable. A lot of ethical issues arise from a lack of clear and effective communication between client and therapist.

ALTERNATE ROUTES

Employees and Independent Contractors

If an incident occurs that makes you uncomfortable from an ethical standpoint—such as a client making sexual overtures, or you accidentally exposing a client while adjusting the drape—the best thing to do is report it to management and to document it in the client's file.

Business Partners

When you have a business partner, that person is like a mirror image of you, as far as the public is concerned. It is critical to choose a partner who shares your business and ethics philosophy. If your partner acts unethically, you must deal with it as swiftly as possible. In your capacity as a manager, if an employee reports an ethical concern to you, handle it fairly and immediately. Your staff members need to know that you take ethics violations very seriously. Partners should present a united front when confronting these types of issues.

EXPLORATIONS

If you are practicing in a state that has licensure, take time to thoroughly read the Massage Therapy Practice Act that governs your location. State massage therapy board meetings, including disciplinary hearings, are open to the public and contain a time period to receive public comments. Attending a meeting of your state board will give you a clear picture of exactly what a regulatory board does in order to carry out their mission of protecting the public.

The Health Insurance Portability Accountability Act

The Health Insurance Portability and Accountability Act (HIPAA), issued by the U.S. Department of Health and Human Services in 1996 and enforced by the Office of Civil Rights, is intended (among other things) to safeguard the privacy of a client's personal identifying information.

All massage therapists should observe the HIPAA Privacy Rule, regardless of whether or not they accept health insurance, when it comes to respecting confidentiality and keeping the client's personal information intact; the code of ethics compels us to do so. HIPAA is even more binding than the code of ethics because it is federal law. Clients should be informed of their right to privacy and your compliance with that expectation. Particularly in today's climate of identity theft, your clients should have the security of knowing their private information is safeguarded.

According to the page on the HIPAA website devoted to small businesses, every health care professional who electronically transmits health or medical information is a covered entity. These transmissions include claims, benefit eligibility inquiries, referral authorization requests, or any kind of e-mail containing the client's information that is sent to a third party. The Privacy Rule covers health care professionals whether they electronically transmit transactions directly or use a billing service or other third party to do so on their behalf. Compliance with HIPAA entails utilizing secure computer transmissions when sending information about a client, keeping written records under lock and key, and even simple but often overlooked things like keeping your computer where others can't see the screen, if client information is visible. If you work in a group practice, for instance, conduct your client intake and exit interviews in the privacy of the treatment room, not in the lobby within earshot of others.

BEYOND THE CODE: THE STANDARDS OF PRACTICE

The NCBTMB developed and adopted the Standards of Practice to provide certificants and applicants for certification with a clear statement of the expectations of professional conduct and level of practice afforded to the public in, among other things, the following areas: Professionalism, Legal and Ethical Requirements, Confidentiality, Business Practices, Roles and Boundaries, and Prevention of Sexual Misconduct. They bear repeating here. Some, such as Standard 1(q), pertain only to certificants, but most of the standards can and should be observed as instructional guidelines for conducting your daily business in a professional and ethical manner, whether you are Nationally Certified or not.

Standard I: Professionalism

Standard I describes the characteristics and expected behaviors of a professional massage therapist. It might be helpful to consider behavior that's unprofessional, just for the sake of contrast. Unprofessional behavior would include any violation of the code of ethics but could also include anything from using slang words for body parts, instead of the correct anatomical terminology, when you're talking with a client, to having a sloppy appearance and a dirty office. The standards for professionalism are detailed in Box 3-1.

BOX 3-1   Standard 1: Professionalism

The certificant or applicant must provide optimal levels of professional therapeutic massage and bodywork services and demonstrate excellence in practice by promoting healing and well-being through responsible, compassionate, and respectful touch. In his/her professional role, the certificant or applicant shall

a. adhere to the NCBTMB Code of Ethics, Standards of Practice, policies and procedures
b. comply with the peer review process conducted by the NCBTMB Ethics and Standards Committee regarding any alleged violations of the NCBTMB Code of Ethics and Standards of Practice
c. conduct him/herself in a manner in all settings meriting the respect of the public and other professionals
d. treat each client with respect, dignity, and worth
e. use professional verbal, nonverbal, and written communications
f. provide an environment that is safe and comfortable for the client and which, at a minimum, meets all legal requirements for health and safety
g. use standard precautions to insure professional hygienic practices and maintain a level of personal hygiene appropriate for practitioners in the therapeutic setting
h. wear clothing that is clean, modest, and professional
i. obtain voluntary and informed consent from the client prior to initiating the session
j. if applicable, conduct an accurate needs assessment, develop a plan of care with the client, and update the plan as needed
k. use appropriate draping to protect the client's physical and emotional privacy
l. be knowledgeable of his/her scope of practice and practice only within these limitations
m. refer to other professionals when in the best interest of the client and practitioner
n. seek other professional advice when needed
o. respect the traditions and practices of other professionals and foster collegial relationships
p. not falsely impugn the reputation of any colleague
q. use the initials NCTMB to designate his/her professional ability and competency to practice therapeutic massage and bodywork, or the initials NCTM to designate his/her professional ability and competency to practice therapeutic massage only
r. respect the traditions and practices of other professionals and foster collegial relationships
s. understand that the NCBTMB certificate may be displayed prominently in the certificant's principal place of practice
t. use the NCBTMB logo and certification number on business cards, brochures, advertisements, and stationery only in a manner that is within established NCBTMB guidelines
u. not duplicate the NCBTMB certificate for purposes other than verification of the practitioner's credentials
v. immediately return the certificate to NCBTMB if certification is revoked
w. inform NCBTMB of any changes or additions to information included in his/her application for NCBTMB certification or recertification

Standard II: Legal and Ethical Requirements

Standard II discusses the legal and ethical practices that should be observed by a professional massage therapist. Two of the most common violations are unlicensed persons practicing in a state that regulates massage therapy, and therapists failing to keep good records. Therapists who practice in unregulated states may have no formal massage education and thus no training in professional ethics or business practices, and that's all the more reason to learn the standards on their own. The legal and ethical requirements of Standard II appear in Box 3-2.

Standard III: Confidentiality

Confidentiality is one of the most important parts of the therapeutic relationship. The connection between therapist and client has to be built on honest communication and mutual trust. A client should feel that his privacy is respected at all times, and be able to feel secure that his personal and medical information are safeguarded. The tenets of confidentiality are discussed in Box 3-3.

Standard IV: Business Practices

Standard IV discusses the principles of conducting business in a manner that's above reproach, exactly what should be expected of a professional health care practitioner. Your professional reputation and your livelihood depend on your conducting business in an honest and ethical manner, according to the standards set forth in Box 3-4.

Standard V: Roles and Boundaries

Standard V is a clarification of the roles and boundaries that should be maintained within a therapeutic relationship. Roles and boundaries are such an important issue

---

BOX 3-2 Standard II: Legal and Ethical Requirements

The certificant or applicant must comply with all the legal requirements in applicable jurisdictions regulating the profession of therapeutic massage and bodywork. In his/her professional role, the certificant or applicant shall

a. obey all applicable local, state, and federal laws
b. refrain from any behavior that results in illegal, discriminatory, or unethical actions
c. accept responsibility for his/her own actions
d. report to the proper authorities any alleged violations of the law by other certificants or applicants for certification
e. maintain accurate and truthful records
f. report to NCBTMB any criminal conviction of, or plea of guilty, nolo contendere, or no contest to, a crime in any jurisdiction (other than a minor traffic offense) by him/herself and by other certificants or applicants for certification
g. report to NCBTMB any pending litigation and resulting resolution related to the applicant's or certificant's professional practice and the professional practice of other applicants and certificants
h. report to NCBTMB any pending complaints in any state or local government or quasigovernment board or agency against his/her professional conduct or competence, or that of another certificant, and the resulting resolution of such complaint
i. respect existing publishing rights and copyright laws, including, but not limited to, those that apply to NCBTMB's copyright-protected examinations

BOX 3-3   Standard III: Confidentiality

The certificant or applicant shall respect the confidentiality of client information and safeguard all records. In his/her professional role the certificant or applicant shall

a. protect the confidentiality of the client's identity in conversations, all advertisements, and any and all other matters unless disclosure of identifiable information is requested by the client in writing, is medically necessary, is required by law or for purposes of public protection
b. protect the interests of clients who are minors or clients who are unable to give voluntary and informed consent by securing permission from an appropriate third party or guardian
c. solicit only information that is relevant to the professional client/therapist relationship
d. share pertinent information about the client with third parties when required by law or for purposes of public protection
e. maintain the client files for a minimum period of 4 years
f. store and dispose of client files in a secure manner

BOX 3-4   Standard IV: Business Practices

The certificant or applicant shall practice with honesty, integrity, and lawfulness in the business of therapeutic massage and bodywork. In his/her professional role, the certificant or applicant shall

a. provide a physical setting that is safe and meets all applicable legal requirements for health and safety
b. maintain adequate and customary liability insurance
c. maintain adequate progress notes for each client session, if applicable
d. accurately and truthfully inform the public of services provided
e. honestly represent all professional qualifications and affiliations
f. promote his/her business with integrity and avoid potential and actual conflicts of interest
g. advertise in a manner that is honest, dignified, accurate, and representative of services that can be delivered and remains consistent with the NCBTMB Code of Ethics and Standards of Practice
h. advertise in a manner that is not misleading to the public and shall not use sensational, sexual, or provocative language and/or pictures to promote business
i. comply with all laws regarding sexual harassment
j. not exploit the trust and dependency of others, including clients and employees/co-workers
k. display/discuss a schedule of fees in advance of the session that is clearly understood by the client or potential client
l. make financial arrangements in advance that are clearly understood by and safeguard the best interests of the client or consumer
m. follow acceptable accounting practices
n. file all applicable municipal, state, and federal taxes
o. maintain accurate financial records, contracts and legal obligations, appointment records, tax reports, and receipts for at least 4 years

BOX 3-5   Standard V: Roles and Boundaries

The certificant or applicant shall adhere to ethical boundaries and perform the professional roles designed to protect both the client and the practitioner, and safeguard the therapeutic value of the relationship. In his/her professional role, the certificant or applicant shall

a. recognize his/her personal limitations and practice only within these limitations
b. recognize his/her influential position with the client and not exploit the relationship for personal or other gain
c. recognize and limit the impact of transference and countertransference between the client and the certificant
d. avoid dual or multidimensional relationships that could impair professional judgment or result in exploitation of the client or employees and/or co-workers
e. not engage in any sexual activity with a client
f. acknowledge and respect the client's freedom of choice in the therapeutic session
g. respect the client's right to refuse the therapeutic session or any part of the therapeutic session
h. refrain from practicing under the influence of alcohol, drugs, or any illegal substances (with the exception of a prescribed dosage of prescription medication, which does not impair the certificant)
i. have the right to refuse and/or terminate the service to a client who is abusive or under the influence of alcohol, drugs, or any illegal substance

for a massage therapist that additional hours of education in this particular area are required for every renewal of National Certification and many state licenses. The rules of roles and boundaries are listed in Box 3-5.

Ethical Dilemmas: Ignoring the Client's Feedback

A client stated during the intake interview that she had received a massage a few days ago from a newly licensed therapist on the other side of town and that she is still very sore. She said the massage was too deep, and when she asked the practitioner to lighten up, the therapist replied, "I can't, because this is what you need." Do you think the other therapist made an error in judgment by ignoring the client's request to change the pressure? Other than giving the massage and working within the client's preference or tolerance for pressure, especially since she is sore, is there anything else *you* should do? Should you call the practitioner in question and discuss it with her? Report her to the massage board, or encourage the client to file a complaint about her?

If the previous therapist happened to be a friend of yours, having a word with her about honoring client requests in general might do some good—but it would be a violation of confidentiality for you to discuss the specific client with her, unless your client had given written permission for her information to be shared. You're not the injured party. It's not your place to file a complaint; that would be up to the client, if she were inclined to do so, but she may not even be aware that it's an option. You could offer her your state regulatory board's contact information and let her know that the massage board exists for the purpose of protecting the public, and that she does have a right to complain if she feels her boundaries have been violated.

A therapist who doesn't listen to client feedback will usually find out soon enough that she's doing something wrong, once she discovers she isn't getting rebooked for future appointments.

Standard VI: Prevention of Sexual Misconduct

The prevention of sexual misconduct is important to any profession that involves therapeutic relationships. It is especially important for the massage therapist, as one of the few practitioners other than a physician to touch partially or fully unclothed people during the course of her work. Anything that sexualizes the relationship, whether in word or in deed by either party, is considered misconduct. The steps for avoiding sexual misconduct are detailed in Box 3-6.

Please note that the massage and bodywork laws in some states and jurisdictions supersede the NCBTMB Standards of Practice pertaining to massage in body cavities or potentially sensitive areas, such as the female breasts. Some states may not allow it under any circumstances; some may allow it with restrictions, such as performing the massage only under a physician's prescription, or when there is a third party in the treatment room. The therapist may also be required to have proof of certification or advanced training in breast or pelvic massage. It's your obligation to know the law as it pertains to you. In any case, this type of invasive bodywork should only be performed by practitioners who have been properly trained in the technique, even if not required by law.

No therapist should rely on verbal consent when performing work on the breasts or in body cavities. Written informed consent that is specific to the procedure should be obtained, after a thorough discussion with the client about what the technique will entail. We must always remember that the client has the right to refuse therapy, including the right to withdraw previously given consent at any stage of the process.

BOX 3-6   Standard VI: Prevention of Sexual Misconduct

The certificant or applicant shall refrain from any behavior that sexualizes, or appears to sexualize, the client/therapist relationship. The certificant or applicant recognizes the intimacy of the therapeutic relationship may activate practitioner and/or client needs and/or desires that weaken objectivity and may lead to sexualizing the therapeutic relationship. In his/her professional role, the certificant or applicant shall

a. refrain from participating in a sexual relationship or sexual conduct with the client, whether consensual or otherwise, from the beginning of the client/therapist relationship and for a minimum of six months after the termination of the client/therapist relationship
b. in the event that the client initiates sexual behavior, clarify the purpose of the therapeutic session, and, if such conduct does not cease, terminate or refuse the session
c. recognize that sexual activity with clients, students, employees, supervisors, or trainees is prohibited even if consensual
d. not touch the genitalia
e. only perform therapeutic treatments beyond the normal narrowing of the ear canal and normal narrowing of the nasal passages as indicated in the plan of care and only after receiving informed voluntary written consent
f. only perform therapeutic treatments in the oropharynx as indicated in the plan of care and only after receiving informed voluntary consent
g. only perform therapeutic treatments into the anal canal as indicated in the plan of care and only after receiving informed voluntary written consent
h. only provide therapeutic breast massage as indicated in the plan of care and only after receiving informed voluntary consent from the client

YOUR OWN CODE OF ETHICS

If you work in a state with no licensure requirements and don't belong to any professional associations, you might not have a code that legally binds you. In that case, familiarize yourself with one of the codes from the National Certification Board, the AMTA, or other professional body.

In addition to the code of ethics set by your profession, you will have your own personal code. For example, maybe your state doesn't have a law governing the draping of clients, but you might decide you want all your clients to be draped, and you have the right to insist on it. You might have other components in your personal code, such as choosing not to work with children unless a parent is in the room during the session. Perhaps you're a person who has a carefully constructed set of boundaries. If so, you already have something to build on. If that doesn't describe you, you'll find the need to develop your own ideas of what's acceptable to you and what's not, in addition to the professional code of ethics you have vowed to observe.

Self-Care for You

Self-care for yourself is part of your own personal code of ethics. It encompasses many things, both inside and outside your business. Taking care of yourself includes the obvious, such as a healthy diet, regular exercise, and adequate rest, but don't forget to make time to enjoy the things you like to do. Getting regular massage should be a part of your personal wellness plan, too. If you're going to encourage your clients to have regular massage sessions, follow your own advice! In terms of conducting your massage therapy business, there are some other important considerations for self-care.

Ergonomics and Body Use Patterns

Sensible ergonomics and body use patterns can prolong your career by many years. First and foremost, setting your massage table at the correct height will maximize your ability to work with the least amount of strain. Be sure to arrange your massage area so that the items you need for performing treatments are within easy reach.

Many therapists suffer career-ending injuries by hyperextending their thumb or wearing out their wrists. Remember that you don't have to go to the bone with every client, even if your practice is based on deep tissue massage. Breaking up your day with a combination of clients who need deep work and those who are seeking a lighter relaxation massage will help you avoid fatigue and repetitive motion injuries.

Body Mechanics for Manual Therapists by Barbara Frye is an excellent guide to working smart instead of working hard. It is a good addition to your office reference library.

Pacing Yourself

Leave ample time between clients for a few minutes of rest. Bear in mind you've got to collect payment and schedule the client, then change the linens. Give yourself time to go to the bathroom, have a drink of water or something to eat, and regroup for the next appointment.

One day of rushing around to catch up can leave you feeling frazzled, but feeling rushed day after day because you aren't pacing yourself will lead to therapist burnout. Many therapists are motivated to go into business for themselves in order to have control over their schedule. If that describes you, then take control!

Words of Wisdom
Run your business—don't let it run you!

BUSINESS ROLES AND BOUNDARIES

While the primary reason for a professional code of ethics is to protect the public, adherence to the code ultimately protects the practitioner as well. Just as clients have boundaries that practitioners shouldn't cross, we, as practitioners, should set our own **roles and boundaries** and enforce them with both ourselves and our clients.

Having clear boundaries can have a big impact on whether or not you become successful in business. When you set boundaries, stay within your clear role as a practitioner and a businessperson, and make your clients and business associates aware of where you stand, you are actually doing them a favor as well as yourself. You want your business relationships to be built on mutual trust and ethical behavior, regardless of what place others have in your life and your business. Fulfilling your own role in the relationship in an ethical way and carefully observing the client's boundaries as well as your own signify you are doing the best you can as a businessperson and practitioner.

The Therapeutic Relationship

The **therapeutic relationship** you have with every client may be even more important than the actual bodywork you perform. This relationship is built on open, honest communication and trust; you must instill the client's confidence in you from the very first contact.

In any therapeutic relationship, there is a **power differential** in favor of the therapist. Massage therapists see people when they are in a vulnerable position, perhaps suffering from pain and/or stress, and that in itself is reason enough for taking extra care with the work we do. We have to remember that it's not just a body on the table, but a body that belongs to someone who has feelings, fears, and insecurities like all of us. Clients have to feel comfortable enough to show you their rolls of fat, their hairy bodies, their scars and warts and imperfections—whatever they perceive to be their bodily faults—secure in the knowledge that you aren't judging them.

Reliability is also an important hallmark of the therapeutic relationship. Your clients should feel secure that you aren't going to cancel an appointment with them unless it's a genuine emergency. Therapists who are chronic cancellers or reschedulers are not successful. Clients should be able to depend on your keeping the agreements you have made with them.

Respecting Client Boundaries

The National Certification Board for Therapeutic Massage and Bodywork, as well as many state boards, has decreed that the CE requirements for renewing certification and/or licensure must include further instruction specifically in the area of roles and boundaries for every renewal period. A policy of professional behavior regarding roles and boundaries is important to every profession that involves a therapeutic relationship. It's something that you'll become clearer about as time goes by and you gain experience confronting various ethical challenges. A basic grounding at the outset of your career is like practicing preventive medicine.

The Practitioner's Role

Whether as a massage therapist or as another kind of holistic health practitioner, you are offering your specific services to people who seek them out. You are not there to be anyone's savior. You are not there to perform the work that another practitioner with different training or a different scope of practice should be doing. Unless you're a counselor, you're not there to give advice on personal problems, and you're certainly not there to discuss yours.

While self-disclosure has its place, keep it within the framework of the therapeutic relationship. For example, "Living with fibromyalgia is certainly challenging. I was diagnosed 3 years ago and I've had to learn to make some adjustments."

Do not be tempted to talk about your own personal problems. If you start using clients as a sounding board for discussing your divorce, for instance, your hormonal teenager, or your worries about your financial troubles, you're putting them in an uncomfortable position. They came to you because they perceived you to be someone who would take care of them, and revealing your personal problems sounds as if you need them to take care of you.

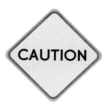

Avoiding Dual Relationships

Having **dual relationships**, such as being friends with people you are seeing professionally, is an ethical dilemma. It sets you up for problems, hurt feelings, and/ or misunderstandings down the road. In addition, dual relationships can become a potential hotbed of financial woes. Family members may have the idea that they're entitled to free sessions. Friends may assume you are going to give them a discount, or that it's okay to say "I'll pay you next Friday when I get my paycheck"; somehow next Friday doesn't come, and you're left in the uncomfortable position of having to ask a friend to pay you money she owes you.

Here's the type of situation that can develop into a problem. You stop in for lunch at a local diner, and one of your clients happens to be there sitting alone and invites you to join her. Suddenly she's talking about making it a weekly thing. That sounds like fun, and it would give you a little break from the office. But once you start going out to socialize, you find that she no longer leaves you the $10 tip you used to get after every session, and she thinks nothing of calling to cancel her appointments on short notice because now she's not just a client, she's a "friend." At the same time, as the practitioner, you might not feel too badly about calling a "friend" to cancel her appointment just because you're feeling a little moody or had some other reason for which you wouldn't cancel a "real client." It's easy to see how boundaries can become blurred.

If you're still in training for your career, and you have to perform a number of practice sessions, beware of performing too many on the people close to you because of the dual relationships issue. Of course, your best friend will probably be glad to get free massages, but when you get your license and you're ready to charge him for a session, won't your feelings be hurt if he never comes? It happens all the time.

Self-Care for Clients

An important part of the therapeutic relationship, and ensuring the continued benefits of therapy, is educating the client about self-care. Remember that as massage therapists, we are not allowed to prescribe, but we can make gentle suggestions, such as encouraging a client to drink more water to keep her muscles hydrated, demonstrating stretches she can do between appointments, suggesting ergonomic changes she might make in her daily work habitat when possible, and reminding her to get enough rest and exercise. You can remind clients to use ice or heat as needed for pain, or to soak in warm Epsom salts baths for soreness, and suggest using topical remedies as long as you don't say that they "must" or "need" to use such-and-such. You could say something along the lines of "I use Bio-Freeze whenever my neck is bothering me."

It is important to document the client self-care portion of each session in your SOAP notes under P (Plan). For example:

P: Demonstrated leg stretches for the client to do several times daily; suggested warm Epsom salts baths for soreness; return within 1 week.

(SOAP notes are discussed in relation to insurance filing in Chapter 5 and explained fully in Chapter 6.)

Maintaining Your Own Boundaries

While money is not the sole measure of success, and for many not even the most important one, most of us in business have the objective that not only will our financial needs be met, but that we'll be successful enough to buy things we want and be secure enough to do things we enjoy. We want to set our own schedule and be the master of our own destiny. Building a successful massage practice not only requires that you respect client boundaries; it requires the client to respect your boundaries, as well.

Let's say you've decided to be home at 6 p.m. every night to have dinner with your family, or that you've chosen to be off on Sundays. Those are boundaries for you and should be treated as such, to avoid finding yourself on a crazy treadmill and setting yourself up for resentment.

A therapist who used to work in my office established Thursday as her day off, and yet I saw her there every single Thursday for 3 years! Her services were in demand, and clients would urge her to make Thursday appointments. Ignoring her own boundaries, she let herself be persuaded. When she came in on Thursdays, she was grouchy and would rush to finish sessions so that she could get on with her plans for her day off. Was she successful? Financially, yes, but it took a health crisis to make her see that she was too accommodating to clients and needed to be firm about her boundaries. Once she started saying "No, Thursday is my day off" with real conviction, she discovered that clients would find another time they could come. She did not lose any clients; they respected her boundaries.

Setting boundaries saves confusion and protects the therapeutic relationship from misunderstandings. Clear communication up front saves scrambled signals later. You can't expect clients to observe your boundaries if you send them mixed messages by allowing violations and then being resentful about it later on. Ultimately, setting your boundaries and making them a working part of your policies and procedures is a smart business move. We'll discuss policies and how to set them in Chapter 9.

Clients are definitely sometimes the guilty party. Sexual comments or behavior of any kind from clients should not be tolerated. If a client makes a sexual comment or overture, and you don't respond right away to let him know the behavior is unacceptable, he might assume you're okay with it even if you aren't. Depending on the nature of the offense, give him the benefit of one verbal warning, and if he continues the behavior after the warning, ask him to leave and not come back.

Online discussions and blogs for massage therapists make it clear that male practitioners are propositioned by female clients just as often as females are by males. One male therapist in his seventies is still practicing massage and energy work; he recently made this comment in an ethics forum: "As old and ugly as I am, you wouldn't believe the amount of women that hit on me during a massage."

Going with the Flow

There are numerous chat rooms and forums on the Internet devoted to the discussion of ethics. Joining one, or at least visiting a few to observe the conversation, is a good way to gain insight about ethical dilemmas experienced by massage therapists from all over the world, and to find out how others handle problems that confront them.

Crossing the line with a client is never acceptable under any circumstances. People seeking any kind of health care, holistic or otherwise, are sometimes those who have been abused or are vulnerable for other reasons. They might be suffering from mental health problems that are not immediately apparent. As a massage therapist, you may be the only person to offer them safe, nonsexual touch. Doing otherwise would open the door to all kinds of problems for both parties.

ETHICS AND OTHERS

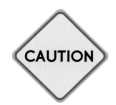

Unless another person's ethics affect you and your business, they are not your concern. Employees or employers, co-workers, business associates, and clients might present you with an ethical dilemma from time to time, getting you involved in something you'd rather not be involved with if you aren't careful. If you practice in a rural area or small town, you already know that word travels fast. That doesn't mean to scrutinize the way other people live, but do be conscious of potential problems that arise and change course when you need to. Here are some examples of how other people's ethics can affect your business:

- A married couple who have both been regular clients are going through a bitter divorce. Each one is spending his or her session time complaining about the other. They're even nagging you to choose between them and to release their partner as a client.
- A divorced mother is bringing her minor child for massage and tells you not to tell the father, who has joint custody of the child and is also a client.
- Your landlord, a pillar of the community, has turned out to have a secret life as an addictive gambler, and some suspicious-looking characters are hanging around in the hallway of your building hoping to catch up with him.

You can be confronted with unexpected problems at any time. While the behavior of others is beyond your control, your reaction to it is entirely up to you. Politely tell the divorcing couple it's inappropriate for you to be in the middle of their problems and you will have to release *both* of them from your practice if they continue to try to place you in that position. Explain to the divorced mother that you don't talk about your clients to anyone, and that she has no right to ask you to tell an outright lie, especially in light of the fact that the child's father has joint custody. Call the police about the loiterers in the hallway.

The People in Your Business

The people in your business include your associates or partners, independent contractors, and employees. If you are in a business partnership with someone, or if you are a sole proprietor who has others working for you or renting space from you, remember that as a business owner, whatever happens at your workplace is ultimately a reflection on you.

If you are considering taking on a business partner, be very careful in your choice. Obviously you want someone who conducts business ethically and who has integrity, but it doesn't stop there. What if you are a stickler for being on time, and your partner is chronically late? What if you are a compulsively neat person, and her grooming or housekeeping is lackadaisical? It's important to be compatible. There must be honest communication between the parties prior to entering into any agreement. (More discussion about partnerships appears in Chapter 4.)

If a practitioner in your premises keeps her treatment room messy, it reflects on your operation. Although it's not an ethics violation, it's still a negative reflection on your business. If an associate is rude to a client, it makes your business look bad. If anyone working in your office is ever accused of a sexual impropriety

REALITY CHECKPOINT

with a client, his or her presence in your business can be both emotionally and financially devastating to you. There may come a time when you find yourself apologizing to a client, or even facing a lawsuit, for something you personally had nothing to do with—because it's your business.

We want to think that all the people with whom we do business are ethical and fair. However, take the time to scrutinize your bills every month. Be sure you're getting what you're paying for, and nothing more or less. Even ethical people with the best of intentions make mistakes. It never hurts to be extra diligent with your own money.

Ethical Dilemmas: The Philandering Business Partner

What can you do when you have a business partner who acts unethically? Let's say you've formed a business partnership with someone you've known for several years, and suddenly she does something totally out of character, like starting an affair with a married client. You can insist that she terminate the therapeutic part of your business relationship, but you have no control over what she does in her personal life. If that behavior is unacceptable to you to the point where you can no longer justify being in business with her, it's probably not going to be as simple as telling her to pack up and leave the premises, especially if joint ownership of the business and/or property is involved. If you have a written partnership agreement (and you should), you would probably have to consult an attorney to find out how to extricate yourself from the agreement with the least amount of damage to your practice.

HANDLING DIFFICULT CLIENTS

Let's expand on the necessity of maintaining roles and boundaries by addressing difficult client situations. Just as the client has the right of refusal when it comes to treatment, you as the practitioner have the right of refusing to take on certain clients.

Even if a client is not being unethical in a literal sense, such as by committing a sexual offense, other behaviors and habits can be unacceptable in a massage business. Most clients are looking for quality services, honest value for their money, and someone who will treat them ethically and with respect; likewise, you as a therapist and business owner should be able to expect the same respect from clients. Is it worth your fee to have a client who acts arrogantly toward you, or acts as if he's doing you a favor by showing up chronically late, or who doesn't respect you or your premises? Here are some typical problematic clients:

- People who are chronically late.
- People who repeatedly cancel appointments at the last minute.
- People who don't call at all and just skip the appointment.
- People who complain that "you haven't fixed the problem" and ask you for extra time when they know the session is supposed to be over.
- People who constantly try to get you to discount your services or ask you for credit.
- People who write bad checks and won't come and pick them up.
- People who litter in the building or the parking lot.
- People who come to their appointments excessively dirty or grimy.
- People who bring disruptive children to appointments and allow them to run wild in your office instead of making them behave or leaving them with a sitter.
- People who bring their dog to appointments because they take their dog everywhere and thought it was okay.
- People who don't *want* to feel better.

The Discount Beggar

Clients who try to regularly get discounts are a problem for any responsible business owner. A person who is in need is one thing, and it's up to you whether or not to help someone. However, a person who is just trying to get a discount so that she can spend money on some luxury at your expense is entirely different. Don't let a client who's driving a new Mercedes, or who has just told you about her fabulous trip to Hawaii, take advantage of you.

Dirty, Smelly Clients

Clients sometimes come to a session straight from work, and if the work is manual labor, they might be dirty. If you're fortunate enough to have a shower in your office, you might have to ask them to shower before a session. Even if you don't have a shower, be sure to have soap and running water they could use. You shouldn't be expected to massage someone who's dirty and sweaty, so don't worry about insulting someone by suggesting he wash up first.

No Dogs Allowed

Unless you are operating a practice devoted to pet massage, heed this warning—particularly if you are practicing in a home office and you think it's okay to have your dog in the treatment area because you're at home. Unless it is an assistance animal, such as a seeing-eye dog, a dog does not belong in your massage or other health care setting, regardless of whether it's in a commercial location or not. The presence of *your* dog may lead clients to believe that it's okay to bring theirs. If your dog barks, even at one person, that might be someone who was bitten by a dog as a child and is afraid of dogs. Your therapeutic relationship will follow her right out the door. Worse yet, if your (or their) dog actually bit someone, you'd have a lawsuit on your hands.

In terms of allowing clients to bring their dog to appointments, you have no way of knowing about the animal's temperament or what kind of care the dog receives. You don't know if it has fleas or ticks or even a disease, and you can't vouch for whether or not a strange dog might bark at or bite someone, like a small child in the waiting room who doesn't know better and pulls its tail. You certainly don't want fleas hopping onto your treatment table or the dog doing his business in the floor. You simply have to tell the client that you can't allow an animal into your premises, even if it's in a carrier.

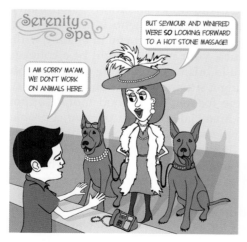

Refusing to Heal

The most difficult client is often the one who won't get well, or who stubbornly finds no benefit from massage. Most clients look forward to their massage. When a client is motivated by a desire to reduce pain, relieve stress, or just feel better overall, the therapeutic relationship is apt to be more open and satisfactory to both parties than with a client who is dragged in by a family member, for instance.

Here's a scenario: Two clients come in, both diagnosed with fibromyalgia. The first one says, "I am really looking forward to this. I've never had a massage before, but Dr. Winker said this will help me feel better." The second one says, "I know this isn't going to help, but my daughter insisted I come." The second client has already decided massage isn't going to help her, and that's beyond your control. Some people are attached to their misery because they get something out of it—sympathy or attention—and it doesn't matter what you do, they won't get better, because they don't want to.

This type of client can suck the oxygen right out of the room, leaving you feeling drained in her wake. If you aren't successful in improving her attitude as well as her pain level within three or four sessions, you might decide to let her go. There's nothing unethical about releasing a client because you feel you can't help her; in fact, as body workers our mission is to provide treatment only when there is a reasonable expectation that the client will benefit. *The client must possess a willingness to benefit*, and some people just don't have that capacity. Fortunately, they're in the minority. Don't take it personally; it isn't about you.

Releasing Clients

Even if one of the categories mentioned above doesn't apply, sometimes a client isn't the "right fit" for your practice, and you want to release him or her from coming to you for massage. You can ask a client to leave if you feel he is constantly abusing your good nature. You can say, for example, "Bob, I realize that I've grown resentful about your chronic habit of showing up late for appointments and then complaining because I can't give you a full session, and my talking to you about it hasn't helped. I'm afraid I'm going to have to suggest that you find a new therapist. A lot of reputable therapists are listed on the AMTA website." At that point, he might decide that he actually does appreciate you and ask you to reconsider, but you should stand your ground.

EXIT AHEAD

YOUR MENTOR

Nothing can help you avoid tricky situations better than having a knowledgeable mentor. A **mentor** is someone who is willing to act as your advisor, a person who has more experience than you in dealing with ethical and business challenges. For instance, your mentor might be a colleague, another therapist who's been successful in business for a long time. A mentor is a good resource whenever you're facing a situation you wish you could avoid, and sometimes, a mentor is invaluable for just plain good moral support. She has probably experienced her own financial struggles, personnel problems, and other issues that new business owners face—and she not only survived, but thrived. It's a good thing to feel like you're not alone, even if you are a lone practitioner. Find a good mentor, and a few years from now when *you* are older and more experienced, return the favor by acting as a mentor to someone who's just starting out.

It's also a good idea to have "distance mentors." These are people you may not have met, but successful professionals whose work you admire and whose career achievements inspire you. Read what they write, listen to their audiotapes, and watch their videos; observe how they advertise themselves, and try to attend their classes as the opportunities arise. Among the therapists at the top in our field, one thing stands out about all of them—their positive attitude. They have the *attitude of success*.

ROADSIDE ASSISTANCE

I was thrilled when I met a very successful internationally known therapist and teacher I admire at a convention, and he said to me, "I'm just a farm boy who was lucky enough to find something I enjoyed doing that I was good at." That is what we all aspire to—finding something we enjoy that we're good at. I was surprised when he told me he constantly attends self-development programs and reads self-help books. I was so much in awe of his accomplishments and his humble attitude that it hadn't dawned on me that even though he's at the top of our profession, he still strives to learn and improve himself. What an inspiration!

POSTCARDS from the HIGHWAY   ## Ralph Stephens

It never was my desire to be a massage therapist until I was 37. I went to college to become a civil engineer. I graduated with a BS in Industrial Education. It would be 17 years before I utilized my teaching degree. After college, I worked as a musician (drummer-vocalist) for 14 years. I played music to help people feel better. As I walked out of my first massage in 1984, I thought, "This would be better for people than playing them music. I could be off the road, self-employed, help people in a much better environment, and live a health-based lifestyle." In September of 1985, I sold virtually everything and moved to Albuquerque to attend the New Mexico School of Natural Therapeutics. After graduation, I returned to my home state of Iowa and opened the first professional office practice of massage therapy in Iowa City on September 15, 1986. I didn't have enough money for next month's rent. In Iowa we say, "If you build it, they will come." They did. I set goals, worked toward them, and accomplished them. I had nothing to start with. I was sleeping in the back of my truck for 5 months, taking showers at the health club, which is where I met a lot of clients. I got involved with my profession through the AMTA, volunteering for state and national offices. Networking with other professionals helped me grow personally and professionally. Successful professionals love to help beginners become successful.

I got involved with my community, joining the Chamber of Commerce and other civic organizations where I met many professional people who could afford massage. Meeting people and selling yourself are the best ways to grow a practice. You get back from your profession and community what you put into them.

I studied with every good teacher I could find. I invested in myself, attending way more than the required number of CE courses. I built up to a full-time practice of 30 people per week, then to a clinic with four therapists and a chiropractor. I work out and stretch everyday and get massage regularly. To give massage you need to get massage. Take care of yourself so that you can take care of others.

I was asked to teach, to share my knowledge and my BS degree finally went to work. I started at a massage school and eventually began presenting CE seminars. I closed my clinic to teach full-time in 1992. Now, I have a limited, home office practice, present CE seminars internationally, write articles and books, and produce training DVDs. I am dedicated to sharing with and passing on my 22+ years of experience and knowledge to other therapists so that together we can help more people gain pain relief and improve the quality of their lives through the power of therapeutic massage.

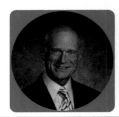

Ralph Stephens is a 2008 Inductee in the Massage Therapy Hall of Fame and the 1997 recipient of the AMTA National Meritorious Award for Leadership, Dedication, and Commitment. He is the author of *Therapeutic Chair Massage* (Lippincott Williams & Wilkins, 2005), has written and produced more than a dozen instructional videos, and is a regular contributor to many massage journals. Ralph teaches a variety of therapeutic techniques all over the world. Visit his website at www.ralphstephens.com.

SUGGESTED READINGS

Bivens TH. *Ethics Worksheet*. Eugene, OR: School of Journalism and Communication at University of Oregon. http://jcomm.uoregon.edu/~tbivins/J397/LINKS/Worksheet.html. Accessed 3/17/2010.

Frye B. *Body Mechanics for Manual Therapists*. 3rd ed. Baltimore, MD: Lippincott Williams & Wilkins, 2008.

Leading Insight.com. *Building Business Relationships*. http://www.leadinginsight.com/business_relationships.htm. Accessed 09/13/2009.

McIntosh N. *The Educated Heart*. 3rd ed. Baltimore, MD: Lippincott Williams & Wilkins, 2005.

National Certification Board for Therapeutic Massage & Bodywork. *Standards of Practice*. http://www.ncbtmb.org/about_standards_of_practice.php. Accessed 07/05/2008.

National Certification Board for Therapeutic Massage & Bodywork. *Code of Ethics*. http://www.ncbtmb.org/about_code_of_ethics.php. Accessed 09/13/2009.

United States Department of Health and Human Services, Office for Civil Rights. HIPAA For Smaller Providers, Small Health Plans, and Small Businesses. http://www.hhs.gov/ocr/hipaa/smallbusiness.html. Accessed 09/13/2009.

Valesquez M, et al. *Thinking Ethically: A Framework for Moral Decision Making*. Santa Clara, CA: Santa Clara University Markkula Center for Applied Ethics. http://www.scu.edu/ethics/practicing/decision/thinking.html. Accessed 3/17/2010.

My Personal Journey

In this chapter, we've discussed the importance of conducting business in an ethical manner. Write down what boundaries are important to you as a therapist, and what your *personal* code of ethics will contain that's unique to you.

My goals _____

_____

_____

What's in my way? _____

_____

_____

What action can I take to remedy the situation? _____

_____

_____

One-year progress update _____

_____

_____

PART 11

Setting Out

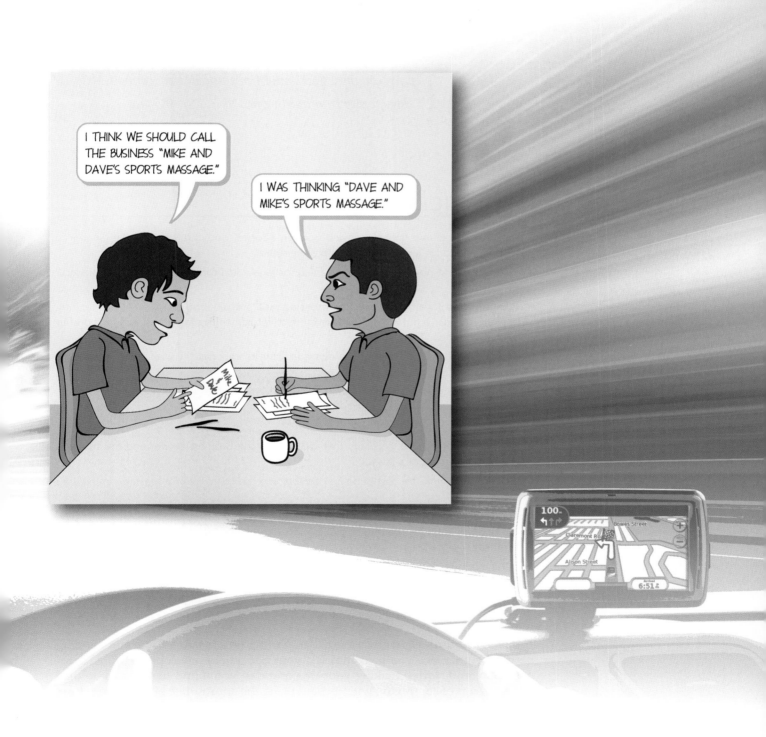

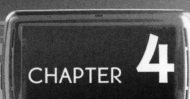

CHAPTER 4

Starting Your Business

*P*lans are only good intentions unless they immediately
degenerate into hard work.

PETER DRUCKER

KEY CONCEPTS

- Obtaining legal and financial advice from an attorney and certified financial planner is recommended for anyone starting a new business.

- Therapists must be aware of the potential for legal ramifications related to the massage profession.

- Inexpensive software programs, Internet sites, and prepaid legal plans are available; they are less expensive but are probably less effective than cultivating a business relationship with an attorney.

- Professional licensure to practice massage may be required in your state; a separate business license may also be required.

- Zoning issues must be a consideration when choosing a business location.

- Careful attention to details when negotiating a lease will produce the most favorable outcome.

- Liability insurance is a necessity that will protect the business owner and the business assets in the event of a lawsuit.

- When setting fees, the cost of doing business and the going rate for massage in the area are essential factors.

- The amount of your capital investment and other initial financial concerns, including paying yourself a salary, require careful planning and close monitoring when starting up a business.

- Setting up your office with the safety and comfort of both client and practitioner in mind is one of the final steps on the countdown to opening day.

- A home practitioner will have many of the same considerations as the therapist who chooses a commercial location, and some that are unique to working in a home office.

Starting a business involves more than putting up a massage table and hanging out a sign. Once you've completed your education, developed a viable business plan, and started making your preparations, you'll find there's a lot to deal with in terms of complying with the law, using the appropriate business structure, obtaining a good location, establishing fees, setting up an office, and getting ready for opening day. The checklists at the end of this chapter will help you be sure you've covered all the bases.

THE LEGALITIES OF BUSINESS

There are many legal matters that go along with being in business, and as an entrepreneur, you might have to seek out professional legal advice at some point. While you may feel comfortable handling a simple rental agreement without legal guidance, you may want to have an attorney look over anything more complex, just to be on the safe side. An important part of operating a successful business is being in compliance with all local, state, and federal laws. Basically, if you are adhering to the laws governing businesses in your state and locality, paying your taxes on time, following ethical business practices, not discriminating against anyone in any way, and working within your scope of practice, you shouldn't have any legal problems. But if you do, it's wise to know a local attorney you can call on for help.

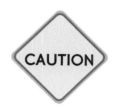

Several factors dictate that massage therapy practitioners should be especially mindful of the potential for legal issues:

- We touch people who are partially or fully unclothed.
- We manipulate soft tissues and affect numerous body systems.
- There are contraindications to be considered in the work we do.
- We obtain private information from people.
- As health care practitioners, we are vulnerable to malpractice lawsuits.

You can't be in compliance with the laws if you don't know what they are. If you're ever faced with a legal situation, pleading ignorance won't help you. It is your responsibility to educate yourself about any local, state, and federal regulations that affect you and your business. You can do this by visiting your local town or city hall. Your state massage board's website is the best place to go for information on state law governing the massage profession. If your state doesn't license massage therapists, check the small business section on your state government's website for general information about operating a business. If you are employing other people, you must follow the Internal Revenue Service (IRS) rules for withholding and paying federal income tax, as well as any state tax for which you're responsible.

Seeking Qualified Advice

When it comes to legal and financial matters, seek out the most qualified, reputable help you can get. Attorneys, for instance, have as many specialty areas of practice as physicians. If you need an attorney for a real estate transaction, hire one who specializes in real estate, not a divorce lawyer. A look through the Yellow Pages will probably yield a lot of possibilities, but a word-of-mouth referral is preferable, if possible. Ask other small business owners for recommendations. You can also check out the American Bar Association for a list of attorneys in your area.

In addition to an attorney, you may want to consult a **Certified Financial Planner (CFP)** when deciding what kind of business structure to set up, and to have him give you a realistic review of your business plan, as mentioned in Chapter 2. Also consult the Chamber of Commerce, SCORE, and the Small Business Administration, as mentioned in the previous chapters, as sources of qualified advice—or at least guidance in where to find qualified advice.

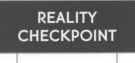

You Get What You Pay For

When it comes to seeking legal advice for your business, there are a number of options available. Spending the money for legal advice up front can save you much more down the road. The old adage "you get what you pay for" is especially true when what you're paying for could mean the difference in the outcome if you find yourself in some sort of legal predicament.

Do It Yourself

There are legal software programs and websites that contain simple do-it-yourself forms for such things as rental and lease agreements, and employee contracts; they basically allow you to fill in the blanks for your particular situation. These make the claim that they are created by lawyers, and they're definitely the cheapest way to go; you may find free simple forms on the Internet, or legal software in the discount bin at office supply stores for as little as $10. But be realistic; you can't expect to get every question answered reliably, or any potentially troublesome legal matter handled, by paying ten bucks for something that comes in a box.

Prepaid Legal Plans

The next step up is a prepaid legal plan. According to the website LegalSurvival. com, as of 2010 more than 45 million Americans use prepaid legal plans, the majority are middle-class consumers who sign up in order to have access to legal services at a steep discount. Although plans vary by the company offering them and the price you pay, most have the following things in common as member benefits:

- A half-hour phone consultation to discuss any legal matter; you can have more than one consultation, but each consultation must be about a different matter.
- Extra time to discuss the same matter, available at an additional charge.
- Discounts averaging 20% to 30% off on hourly rates or flat fees for specific services, such as real estate closings.
- The writing of a simple will, usually at no extra charge.
- A review of legal documents.
- An attorney letter-writing service, which might come in handy when a communication from a lawyer may be enough to get the results you need, such as threatening someone with legal action if he doesn't pay you or fails to honor a contract.

Consultations for prepaid legal plans often take place by phone; you may never meet the attorney who represents you. There may also be local attorneys in your area who participate in such plans, and in that case, you may have face-to-face meetings when called for. Individual plans, family plans, and business plans are available. The American Prepaid Legal Services Institute (APLSI) is a good source of information about prepaid plans because they neither sell nor endorse any plans; they exist to disseminate information to the public and act as a professional association for their provider members, much the same as AMTA and ABMP do for massage therapists.

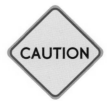

According to a survey conducted by APLSI in 2008, 57% of their membership joined because it was a benefit offered by their employers; some companies are offering prepaid legal insurance that is subsidized for employees, the same as medical insurance. According to APLSI's latest statistics, prepaid legal plans usually cost from $70 to $400 per year, depending on the level of service the consumer chooses.

One caveat to both do-it-yourself aficionados and those who decide to use prepaid plans: No matter what they promise you, software, legal advice websites on the Internet, and prepaid plans all pertain to law that is subject to regulation by the courts, both state and local. Plans that resemble insurance arrangements are subject to regulation by your state's insurance commissioner. What works in one state may not work in another. Be certain that any plan you participate in has registered with your state bar association, a sign that they are selling plans that comply with the laws in your state.

A Professional Relationship

Neither of these avenues will be as satisfactory as cultivating a professional business relationship with a local attorney. You don't have to keep one on retainer; most attorneys will handle matters for you from time to time and just charge you by the hour or the job. You may already have a lawyer who has handled personal or business matters for you in the past. If she doesn't handle the particular type of law you need for your massage business, perhaps she can recommend a colleague to help you.

There is something to be said for building a relationship with someone you know and trust and someone who has the particular expertise you are looking for, even when it costs more. Remember that you get what you pay for.

PROFESSIONAL LICENSURE

As of 2010, 44 states, the District of Columbia, and Puerto Rico have adopted regulations governing the licensing of massage therapists, including education and examination requirements that must be met prior to receiving a license to practice, and in most states, requirements for continuing education in order to renew licensure. Other fields of holistic health, including acupuncture and chiropractic, and in some states naturopathy, are also subject to licensure laws in most places.

If you live in a state that does not regulate massage therapy, you may have a harder time separating yourself from the "recreational" massage therapists. It is archaic that in some places, massage continues to be equated with adult entertainment and is not recognized for its therapeutic value. Due to that outdated perception, there are still places with laws stating such rules as "No massage performed between the hours of midnight and 8 a.m." or "No massaging members of the opposite sex." It's sad but true. There is strength in numbers, and the professional massage therapy associations are working hard to change that image.

Even if it is not required by your state, take one of the examinations currently offered by the National Certification Board for Therapeutic Massage and Bodywork (NCBTMB), the Massage and Bodywork Licensing Examination (MBLEx) offered by the Federation of State Massage Therapy Boards (FSMTB), or the Asian Bodywork Therapy (ABT) Examination offered by the National Certification Commission on Acupuncture and Oriental Medicine (NCCAOM). Establishing your credentials by being licensed or certified, along with belonging to a professional association, will set you apart from nonlegitimate practitioners.

ROADSIDE ASSISTANCE

Recently, I wrote a letter to the editor of our local paper detailing the legal requirements for practicing massage in my state because we have had an ongoing problem in my town with unlicensed people practicing massage. A friend later told me he had read my letter and said he hated the government's interfering in every facet of people's

(continued)

lives. He reasoned that if he wanted to do massage, and made it plain to people that he was an intuitive therapist who didn't have training or a license, why shouldn't that be okay? I told him that the general public is uneducated about the many contraindications of massage and pointed out the danger that an untrained person could really hurt someone. Just as I would have suspected, he was unaware of any contraindications and surprised to hear that they exist. I personally don't like government interference in every facet of my life anymore than my friend, but I recognize the value of licensing massage therapists as a measure of quality assurance. First, do no harm, and we can't stop at just giving massage; it's up to us to educate the public, too.

Obtaining professional licensure, registration, certification, or whatever requirements apply to you is a sign that you have invested the time and money to get professional training and passed an exam to prove competence. It reassures the public of your commitment to provide services while abiding by a code of ethical professional behavior in the framework of the therapeutic relationship.

If massage is regulated in your state, you should make it your business to know every word of your state practice act and any accompanying rules and guidelines because you are subject to those laws.

BUSINESS LICENSES, ZONING, AND LOCATION

Business licenses, zoning laws, and location are all important considerations when you're planning to open a business. The city or town hall in your locale is the source for information about the requirements for your proposed location.

A Business License

In addition to obtaining professional licensure from your state, you might need to obtain a business license. There may be state, county, and/or local licenses required of businesses in general. These requirements vary widely from place to place, so check carefully to be sure you're in compliance.

Zoning Laws

In certain localities, the zoning laws can drastically affect your business, and you need to research locations ahead of time. You wouldn't want to sign a 3-year lease on a building in a zoned area where massage is prohibited and find it out after the fact.

If you intend to conduct your practice at home, you must also make sure you are in compliance with any local zoning laws. Your neighborhood association may prohibit having any signage, or, for that matter, operating any type of business from home, particularly if you live in an upscale community.

If you haven't yet decided on a location for your massage business, bear in mind that you can't construct a concrete business plan and preliminary budget without knowing where you'll be and the cost of the rent or mortgage and the utilities.

A Good Location

Your location can make or break your business. When looking for office space, keep several things in mind besides the expense. There should be ample parking. The entire place, including entranceway, treatment rooms, and the bathroom, should be handicapped-accessible, and this means a ground-floor location or a building with an elevator.

Having an office on a busy road with a lot of foot traffic is obviously better than being located on a dead-end street. You need to have a visible sign, either at the driveway entrance or on the building itself, or both, unless you intend to operate solely by word-of-mouth.

If other busy businesses are nearby, that's a plus for your business. Busy shopping centers and strip malls are good places. A medical park with physicians and/or other health care practitioners conveniently located is desirable for making mutual referrals, something else that will help your business grow.

Any place that's highly visible is great—with a few exceptions:

- Avoid locating your business next to another business that's noisy, like a sheet metal fabrication shop or car garage.
- Don't locate near an adult bookstore or x-rated movie theater. You don't want to reinforce the tired old "massage parlor" image by being located near such a place.
- Having a bar next door will be noisy, and intoxicated people might be hanging out on the street.

Negotiating a Lease

Many massage therapists who are just starting out do not have the money to purchase property for their business, so they either rent or lease space for their massage setting. A rental contract may be from month to month, while a lease obligates you to stay for a certain amount of time, usually at least 1 year. With a lease, you are obligated to pay for the stipulated period of time, even if you move out. Most commercial properties are leased instead of rented, particularly those in prime locations, because landlords generally want to avoid the trouble of having tenants move in and out every few months.

Whether you are renting or leasing, you need to have a written agreement with the landlord, spelling out the terms and each party's responsibilities. Paying close attention to the details when negotiating the lease for your business location will pay off. Some of the crucial components of such an agreement are the following:

- The names of the individuals involved in the lease agreement.
- The property to which the lease refers.
- The period of time the agreement covers, and whether or not there are options to renew.
- The monthly payment expected, and the due date.
- The amount of the penalty, if any, for paying late.
- Any required deposits, such as first and last month's rent, or other form of security deposit.
- The person responsible for repairs and maintenance.
- A statement about whether or not the landlord is allowed to enter the property without permission.
- A statement about whether or not the tenant is allowed to sublet.
- Any other stipulations and rules imposed by the landlord, and/or special considerations given to the tenant.
- A statement about how the lease could be affected if the property is sold.

An example of a standard lease agreement appears in Figure 4-1. Be aware that your own lease may be short and simple, or substantially longer and more detailed, depending on the terms agreed upon between you and the property owner. Don't assume that any verbal agreements you may have discussed are in the written lease; be sure to read every word before you sign on the dotted line.

Lease Agreement

This is a legally binding agreement between James Sorenson, hereafter referred to as the Lessor, owner of the property located at 300 Northern Star Avenue, Cookville, KY 98765, and Karina Lebovitz, hereafter referred to as the Lessee.

Lessee agrees to pay the Lessor the sum of $1000 per month, due and payable on the first day of the month, commencing April 1, 2011, and ending April 1, 2012. Lessee acknowledges that payments received later than the 5th day of the month are subject to a $50 late fee.

Lessee further agrees to pay a security deposit of $2000, to be held in escrow by the Lessor, with the understanding that it will be refunded to the Lessee upon termination of this agreement, providing the property is left in its original condition or better.

Lessor agrees to review the lease on April 1, 2012, and annually on April 1 thereafter, and will give Lessee first opportunity to renew the lease, assuming that the premises have been kept in the condition agreed to by the Lessee, to be ascertained by an annual inspection of the premises.

Lessor agrees to be responsible for the following maintenance on the property: repairs as necessary on plumbing, electrical, heating, and air conditioning systems. Lessee agrees to inform Lessor immediately of any maintenance problems.

Lessee agrees to be responsible for grounds maintenance, including the obligation of mowing the lawn once a week during the months from March-October, and keeping sidewalks and entryway free from snow and ice during the months November-February.

Lessee agrees to be responsible for the removal of trash from the premises, using containers provided by the town of Cookville. Regular business trash pickup occurs on Monday and Thursday. Lessee agrees to abide by the recycling laws of the town and will separate trash accordingly.

Lessor agrees not to enter the leased property without the Lessee's permission, with the exception of an annual inspection to be conducted with 7 days prior notice, to occur on or near the renewal date of said lease.

Lessee acknowledges that no subletting of premises is allowed.

Lessee acknowledges that no smoking is allowed inside the building. Lessee acknowledges that no pets are allowed inside the building.

Lessee agrees to purchase rental insurance and to provide Lessor with a a copy of said policy no later than seven days after the commencement of this agreement.

In the event Lessor decides to sell the property, first right of refusal shall be offered to Lessor. If Lessor decides not to purchase said property, Lessor acknowledges that this lease is not transferable, and that the sale of said property is cause to terminate the lease. Lessor agrees to give Lessee 90 days notice in the event said property is sold.

Lessee agrees that any violation of the terms of this lease is cause for termination of the lease.

This is a binding legal agreement between Lessor and Lessee, acknowledged and witnessed this date of April 1, 2011.

Lessor's Signature_____

Lessee's Signature_____

Witness's Signature_____

FIGURE 4-1   A standard lease agreement.

There may be other stipulations as well, such as not allowing pets into the building, not allowing smoking in the building, and allowing periodic inspections by the landlord.

Before you sign any agreement, be sure you are comfortable with the terms. If the building is relatively new, you might agree to doing your own maintenance in exchange for a lower rent, but you wouldn't want to risk that in a 50-year-old building that might have leaky plumbing and faulty wiring. What if the building needs painting or the carpet needs to be replaced, who is going to do that? It's impossible to be too careful in spelling things out so that there are no surprises later on.

EXPLORATIONS

Try this exercise *before* you rent or lease a building. Make a list of the specifics about your ideal property, and the terms you'd like to have. For example, write down the location you desire, the type of building you'd like to have, the amount of square footage you need, what amenities you require, and the amount of rent you're prepared to pay. Do you want a full kitchen, or is a small break area going to suffice? Do you require a tub or shower, or will a bathroom with a toilet and sink be enough? Do you prefer tile floors, or carpet? Do you need retail space? Be specific about what you're looking for; your list can be a bargaining tool when you're negotiating with a landlord.

LIABILITY INSURANCE

The safest course of action is not to place your hands on a client until you have obtained liability insurance, even though there may be no law requiring you to have it. In most circumstances, if you are still a student, you are covered under the liability policy of your school while you are on their premises, or while participating in school-sponsored events, such as performing community service or doing an internship. You might be in a school that requires you to buy your own insurance. However, in states that do not regulate massage, you might be attending a school that doesn't even have liability insurance or any requirements for you to provide your own. You need to check that out. Someday, a client may get up from your massage table and claim that you injured him in some way. Your table might collapse in a heap on the floor and hurt someone. It's something we all hope will never happen, but definitely something we should be prepared for.

The National Practitioner Databank (NPD) posted a summary of malpractice actions taken against massage therapists during the period from September 1, 1990 through May 12, 2008. According to the report, 35 massage therapists were sued for medical malpractice during that time. It's doubtful that these statistics represent the total number of therapists who were actually sued because the NPD is entirely dependent on professional associations reporting voluntarily; therapists practicing without benefit of professional membership—and thus possibly without liability insurance—were not included. The statistics also do not reflect the number of civil lawsuits that may have been filed against therapists for reasons other than injury to a client, such as sexual or other ethics violations.

Although the statistics aren't high, and many therapists think they're exempt from the need for liability insurance, in addition to protecting yourself, it's another way to say, "I'm a responsible member of the health care profession." The liability insurance that is available from a professional association costs less per year than most therapists would make from doing a half-dozen massages. Don't get caught without it!

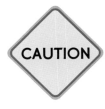

ROADSIDE ASSISTANCE

An attorney asked me a couple of years ago to act as an expert witness in a lawsuit. He was representing a woman who claimed that a massage therapist had broken her clavicle. After reading through a massive pile of documents, I called the attorney and told him if I was going to testify on behalf of anyone, it would be the massage therapist. The woman's family physician had signed an affidavit stating that she was taking a medication that had the side effect of making bones brittle and that a bone could break spontaneously with no pressure whatsoever. The client did not give this information to the massage therapist during the intake interview. She had gone to numerous doctors trying to get one to say it was the therapist's fault, and none of them would. The attorney took my advice and got her to settle the suit.

As a business owner, you need a comprehensive liability insurance policy that covers "slip-and-fall"—an instance of a client falling down and getting injured while on your property—as well as malpractice coverage. Be sure to get vandalism covered in your policy, and damage protection from uninsured motorists. Hopefully, no one will ever drive through your front door, but weirder things have happened. If you are the owner of your premises, your comprehensive coverage should include fire and damage insurance. If you are renting your office space, you'll need renter's insurance to cover the replacement cost of your equipment and other belongings in the event of a fire. If you are working for someone as an independent contractor, or even an employee, the owner might require you to have proof of your own liability coverage.

One thing that has attracted a lot of attention in the years since Hurricanes Katrina and Rita devastated New Orleans and Mississippi is the fact that comprehensive insurance does not cover floods. Hurricanes, melting snow, and heavy rains can all cause floods, and many people have suffered devastating loss after discovering that their regular insurance didn't cover damage and loss caused by a flood. The National Flood Insurance Program is the primary source of flood information and insurance coverage in the United States. Your insurance agent will be able to direct you to the right place.

Insurance policies tend to be pages and pages of legalese and jargon—and you should read every word. If you don't understand it on your own, then have your agent sit down and spell everything out to you.

Words of Wisdom
Being prepared for a crisis is better than trying to fix one after the fact.

CHOOSING YOUR BUSINESS STRUCTURE

Choosing the business structure that's right for you requires some thought, and perhaps, as mentioned earlier, professional advice. You may be required to register your business with local and state governments; in many places, you can do so on the Internet.

Consult with an accountant, a CFP, a tax professional, or an attorney specializing in financial and company matters to help you decide the best structure for your particular business. Maybe you happen to have a degree in business. If you feel savvy enough, and do enough research on the IRS website, you may decide for yourself without benefit of outside help, but if you don't feel 100% confident about your choice, get professional advice. The choice you make will have an impact on many aspects of your business, including taxes, personal liability, and rights of ownership succession.

Certain structures may not be available in every state. Ideally, you want to start out with the right structure because changing it later will create a lot of extra work, changing employer identification numbers (EIN), notifying concerned agencies like the IRS, and so forth. Table 4-1 summarizes the primary characteristics of each type of business structure. The tax obligations and forms associated with the various business structures will be discussed in Chapter 7.

Sole Proprietorship

If you are an individual opening a business owned by you alone, you are operating a **sole proprietorship**. Your Social Security number is all you need to identify yourself to the IRS. As a sole proprietor you may also elect to refer to your company as

TABLE 4-1	Business Structures				
	Sole Proprietorship	Partnership	C Corporation	Subchapter S Corporation	Limited Liability Company
Owner has limited personal liability for business debts			X	X	X
Can be owned by another business entity			X		X
Owner must be a U.S. citizen or resident	X	X	X		X
Must hold annual meetings and record minutes			X	X	
Company can issue shares of stock			X	X	
Owners can report business profit and loss on personal tax returns	X	X		X	X
Owners can split profit and loss with business entity for lower tax rate			X		
Business may have unlimited number of owners		X	X		X
State registration protects the company's name			X	X	X
Business duration may be perpetual, having successive owners			X	X	X

a **DBA (Doing Business As)**; for example, Jim Smith, DBA Triad Sports Massage. A DBA is not a formal business structure in itself; it is just an identifier.

Partnerships

A **partnership** is the legal relationship resulting from two or more people in business together. Each person contributes money, labor, property, or expertise to the business and expects to have a share in the profit or loss of the business. The business is subject to income, losses, investments, and deductions resulting from its operations but does not pay tax as a business. Instead, the profit and loss are passed through the partnership and divided among the partners, who must report their share of income or loss. A partnership requires a federal tax identification number, also known as an **Employer Identification Number**, which can be obtained online from the IRS website.

C Corporation

In forming a **C corporation**, the partners exchange capital or property or both in exchange for certificates of stock in the corporation. People who own stock in a corporation are its **shareholders**. A C corporation must also have an EIN. Check with your attorney or tax professional to see if this is the appropriate setup for your particular situation. This type of business structure offers protection of personal assets, so if you're already well-off financially and own a lot of property, it may serve you to incorporate this way. A C corporation can be owned by another business entity.

Subchapter S Corporation

An eligible corporation can elect to be treated as a **subchapter S corporation**, which makes a difference in the way taxes are handled for the corporation and its shareholders. A subchapter S corporation also has an EIN and offers protection of personal assets, but it differs from a C corporation in that it cannot be owned by another business entity.

Limited Liability Company

A **limited liability company (LLC)** enjoys a limited protection of personal assets and debt liability similar to that of corporations. LLCs have members rather than shareholders, and the members may be individuals, corporations, or other entities. In some states, an LLC can consist of only one member. There are other advantages similar to those for sole proprietorships and partnerships; the LLC is a pass-through for profit or loss, which is then assigned to the members for taxation purposes. An LLC is a relatively recent business structure that combines the features of the other ones.

SETTING FEES

Although we will explore this topic more fully in Chapter 12, let's take a brief look at setting fees. Your fees should be based on several factors. First and foremost, what are other people charging in your area? If you're the first massage therapist in a small town or rural area, charge as you please. If you're not the only therapist practicing, the best policy is charging what the market will bear—whatever is standard and customary in your area.

If you're charging way more, or way less, than other area therapists, there ought to be a good reason. Maybe you want to have a low-cost, or sliding fee, clinic serving the poor or senior citizens on fixed incomes—go ahead, and ignore anyone who criticizes you. If that's not the case, don't price your services a lot lower than the norm with the intent to take business away from other therapists. That won't serve you in the long run. At the same time, if you're charging more than other people, be prepared to give a reason such as "I just don't do hour sessions; it takes at least an hour and a half to do the work I do with people, so I charge more for the session." That sounds reasonable.

If you're an experienced therapist who's been in business for years, you may feel justified in charging more than someone fresh out of massage school. The reality, for people who are employees of someone else, is that most employers pay hourly or pay a commission on massage, and each employee is apt to get the same amount of money regardless of experience. If you are looking for a job, don't hesitate to use your experience as a marketing tool: "I've been licensed for 10 years and have certifications in myofascial release and advanced medical massage."

Words of Wisdom
Make yourself sound valuable. You are! If you don't toot your own horn, who will?

When you make your preliminary budget for your business plan (see Chapter 2), your fee structure, and thus your expected income, has to be a factor. In order for you to know whether or not your plan is feasible, you have to know what your break-even point is, and how many massages you have to perform each month in order to meet it. If you set your fee at $50 for a massage, and budgeted expenses total $3000 per month, that means the first 60 massages each month have to go to pay business expenses and the rest is yours. But if you raise the price $10 and charge $60 for a massage, only the first 50 massages each month have to go to pay the bills, and the rest is yours.

In addition to knowing your break-even point and knowing what the market will bear, establishing fees involves asking yourself *what value your customers get out of the total experience they have at your business.* The atmosphere and the comfort of your massage setting, and the level of service clients receive, are just as important as your skill as a therapist, and should be factored into your fee structure.

If you practice at home, or do outcalls, you won't have the same overhead as a therapist practicing in a nice professional office. That doesn't mean that your skill and your time are worth any less, but it does mean you could charge a little less than someone who's paying a premium for real estate. Use your discretion.

CAPITAL INVESTMENT AND INITIAL FINANCIAL CONCERNS

While your sweat equity is certainly an investment, the actual money you sink into your business is your real **capital investment**, and it's obviously important to keep track of this. It's doubly important if you are in a partnership or have incorporated your business. Your financial software can do it as long as your entries are accurate and up-to-date.

There are many places you have to spend money prior to your actual opening date of business. If you own the building you are operating in, ask your financial advisor about the best way to handle the mortgage, either personally or through the business. You might be advised to rent it to your corporation.

If you're renting, you'll have to pay a security deposit and deposits for all your utilities. Furnishings and office supplies, décor, signage—all those things you lay out money for constitute your capital investment. Record every penny of it. Your capital investment, plus any money you invest at any time, is your tangible equity in your business. That figure will be important in the future, if you should need to borrow money, decide to take on a partner, or sell your business.

Your capital investment is also vitally important to your tax situation. Say you've invested $25,000 in starting up your business. Until such time as you draw out that $25,000 you initially invested, the money you take out of your business is a reimbursement of what you've put in.

Your Salary

When your business begins to bring in enough money to pay the expenses and have some left over, you can begin to take a salary or draw. In the meantime, let's say you file taxes the first year, and you've earned $10,000 for the massages you've done during the year. That $10,000 is not technically profit because you haven't made the total $25,000 you invested back yet. Be sure your tax preparer knows the situation because it will make a huge difference in the amount of tax you owe. Keep track of every penny you put in, and every penny you draw out. It's as simple as that. There are many tax software programs available for the do-it-yourself business owner, but just like the attorney versus the legal software, you get what you pay for.

Don't plan on writing yourself a big check every week; it isn't realistic. Your ability to bring in business, coupled with your ability to budget wisely, recover your investment, and cover your operating expenses on an ongoing basis will determine your salary. All the money you take in is your **gross income**. The money that's left after you cover expenses and pay taxes is your **net income**—your profit, your salary. Obviously, you have to have something left before you can get anything. Once you have enough business coming in to cover your expenses and have some income left over, you may opt to pay yourself a set rate every week or month, and leave the rest of your profit in the business as equity. Or you could pay yourself varying amounts based on how much money is coming in and flowing out at any given time, if necessary. There are busy periods and slow periods in all service-based businesses. Drawing a regular salary instead of various amounts here and there does allow you to budget for your salary, and of course you can adjust it as business increases.

It is essential to consult a tax professional. The IRS code covers thousands and thousands of pages. You will be busy enough trying to run your business and cannot possibly keep up with all the latest tax developments. Let a professional who is in the business of keeping up with it do the job, so you can focus your energies on making enough money to pay your taxes!

EXPLORATIONS

If there are successful massage and bodywork businesses already established in your town, pay attention to the advertising venues they are using. Most business owners who have been operating for a few years have already figured out where it pays to advertise and where it doesn't, and they won't keep pouring money into something that isn't bringing in any return.

SETTING UP YOUR OFFICE

Finally, the countdown to opening day has arrived. You've obtained a space, and now you need to set it up. Consider equally the comfort and safety of your clients, and the comfort and safety of *you*.

Ergonomics

The primary consideration is that your office is ergonomically comfortable for you and your clients in every way. If you're a lone practitioner, a small desk or table, a chair for your client to sit in while waiting, and a filing cabinet may be enough for you. Be sure tables and surfaces are at a good height for you so that you don't have to strain to reach anything. If you're using a computer, set it up so that your wrists are in a neutral position and the monitor is right in front of you.

Arrange the treatment room so that everything you need is within easy reach. The floor should be clear of any obstructions. The bathroom door should lock, and keep the bathroom fully stocked with dispenser soap, paper towels, tissues, and extra toilet paper. A mirror above the sink is a necessity. If you have bath or shower facilities clients may be using, provide a blow-dryer. A robe for clients to wear on the way to the bathroom is also important.

Decoration

When choosing the decor for your office, it's best to have an uncluttered style. Avoid the temptation to decorate with every picture of your child from kindergarten through the wedding. A personal memento or two is okay, but don't overwhelm clients by displaying your vast collection of Star Trek memorabilia. They're there for a relaxing experience, not a stroll down (your) memory lane.

Going with the Flow

Spas are enjoying more popularity than ever. Even if you're running a medical massage practice instead of a spa, incorporating some elements of spa decor into your office can work for you. A bubbling fountain, candles or ambient lighting, an aromatherapy diffuser, a soothing color scheme, and a few lush green plants are inexpensive ways to create an inviting, relaxing atmosphere.

Opening Day

The checklist in Box 4-1 will guide you from the moment of inception of your massage business to opening day and beyond.

Working at Home

Let's examine the concept of working at home because not every practitioner is going to approach it in the same way. Maybe you're thinking of "flying below the radar"—operating strictly by word-of-mouth referrals, not having any signage, not doing any advertising, not registering your business in any way. That approach

---

BOX 4-1   Opening Day Checklist

- Write down your wish list.
- Do a market study; find out how many practices of your type are in the area; try to obtain their menu of services and prices.
- Refine the wish list into your business objectives.
- Find a suitable location. Pay the deposit or down payment if you're buying; sign the mortgage papers, lease or rental agreement. (Box 4-2 is a separate checklist for the home practitioner.)
- Visit the Small Business Administration in your area for an information packet for new entrepreneurs.
- Visit the Chamber of Commerce for a membership packet.
- Revisit your household budget so that you'll know where you stand financially as a preliminary to writing your business plan.
- Write your mission statement.
- Arrange for telephone service, Internet service if needed, and a Yellow Pages advertisement.
- Once you know your location, investigate the historical cost of the utilities so that you can budget for them.
- Order signage (see Chapter 14).
- Develop your business budget.

(continued)

BOX 4-1 Opening Day Checklist

- Pull all the facts and plans together into a cohesive written business plan that you can take to the bank; even if you're not going to borrow money, write the plan so that you'll have it to follow.
- Research local banks for the most favorable rates, and open a business checking account. Order checks and deposit slips.
- Set a budget for purchasing equipment and furnishings, and shop for the best deals.
- If you are going to have associates, start looking for them through word-of-mouth or classified ads.
- Consult an attorney or financial planner for advice regarding your business structure (sole proprietorship, corporation, etc.).
- Obtain the necessary business licenses and permits.
- Obtain your EIN from the IRS.
- Obtain your practitioner's identification number if you are going to accept health insurance (see Chapter 5).
- Apply for a business loan, if that is a necessary part of your plan.
- Start planning your grand opening.
- Pay the utility deposits and get the utilities turned on.
- Set up credit card processing if you intend to offer that payment option (see Chapter 6).
- Do necessary repairs, painting, and cleaning in the office before moving in furniture and equipment (or have the landlord do it if appropriate).
- Move into the office and decorate. Nice green plants are an inexpensive way to make your office look nice.
- If you intend for your business to have an Internet presence, obtain your domain name and build (or hire someone to build) your website. Many web hosts have very simple templates you can use to build your own site. Do this *before* ordering literature so that you can include your website address on your business cards and brochures.
- Have your business forms and literature designed and printed—cards, brochures, menu of services, intake forms. The intake form should contain the HIPAA privacy statement, or else you should obtain separate HIPAA brochures as required by law (see Chapter 3).
- Decide on your initial marketing strategies. Contact local newspapers and other media outlets to announce your grand opening. Most will cover a business opening at no charge.
- Join the Chamber of Commerce and enlist their help with your grand opening and ribbon-cutting ceremony.
- Obtain necessary office and janitorial supplies.
- Obtain any items you will be retailing.
- Make arrangements for laundry service, if needed.
- Obtain necessary insurance policies: liability insurance and renter's or mortgage insurance.
- Put a professional-sounding message on your answering machine.
- If you're employing staff, do the hiring and bring them in for orientation prior to opening day.
- Order name tags and/or desk plates for yourself and staff, as needed.
- If you are wearing a uniform or requiring staff members to do so, obtain them and/or inform staff of where to get them.
- Arrive early on opening day for last-minute straightening up.
- Turn the sign to "Open" and get ready to greet your first customer!

isn't recommended; flying below the radar often means running a cash business, avoiding income tax, and other issues that we do not encourage.

Challenges for the Home Practitioner

People want to work at home for many reasons. Starting out at home can be a way to get your business established while saving money for a real office in a better location. Some therapists work at home to be near their children or a family member who needs caretaking.

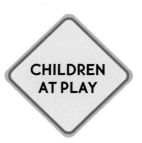

However, consider this: If you have noisy young children, how is that going to work out for you if you're in the middle of giving a massage or an acupuncture treatment and your 2-year-old goes ballistic? You may want to plan your office hours when your spouse or other babysitter is at home to take care of such situations, or in the evenings after the little ones are in bed. You also have to take extra care to present a professional front—no toys in the floor, no pail of smelly diapers in the bathroom. Your home needs to be clean and neat if you are going to practice massage there. Working at home is a convenience in some ways but requires just as much or more work as having an office elsewhere.

Most people's homes are not handicapped-accessible. Yet in any type of health care business, the possibility is very real that some clients might be handicapped. If you own your property, you can go to the expense of installing a wheelchair ramp and making the bathroom handicapped-accessible; if you're renting, ask your landlord if he would be willing to do so.

A Dedicated Phone

Why go to the expense of a separate phone line for your business if you already have one at home? Unless you live alone, and unless you're always willing to answer the phone in your business persona, you'll find having a business phone line is a smart move. If you have children at home, you don't want your child saying "Oh yeah, Dad, some guy wanted an appointment tomorrow but I didn't ask his name or number," or your teenager answering the phone with a "Yo, whassup." People may call you at all hours of the day and night—another reason to have a separate phone line and an answering machine or voicemail that can pick up calls after your workday is over.

I'm Not at Home, I'm at Work

Another consideration is that because you are at home, some people have a hard time thinking you're actually working. You might have to explain to friends and family who have been used to calling anytime or stopping by at will that you are working between the hours of such-and-such and are not available for socializing during those times. You might also have a sign you can put on the outer door that says "Massage in Session" or something similar, to discourage would-be visitors from dropping in.

If you own your home, you may want to consider creating a separate entrance for your massage setting. If you have an area where your treatment room has an adjoining bathroom, and you have a separate entrance, that will eliminate the need for clients to walk through the rest of your private living space.

Avoiding Isolation

You can be successful working at home; success is all about your goals and your personal definition of success, and making money while staying at home may well define that for you. Just remember that if you work at home, you never really leave the office. In addition, people who practice alone sometimes feel isolated. You'll have to make

---

BOX 4-2   Opening Day Checklist for Home Practitioners

- Write a business plan for working at home.
- Check with your local government to see if the zoning laws allow home businesses.
- Check with your local government to see if signage is allowed or restricted; order signage, if desired.
- Obtain the required licenses and permits.
- Obtain an EIN from the IRS if needed; the majority of home practitioners act as sole proprietors and will not need one.
- Research local banks for the most favorable rates, and open a business checking account.
- Order checks and deposit slips.
- Set up credit card processing if you intend to offer that option for payments.
- Obtain liability insurance.
- Check with your insurance agent to see if additional homeowner's insurance is required.
- Visit the local Small Business Administration for an information packet.
- Visit the local Chamber of Commerce for a membership packet.
- Install a separate phone line or obtain a cell phone with a business number.
- Set up a Yellow Pages ad if you intend to have one.
- Set aside a work area in your home; clean and decorate it as needed.
- Be sure the yard and grounds are clean, groomed, and free from obstruction.
- Obtain any necessary supplies and equipment you don't already own.
- Decide how you are going to advertise, and place opening ads.
- You're in business!

---

an extra effort to get out and spend some quality time away from that environment so that you won't become stagnated. Make it a point to have lunch out, or go to the park or window-shopping, or some other excursion every week. Take time to have a social life. Don't become a hermit just because you're working at home.

Box 4-2 is a checklist for opening day for home practitioners.

POSTCARDS from the HIGHWAY   ### Joel Tull

In 1957, my grandmother gave me a dollar for rubbing her feet, partly to reward my willingness to touch her gnarled and calloused feet but mostly to teach my brother a lesson for refusing a nickel for the same task. That was the beginning of my path to becoming a massage professional with million-dollar hands.

Accomplishing this was simple but not easy. In the 1970s, I charged $10 for a 1-hour outcall and counted myself lucky if I saw four people in a week. In the 1980s, I practiced full-time and slowly learned the lessons that brought me success. I had always seen massage as an art form but now began to see it as a sacrament as well. Massage was a "calling" like the ministry chosen by my siblings. They preached; I laid on hands.

I came to massage with experience that gave certain advantages. Years of working in building trades gave me physical stamina and much of the manual dexterity needed. I also knew that any work was better than no work. A contractor out of work is not in a position to showcase his talent or get referrals. A failed retail business taught me the value of keeping records and keeping in touch with customers. My connection to the arts proved more important than either of these insights.

My first clients were professional dancers. They tortured their bodies for little or no pay for the love of the act of dancing. Other clients were professional musicians who

(continued)

Joel Tull *(Continued)*

practiced for years to get a $50 wedding gig. I realized that I must practice, practice, practice. I was astounded when new massage graduates who 2 weeks prior had been paying for the privilege of giving practice sessions, now insisted on $60 to touch a client. No musician locks up his violin until a paying customer is within earshot.

I resolved that I would keep my hands on bodies at whatever fee to learn my craft. The sheer numbers created a huge referral network, eventually landing me at the Olympic Games in Australia. Over the next two decades, I filled my appointment book with paying clients, "comps," and over 2000 massage exchanges. I tracked every dollar generated in a little ledger book and then spreadsheets in multiple generations of computers. The numbers were a source of assurance when clients left or switched to one of the dozens of new therapists who seemed to graduate each week. A couple who booked weekly could relocate and cost you one tenth of your income.

Records accurately predict income and do not flatter or make judgments. Armed with information, one can negotiate fee schedules, discounts, and cancellation fees confident that the mortgage is paid. When a therapist is conflicted in a client-therapist relationship because the therapist needs the income, the outcome is seldom happy. Armed with information, you can decide when to direct income or time to continuing education, marketing, or to balance personal life if your "stats" indicate an imbalance. Set your sights on million-dollar hands, and never regret a massage you "give."

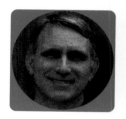

Joel Tull began practicing massage in Saratoga Springs, New York, in 1974, working with the dance faculty of Skidmore College and members of the New York City Ballet. He moved to Greensboro, North Carolina, in 1976, and in 1987, he expanded his private massage practice into a group practice, The Human Touch. For over 30 years, Joel has worked with hundreds of athletes, dancers, and performing artists from around the world. He has provided massage at the Olympics in Sydney, Australia; the Goodwill Games in Brisbane, Australia; and the World Track and Field Championships in Japan, Canada, Spain, France, and Hungary. In 2004, he was a featured speaker to the Medical and Coaching Staff of the Slovenian Olympic Committee in Ljubljana, Slovenia. He has received the Meritorious Award from the American Massage Therapy Association. Joel teaches workshops for massage professionals throughout the United States. Visit his website at www.joeltull.com.

SUGGESTED READINGS

American Bar Association. *Lawyer Locator.* http://www.abanet.org/lawyerlocator/searchlawyer.html. Accessed 09/22/2009.

American Prepaid Legal Service Institute Online. *How Much Does a Legal Plan Cost?* http://www.aplsi.org/legal/#cost. Accessed 09/22/2009.

Certified Financial Planner Board of Standards, Inc. http:www.cfp.net. Accessed 09/22/2009.

Friedman B. *Prepaid Legal Plans: Information on Prepaid Legal Plans for Individuals, Families, Business & Commercial Drivers.* http://www.legalsurvival.com/discount_legal_plans.html. Accessed 03/09/10.

Gegax T, Bolsta P. *The Big Book of Small Business: You Don't Have to Run Your Business By the Seat of Your Pants.* New York, NY: HarperCollins Publishers, 2004.

La Plante C. *A Guide to Starting Your Own Business.* http://www.amtamassage.org/journal/spring05_journal/GuideToStartYourOwnBusiness. pdf. Accessed 09/22/2009.

National Practitioner Database Summary Report. http://www.npdb-hipdb.hrsa.gov/pubs/stats/NPDB_Summary_Report.pdf. Accessed 09/21/2009.

O'Berry D. *Small Business Cash Flow: Strategies for Making Your Business a Financial Success*. New York, NY: John Wiley & Sons, 2007.

The Company Corporation. *Selecting the Right Business Structure*. http://www.incorporate.com/business_structures.html. Accessed 03/0910.

My Personal Journey

In this chapter, we've discussed obtaining professional legal and financial advice, choosing the right business structure, and setting up an office. Visit the IRS website at www.irs.gov to read the full details of each type of business structure, and choose the one you feel is right for you. Then, check out the small business section on the official government website for your state, and take care of any registrations that are necessary for your business. If you feel you need legal help, make an appointment with an attorney.

My goals _____

_____

_____

What's in my way? _____

_____

_____

What action can I take to remedy the situation? _____

_____

_____

One-year progress update _____

_____

_____

Managing Obstacles and Steering Toward Success

CHAPTER 5

If you can find a path with no obstacles, it probably doesn't lead anywhere.

FRANK A. CLARK

KEY CONCEPTS

- Any business owner must be prepared to deal with setbacks and obstacles.
- A financial crisis is the most common problem for a small business.
- A setback is a normal part of the business process, and using it as a learning experience is crucial to success.
- Having a contingency plan in place for emergencies or times of economic downturn is a smart business strategy.
- A successful entrepreneur will always arrive at a point where the decision must be made to grow the business or to remain static.
- Expanding a business means taking on new and different responsibilities than the ones you started out with and it might mean revising your business plan.
- Growing your business can include offering additional services, expanding hours of operation, or adding more practitioners.
- Accepting health insurance is a sure way to increase business and can be a buffer against an economic downturn; it requires a lot of preparation, paperwork, and attention to detail.

Since every business will go through some sort of change or setback at one time or another, it's important to be able to look past the obstacle and plan your future strategies. In order to develop your new business focus, ask yourself these questions: "What is the big picture I have for my business?" "What can I do differently to keep this setback from occurring again?" "What goals do I want my business to achieve in the next 3, 6, and 12 months?" "How can I use this setback as a learning experience?" The answers to these questions are guidelines for revising your goals and developing a plan to help you meet them.

Surviving setbacks and making a long-term commitment means you'll eventually come to a crossroads, when it's time to decide whether to grow your business or keep it the same. Accepting health insurance is one way to make your business grow, even in times of economic downturn; it can cause a dramatic increase in clientele and provide a buffer against inflation.

DEALING WITH ROADBLOCKS

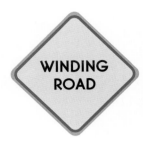

People who have been in business more than a year or two can probably vouch for the fact that it isn't an easy road, and they can also tell you how rewarding it is to face an adversarial situation and come out on top—ready to make their business survive and thrive. Having a contingency plan is good in theory, and you should certainly have one for certain circumstances, such as not getting as many clients as you had planned for during your first year. However, it's important to recognize that things may happen that you really can't anticipate. When a setback occurs, it's crucial to take action and not react negatively. View it as a bend in the road, not the end of the road.

In the previous chapters, you were encouraged to seek professional advice from the many avenues that are available to small businesspeople: SCORE, the SBA, the Chamber of Commerce, a mentor, and professionals such as attorneys and financial advisors. While it's better to get help at the outset, it's not too late to seek advice during a time of crisis. Your mentor may have been through the very same thing. A financial advisor may be able to help you dig out of a hole that you feel is bottomless. Don't be too stubborn to ask for help.

Financial Setbacks

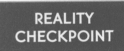

The first setback you should be prepared to face is the one that probably occurs with the most frequency—a financial setback. It takes money to start a business, and it takes money to maintain a business. A financial reversal is, obviously, something a business owner hopes never happens, but it is necessary to be prepared. You don't want to risk losing your business because of some unforeseen circumstance, like unanticipated costs or a downturn in the economy.

Unanticipated Expenses

Sometimes things happen unexpectedly. For instance, if your car requires a repair that costs $1000 when your business has only been open for a month, can you afford it? If you created your business plan and budget projections based on having 30 clients a week, and you only get 20, can you still cover your expenses? No one plans to be sick or injured. If you were out of work for 2 weeks, would it throw you into a financial frenzy? What about 2 months? Many professional associations, such as the AMTA (American Massage Therapy Association) and Associated Massage & Bodywork Professionals (ABMP), offer disability insurance for such emergencies.

Economic Downturn

Sometimes your business will be affected by external factors beyond your control. When the economy takes a downturn, small businesses that are service providers are often one of the first sectors to suffer. When people have less discretionary money to spend, they tend to cut back first on those things they don't view as necessities. During a recession, you may have steady clients who lose their jobs, which by default will affect *your* business.

We all hope a financial setback—falling short of our projections—will only be temporary. Stepping up your marketing efforts, getting your own name and your business name out to the public, and other strategies can help minimize the difficulties of small business ownership during an economic downturn (see Chapter 13). When financial security is at risk, it's more important than ever to scale back your expenditures and to stay in close contact with your financial planner or accountant.

Being Prepared

Here's an example of being prepared, being flexible, and having a backup plan. A friend found herself in a terrible bind when the county decided to widen the highway in front of her massage therapy business—a construction project that lasted for 2 months. Unaware it was going to happen, she arrived at work one morning to find construction barrels in front of her parking lot, heavy machinery blocking the road, and a worker directing traffic to make a detour around her place. Although access was allowed for people who had an appointment, noise was a problem; the constant sound of jackhammers, bulldozers, and dump trucks is not conducive to a relaxing massage. She was able to handle the situation by forwarding her business calls to her cell phone, converting some of her appointments to outcalls, and by seeing clients at her home temporarily.

Most setbacks, like this one, are temporary. Having both a contingency plan and a nest egg can keep you from going into panic mode if an emergency arises.

Other Types of Setbacks

Not all setbacks are financial in nature. Staff problems, dissatisfied clients, and ethics violations are other types of setbacks that you may be facing one day, and it's a good idea to try to anticipate them. There's a solution to every problem, so don't get discouraged.

Staff Problems

If you have employees or independent contractors, issues with staff members are inevitable. There is no guarantee that someone won't get mad and walk off the job, and maybe even steal your clients on the way out the door. You can be somewhat protected by having staff members sign contracts listing the terms of their employment, including a noncompete agreement if they leave (see Chapter 8); however, such provisions usually don't stand up in court.

In the medical world, client files are client property. If your massage business is a health care business, bear in mind that client files actually belong to the client, not to you, and not to other practitioners who work in your office. Make this clear to staff members. (See Chapter 9 for a further discussion of policies and procedures.) Departing practitioners should never be allowed to take client files, but if the client requests her own file, you must give it to her. If a client really wanted to follow a departing staff member, it wouldn't endear you to the client if you acted ungraciously about it.

Dissatisfied Clients

If you learn that a client is dissatisfied and speaks poorly of you, obviously it's not good for business. Ask yourself what the complaint might be. Were you chronically late for appointments? Did the client feel she got value for her money when she saw you for massage? Did you check with her about pressure or discomfort during sessions? Is your office as clean as a health care setting should be? Be honest with yourself. If you know beyond doubt that you provided the best of care and service in a nice clean environment, then accept the possibility that certain clients won't be satisfied no matter what you do. Don't take it personally, just let it go.

Ethics Violations

An ethics charge made by a client against you, or someone in your office, is a serious professional setback. If you have employees or independent contractors, naturally you will have made an effort to get the best people you can. While it may sound gloomy to suggest that you should do a criminal background check on everyone who works in your office, it's a wise business practice to do so (see Chapter 8). If your state licenses massage therapists, be sure to check with the licensure board to make sure your staff members' licenses are in good standing, and that none of your employees has had any reprimands or ethics charges. Some states require their own criminal background and/or fingerprint checks before issuing a license to practice massage.

If you or someone you employ is accused of an ethics violation, you have to meet the situation head-on. The accused party will be given an opportunity to have legal representation and character witnesses at a disciplinary hearing. The rules governing a licensure board disciplinary hearing are different from a criminal hearing in a court of law; in some cases, hearsay is allowed in as corroborating evidence. Licensure boards tend to err on the side of caution whenever someone is accused of a violation, especially if it is a charge of sexual impropriety.

A sexual or other assault charge may be reported to the police instead of, or in addition to, a licensing body. An arrest for sexual molestation is the type of thing that ruins a business. Your name, or the name of your business, in the news in a negative story of any kind is never a good thing, and the damage multiplies exponentially when it happens in a small town. Again, remember that you cannot be too careful in checking the background of potential staff members, keeping in mind the need to avoid future setbacks.

ROADSIDE ASSISTANCE

During my 5-year term of serving on a state massage therapy board and participating in many disciplinary hearings, I was shocked at the number of ethics violations in which one massage therapist was accusing another of a sexual impropriety. In most cases, these were therapists who barely knew each other; maybe they had met at a class and decided to set up a massage trade. I believe there was usually no real intent to cause harm; I think the accused therapist may have viewed the person on the table as a colleague instead of a client and been too casual about draping or making an inappropriate comment. That doesn't matter to the public; if such an accusation is made and word gets out, the negative effect on your business is just as damaging. The commonsense and ethical path to take is to treat everyone on your table with the same respect and ethical behavior, no matter how well you know them.

Words of Wisdom
I can accomplish any task I set my mind to.

Real Obstacles Versus Imaginary Obstacles

The purpose of the exercise at the end of the chapter, *My Personal Journey*, is for you to write a list of the *real* obstacles that are standing in the way of reaching your goals, and then brainstorm about what you can do to overcome them. You may want to share them with your mentor; a fresh pair of eyes can sometimes see things that you can't. A financial advisor may be able to tell you how to rearrange your finances by consolidating a debt or getting a loan in order to start your business. A banker will look not only at your credit score and what assets you have right now, but at your future earning potential when considering giving you a loan. The point is, if you think you don't have the money, don't stop there; you'll be getting in your own way if you do. Seek professional advice to help you move forward.

One of the biggest detriments to success, besides negative thinking, is procrastination—putting off until tomorrow what you can do today. Somehow, it seems, tomorrow never comes. If you're a lifelong procrastinator, being an independent businessperson may not be the road for you to take. You might be better off working for someone else, and letting your employer worry about the business end of things while you focus on doing massage.

ROADSIDE ASSISTANCE

I once read a Dear Abby column in which a man wrote to say he was 50 years old and had wanted to be a doctor all his life. Now he had enough money to go to medical school, but in the 8 years it would take him to finish, he would be almost 60 and his family was discouraging him by telling him he was too old. Abby's reply was that if he didn't go to medical school, in 8 years he would still be almost 60—and he wouldn't have done what he truly wanted to do. Don't get in your own way by thinking you're too old, too shy, too lacking in self-confidence, too obligated to this or that person or thing. Those aren't real obstacles. They're just baseless fears hanging around taking up space in your brain. Take a deep breath and let them go.

If you've carefully constructed your business plan and done everything you're supposed to do, it's all going to turn out great, isn't it? We certainly hope so. In reality, though, sometimes things happen that are beyond our control; even the best-laid plans go wrong. At other times, things happen that we *could* have controlled, but we dropped the ball. You have to pick yourself up and dust yourself off and start all over again—that's *perseverance*.

We've all heard of overnight success stories, but those are few and far between, and usually it turns out that the "overnight success" had actually taken years of plugging along in obscurity until a big break came. Most success stories are filled with a background of years of hard work and the occasional heartache. Everyone, no matter what the business is, suffers through illness, death of a loved one, accidents, and other personal tragedies. Hurricanes, floods, fires, and other disasters have closed hundreds of businesses in the blink of an eye. You have to think of any obstacle as a challenge, find a way to meet it, and learn something from the experience.

GROWING YOUR BUSINESS

Every business that succeeds eventually reaches a point where you have to make a decision: *to grow or not to grow*. If your list of objectives included getting 25 clients a week, and you've done that, what are you going to do next? When you've met your goal, it's time to choose between setting the bar higher, or letting it stay where it is. When you get to that point, you can choose to stop taking new clients, or you can choose to expand your business. You can tell people you'll put them on your waiting list, but if they're in pain and looking for relief, they may not be willing to wait for one of your clients to leave or move away.

Deciding to expand your business when you've gotten used to being a solitary practitioner is a big step—almost as big as going out on your own. It presents new opportunities and involves new responsibilities at the same time. If you decide to expand, you have to decide whether you want to bring in an independent contractor or an employee. Another practitioner might be treated as an independent contractor, but if you need a receptionist, that person will probably be an employee drawing a salary. (Employees and independent contractors are discussed in Chapter 8.)

ROADSIDE ASSISTANCE

When I started my business, circumstances dictated that I expand almost immediately. My husband and I were asked to go into business with two other practitioners, and when they decided to leave after only 2 months, we were left with two empty treatment rooms—a totally unacceptable state of affairs. My goal immediately became to fill those rooms with other professionals who could help pay the rent. I called two practitioners I knew who worked together at another business that I'd heard might be closing down. On the first call, they said thanks but no thanks; they were happy where they were. Two days later, they called me back and said they'd revisited that decision after having an honest talk with the business owner, finding out the place was indeed going to go out of business. There was no issue of stealing clients; the business was closing, and all their clients followed them right down to our office. Sometimes an opportunity just presents itself. Deciding to expand was a no-brainer for me; I had empty space I needed to fill.

Expanding Your Horizons

When one business goal is met, other opportunities arise. If you're thinking of expanding, do some research—another market study or a customer survey—to find out where there is a need, and *fill that need*. It may be that there's a demand for massage in the evenings or on weekends that you could get another practitioner to fill, if you haven't been operating during those hours, and don't want to work at that time yourself. Look at it this way: You're paying for your space 365 days a year. If you are closed every Saturday and Sunday, that's 114 d/y that your business isn't bringing in any money to cover the overhead. This is not meant as an encouragement for *you* to work 365 days a year. Many prospective clients are off work on the weekends and that might be a convenient time for them to get a massage; the same logic goes with evening hours. Somewhere in your town is a therapist who wants to build a clientele, and who would be willing to work those hours. Try running an ad or calling your local massage school to find her.

Enhancing Your Menu of Services

There are many spa techniques and variations on massage you could add to your menu of services, even if you don't have a fancy wet room equipped for hydrotherapy treatments. For instance, heat your massage oil, and your massage is no longer just a massage, it's a hot oil massage. If you have a kitchen crock-pot and running water, you can easily do salt scrubs and even mud treatments. Try sprucing up your menu and adding a few things to your repertoire. The NCBTMB lists more than 300 hands-on and home study classes in spa techniques that are available for approved continuing education; many are specifically about spa techniques that can be done without special equipment. Be sure to check your massage board's regulations to make sure spa treatments fall within the scope of practice in your state.

ROADSIDE ASSISTANCE

When I opened my business, I wasn't even considering offering spa treatments. Then the phone started ringing with people wanting to know what kind of spa treatments we offered. I quickly realized if they couldn't get it here, they'd go somewhere else, and I've offered body wraps, mud wraps, and salt scrubs ever since. They're all simple to do, and they have the added benefits of putting a little variety in your day and saving your hands for deep tissue massage.

Collaboration with Other Practitioners

If you started out offering just massage and bodywork, you may choose to complement those with other services by asking a practitioner of another discipline, such as an acupuncturist or an aesthetician, to join your staff. One of the great things about holistic health care is how complementary one practice is to another. Massage goes hand in hand with acupuncture and chiropractic. Energy work could fit in with any other holistic practice, as could other disciplines, such as midwifery, homeopathy, or naturopathy. We're all in the position to work together and to help each other grow and prosper. If you help someone in a complementary field get started in business, or take in another massage therapist, ultimately it helps you expand the services to your clients and thereby increase your bottom line.

Accepting Health Insurance in Your Business

Accepting health insurance is a sure way to grow your business. Most massage therapists don't even consider accepting insurance because they have the mistaken idea that no health insurance companies will pay for massage. That is simply not true, but you have to do some research to find out which companies will pay and which ones won't.

Accepting health insurance can be a buffer against an economic downturn. When people can get massage for no payment at all, or the price of a copayment, instead of having to pay full price, they will be less likely to cut back on massage as a way of reducing their expenses.

Dealing with the paperwork associated with filing insurance claims is something you have to learn, and it isn't taught in most massage schools. Familiarity with the jargon of the insurance industry, attention to detail, a commitment to timeliness in filing claims, the correct use of medical terminology and coding, and keeping professional SOAP notes are all essential (See Chapter 6 for a full discussion of SOAP notes.) There are several types of insurance that could help you expand your business.

Remember to abide by HIPAA (the Health Insurance Portability and Accountability Act) and the rules that govern the safeguarding of client information, discussed along with confidentiality, in Chapter 3. In fact, you need to remember to follow those guidelines, regardless of whether you're accepting insurance.

EXPLORATIONS

Attend a continuing education class on insurance billing. If you aren't sure whether you want to accept health insurance for your clients, attending the class will give you a realistic picture of what the insurance companies require and the paperwork involved. This exploration will help you make up your mind about whether to take your business in that direction or not. Education is never wasted.

Medical insurance plans vary greatly from state to state, and from policy to policy. Calling the customer service number on the back of each client's insurance card is the only way to find out if his particular plan will cover massage therapy. Even people who work for the same company may have different plans, and one plan may pay and one may not. Some companies require a doctor's referral for massage, and some stipulate that the massage must be performed in a physician's office or a chiropractic office. Therapists working in states where massage is unregulated will probably not be eligible to accept insurance at all, although it doesn't hurt to call the insurance company to ask. Otherwise, you don't have to be working in a big clinic; even a lone practitioner can successfully bill insurance, if you follow all the steps correctly.

Your number one consideration should be the following: Don't make this move until you are sure you have enough cash built up to wait for payments from the insurance company. There might be times when the insurance companies owe you a lot of money for massage that you have personally performed, if you're a solo practitioner, or that you may have already paid staff members to do. As the owner of the business, you have to pay your employees, even if it means you're not getting paid yourself.

Sometimes it takes months for insurance reimbursements to arrive, so keep that in mind when deciding how much insurance you can feasibly accept and still have enough regular cash flow to keep your business afloat.

ROADSIDE ASSISTANCE

I announced that I would accept health insurance the day I opened my business. At first, there were only a few clients with insurance, but word-of-mouth caused that to change quite suddenly. I got more than 150 regular insurance clients within a couple of months; the growth was so fast that it was actually scary. Accepting insurance made my massage clinic accessible to those who couldn't afford to pay for services out of pocket, and that's a lot of clients.

One local company I know with more than 300 employees started allowing their employees $1000 per year for massage and acupuncture. When the owner saw the effect that amount had on the overall health and wellness of his employees, resulting in less time off work and a substantial reduction in claims against major medical insurance, within 2 years he decided to raise the amount to $5000 a year. This has been a great boon to my business. You have to be prepared to deal with the extra paperwork, but accepting health insurance can mean a huge increase in your income.

ROADSIDE ASSISTANCE

There are several dozen massage therapists in my county, but with the exception of one business specializing in physical therapy and injury rehabilitation that is affiliated with our local hospital, none of them accepts insurance. As a result, all that business comes to my door. I saw a need, and filled it—or you could say I saw an opportunity and grabbed it. You can do the same!

Major Medical Insurance

Major medical insurance is the type with which most people are familiar; it's the insurance most frequently offered by employers and the type that many self-employed people buy on their own. Major medical insurance is often subject to a **deductible**, a set amount of money policy holders must spend themselves before the insurance company will pay. Policy holders may also have a **copayment**, a specified amount they must pay at the time of each visit to a medical office or other health care setting. The copayment may be a set fee, or it may be a percentage of the total charge. In some instances, there may be a copayment and an additional percentage the client has to pay. For example, a client may hold an 80/20 policy, meaning that the insurance company will pay 80% of the charges, and the client is responsible for the remaining 20%.

Major medical insurers typically want health care practitioners to belong to their **provider network**, and there is usually a different **fee schedule** for providers who are in the network and those who are not. When you join a network, you agree to abide by the fee schedule set by the network, which usually means discounting your services, and you are prohibited by law from billing the client for the difference. For example, if you charge $75 for massage but the network agrees to pay only $60, you are not allowed to bill the client for the remaining $15.

You should contact the insurance company you are dealing with prior to accepting a client to find out if the above scenario is the case. The insurer usually sets a limit on the amount you may charge for massage, and sometimes includes fees for adjunct therapies, such as using hot or cold packs. It is your responsibility to get the details from any insurance company with which you want to do business.

Insurance companies require health care practitioners to have a National Provider Identifier (NPI), a number issued by the National Plan and Provider Enumeration System (NPPES). You can apply for your NPI on the NPPES website. Insurance companies also require that you have an Employer Identification Number (EIN), available online from the IRS. You do not have to be an employer or have others working in your office in order to obtain an EIN; it simply serves as an identification number for your business, just like a Social Security number serves as your personal identification number.

Insurance claims are filed on a **Health Insurance Claim Form (HICF)**. An example of a properly filled-in form appears in Figure 5-1. Paper forms are available from any medical supply store and the larger general office supply stores. Many insurance companies and networks have websites where providers may file electronic forms, to reduce paperwork and expedite payment. Medical office software is also available; it's expensive, but if you find your business starts overflowing with insurance clients, it may be worth the investment.

Going with the Flow

There is a slowly but surely growing trend for companies to offer massage in the workplace as an employee benefit. According to statistics from the Society for Human Resource Management quoted on the ABMP education website, in 2000, 8% of their 200,000+ member companies offered massage as an employee benefit. By 2007, that number had increased to 13%. Interestingly, ABMP reports that 77% of the top 100 U.S. companies offer workplace massage as an employee benefit.

Worker's Compensation

Worker's compensation is insurance provided by employers in the event an employee is injured on the job. In the United States, all 50 states currently allow massage therapy to be covered under worker's compensation, but it must be prescribed by a physician, and preauthorization must be obtained. Worker's compensation is administrated by each state, and the industrial commission in each state sets the schedule of fees for reimbursement. There is a separate program for employees of the federal government. As with major medical insurance plans and networks, when you accept worker's compensation, you agree to work for the fee they have set, and you are prohibited by law from billing the client for the remainder. Worker's compensation claim forms must be filled out by the client and the practitioner. These forms are available as free downloads on the individual state websites.

Personal Injury Clients

Personal injury cases are risky business. When you take on a personal injury case, you are agreeing to treat a client who has been injured through the fault or negligence of another person or entity; the client is involved in a lawsuit, and you are agreeing to wait for payment until the civil lawsuit has been settled. There are

1500

HEALTH INSURANCE CLAIM FORM

APPROVED BY NATIONAL UNIFORM CLAIM COMMITTEE 08/05

PICA — PICA — CARRIER

1. MEDICARE (Medicare #) / MEDICAID (Medicaid #) / TRICARE CHAMPUS (Sponsor's SSN) / CHAMPVA (Member ID#) / GROUP HEALTH PLAN (SSN or ID) [X] / FECA BLK LUNG (SSN) / OTHER (ID)

1a. INSURED'S I.D. NUMBER (For Program in Item 1): 268591402

2. PATIENT'S NAME (Last Name, First Name, Middle Initial): Client, Joe M.

3. PATIENT'S BIRTH DATE MM DD YY: 01 15 55 — SEX M [X] F

4. INSURED'S NAME (Last Name, First Name, Middle Initial): Client, Mary J.

5. PATIENT'S ADDRESS (No., Street): 120 Fox Trot Dr.

6. PATIENT RELATIONSHIP TO INSURED: Self / Spouse [X] / Child / Other

7. INSURED'S ADDRESS (No., Street): 120 Fox Trot Dr.

CITY: Anytown — STATE: NC

8. PATIENT STATUS: Single / Married [X] / Other

CITY: Anytown — STATE: NC

ZIP CODE: 24111 — TELEPHONE (Include Area Code): (291) 615-4021

Employed [X] / Full-Time Student / Part-Time Student

ZIP CODE: 24111 — TELEPHONE (Include Area Code): (291) 615-4021

9. OTHER INSURED'S NAME (Last Name, First Name, Middle Initial)

10. IS PATIENT'S CONDITION RELATED TO:

11. INSURED'S POLICY GROUP OR FECA NUMBER: SL200

a. OTHER INSURED'S POLICY OR GROUP NUMBER

a. EMPLOYMENT? (Current or Previous) YES / NO [X]

a. INSURED'S DATE OF BIRTH MM DD YY: 04 06 60 — SEX M / F [X]

b. OTHER INSURED'S DATE OF BIRTH MM DD YY — SEX M / F

b. AUTO ACCIDENT? YES / NO [X] — PLACE (State)

b. EMPLOYER'S NAME OR SCHOOL NAME: ACME Paint Supply

c. EMPLOYER'S NAME OR SCHOOL NAME

c. OTHER ACCIDENT? YES / NO [X]

c. INSURANCE PLAN NAME OR PROGRAM NAME: Blue Options

d. INSURANCE PLAN NAME OR PROGRAM NAME

10d. RESERVED FOR LOCAL USE

d. IS THERE ANOTHER HEALTH BENEFIT PLAN? YES / NO [X] *If yes,* return to and complete item 9 a-d.

READ BACK OF FORM BEFORE COMPLETING & SIGNING THIS FORM.

12. PATIENT'S OR AUTHORIZED PERSON'S SIGNATURE I authorize the release of any medical or other information necessary to process this claim. I also request payment of government benefits either to myself or to the party who accepts assignment below.

SIGNED: Joe M. Client — DATE: 09/05/2009

13. INSURED'S OR AUTHORIZED PERSON'S SIGNATURE I authorize payment of medical benefits to the undersigned physician or supplier for services described below.

SIGNED: Joe M. Client

14. DATE OF CURRENT: ILLNESS (First symptom) OR INJURY (Accident) OR PREGNANCY(LMP) MM DD YY: 09 01 2009

15. IF PATIENT HAS HAD SAME OR SIMILAR ILLNESS. GIVE FIRST DATE MM DD YY

16. DATES PATIENT UNABLE TO WORK IN CURRENT OCCUPATION MM DD YY FROM — TO

17. NAME OF REFERRING PROVIDER OR OTHER SOURCE: Dr. David Harris

17a. — 17b. NPI: 1852383940

18. HOSPITALIZATION DATES RELATED TO CURRENT SERVICES MM DD YY FROM — TO

19. RESERVED FOR LOCAL USE

20. OUTSIDE LAB? YES / NO [X] — $ CHARGES

21. DIAGNOSIS OR NATURE OF ILLNESS OR INJURY (Relate Items 1, 2, 3 or 4 to Item 24E by Line)

1. 729.1
2.
3.
4.

22. MEDICAID RESUBMISSION CODE — ORIGINAL REF. NO.

23. PRIOR AUTHORIZATION NUMBER: 140105

	24. A. DATE(S) OF SERVICE From MM DD YY	To MM DD YY	B. PLACE OF SERVICE	C. EMG	D. PROCEDURES, SERVICES, OR SUPPLIES (Explain Unusual Circumstances) CPT/HCPCS	MODIFIER	E. DIAGNOSIS POINTER	F. $ CHARGES	G. DAYS OR UNITS	H. EPSDT Family Plan	I. ID QUAL	J. RENDERING PROVIDER ID. #
1	09 05 09	09 05 09	11		97124		1	75 00	3		NPI	1852383850
2											NPI	
3											NPI	
4											NPI	
5											NPI	
6											NPI	

25. FEDERAL TAX I.D. NUMBER: 56-0000000 — SSN / EIN [X]

26. PATIENT'S ACCOUNT NO.: 4130

27. ACCEPT ASSIGNMENT? (For govt. claims, see back) YES [X] / NO

28. TOTAL CHARGE: $ 75 00

29. AMOUNT PAID: $ 20 00

30. BALANCE DUE: $ 55 00

31. SIGNATURE OF PHYSICIAN OR SUPPLIER INCLUDING DEGREES OR CREDENTIALS (I certify that the statements on the reverse apply to this bill and are made a part thereof.)

SIGNED: KD Smith LMT — DATE: 09/05/09

32. SERVICE FACILITY LOCATION INFORMATION: KD Medical Massage, 30 Main St., Anytown NC 24111

a. — b.

33. BILLING PROVIDER INFO & PH #: (910) 426-4777 — KD Medical Massage, 30 Main St., Anytown NC 24111

a. — b.

PATIENT AND INSURED INFORMATION — PHYSICIAN OR SUPPLIER INFORMATION

NUCC Instruction Manual available at: www.nucc.org

APPROVED OMB-0938-0999 FORM CMS-1500 (08/05)

FIGURE 5-1 A properly filled-in HICF.

several things to consider when accepting a client involved in a personal injury case:

- The lawsuit may not go in favor of the client, and he will not get any money.
- If the lawsuit does go in favor of the client, there is no guarantee that he will get enough money to pay all his bills.
- Massage therapists tend to be at the bottom of the payment list when other health care providers, such as hospitals and physicians, are ahead of them.
- It is common for personal injury lawsuits to drag on for several years.

Personal injury cases can be lucrative if you have the time and resources to wait for remuneration. If the client does not win the case, he can be held personally responsible for the payment, as long as you have had him sign a **practitioner's lien**, like the example in Figure 5-2. However, in the case of someone who has run up thousands of dollars of medical bills in the hope that he'll collect enough money from the lawsuit to pay it all off, and then doesn't win, you may be subject to the old adage about squeezing blood out of a turnip. It's a risk you take when you choose to take on a personal injury case.

THERA-SSAGE
431 S. Main St., Ste. 2
Rutherfordton NC 28139
828-288-3727

PRACTITIONER'S LIEN

Name: _John O'Sullivan_   File # _2112_

Address: _1999 Shadyside Circle_ City: _Rutherfordton_ State: _NC_ Zip: _28139_

Home phone: _828-704-1881_ Cell: _828-988-4321_ Work: _828-098-7653_

I, _John O'Sullivan_ , hereby acknowledge that I am receiving massage therapy services from THERA-SSAGE, and that THERA-SSAGE is filing insurance on my behalf with _Farmer's Insurance_ .

I hereby acknowledge that all monies due and payable to THERA-SSAGE are my sole responsibility, and in the event that my insurance company declines payment of all or any part of the fee, I agree to pay THERA-SSAGE in full upon demand of payment.

Signature: _John O'Sullivan_ Date: _09/05/2009_
Witness: _Laura Allen_ Date: _09/05/2009_

FIGURE 5-2 A properly filled-in practitioner's lien.

Health Savings Accounts and Flexible Spending Accounts

Unlike a traditional insurance plan, a Health Savings Account (HSA) is a tax-free savings plan that can be used to pay for current and future medical expenses. It is owned by the individual and is used in conjunction with major medical plans that have a high deductible, or it can be used by those not covered by another plan. In 2008, the federal government considered a high deductible to be $1100 for an individual or $2200 for a family.

HSAs and a similar plan, the medical expense Flexible Spending Account (FSA), sometimes referred to as a flex plan, allows employees to have funds deducted from their paycheck and deposited into the account, without having to pay payroll taxes on the money. These plans are gaining in popularity because they can be used for wellness-based expenditures, such as massage therapy, or vitamins, over-the-counter drugs, and preventive health screenings. When a client has an HSA or an FSA, he is usually given a debit card that can be processed like a credit card. If you do not accept credit cards, you may provide the client with a copy of your bill so that he can get his own reimbursement. Some employers match contributions. In 2009, the maximum contribution allowed was $3000 for an individual and $5950 for a family. Although there are many rules governing HSAs and FSAs, there aren't any details for you to worry about as far as accepting them in your business, other than processing the debit card or giving your client a receipt for reimbursement purposes.

Medicare/Medicaid

At this time, neither Medicare nor Medicaid will pay for massage therapy unless it is performed in the office of a medical doctor or chiropractor. The number of physicians who have a massage therapist on staff is relatively small, and even chiropractors with a practitioner on staff generally will not include massage on a Medicare/Medicaid claim because of the very small amount the chiropractor is allowed to bill. In 2009, Medicare allowed a chiropractor to bill $28 for an adjustment. Since they are not allowed to bill for consultation time, most chiropractors don't consider it worth their while to provide adjunct therapies for a Medicare client.

Another issue with people who qualify for Medicare and/or Medicaid is that even if they have secondary insurance that would normally pay for massage therapy, the secondary insurance company will not pay until Medicare or Medicaid does. Since neither program will pay for massage therapy except for the isolated circumstances mentioned above, the secondary insurer won't pay, either. Maybe someday the amount of money that could be saved on medications and surgery because of the benefits of massage will change these policies.

Processing Claims

There are many steps involved in collecting the information required for processing and filing an insurance claim.

1. Copy the client's insurance card and one other form of identification, and call the insurer to find out whether or not the client is covered for massage, if he needs a physician's referral or preauthorization, or has any restrictions on his benefits, such as a certain number of visits allowed per year. Ask whether the client is subject to a deductible and copayment, and record the amounts. Of all the steps, this is the most important.
2. When an insurance client comes in for the first time, have him fill out the **intake form**. An example of a properly filled-in intake form appears in Figure 5-3.

Name _Cathy Lynn Festus_ DOB _09/05/1959_ FILE # _5631_
Mailing Address _725 Old Fairgrounds Road_ City _Parkertown_ ST _TX_ ZIP _54312_
Home phone _877-925-5346_ Cell _877-995-9955_ Work _877-519-4876_
E-mail if you want to be on our newsletter list and to be notified of
events and specials _clfestus@parker.net_
Emergency Contact Person _Samuel James Festus_ Phone _877-995-9954_

EVERYONE FILL OUT INFORMATION BELOW:

General & Medical Information

Have you ever had a professional massage?	Yes ☐	No ☑
Do you experience frequent headaches?	Yes ☐	No ☑
Are you pregnant?	Yes ☐	No ☑
Are you diabetic?	Yes ☐	No ☑
If yes to the previous question, is it under control?	Yes ☐	No ☑
Do you have a seizure disorder or epilepsy?	Yes ☐	No ☑
Do you suffer frequently from stress?	Yes ☐	No ☑
Have you had any broken bones in past 2 years?	Yes ☐	No ☑
Do you have tension or soreness in a specific area? _Lower back_	Yes ☐	No ☑
Do you have cardiac or circulatory problems?	Yes ☐	No ☑
Do you suffer from back pain?	Yes ☑	No ☐
Do you have numbness or stabbing pain anywhere?	Yes ☐	No ☑
Are you sensitive to touch or pressure anywhere?	Yes ☐	No ☑
Have you ever had surgery? If so, explain.	Yes ☐	No ☑

Hysterectomy 2002

Is the pain you are in due to an injury? If so, explain.   Yes ☐   No ☑

Please list any medications you are taking:

We require a twenty-four hour notice in the event of a cancellation or
you will be billed for the appointment at the practitioner's discretion.
You are free to send a friend or family member in your place. Please
initial here to indicate that you have read and accept this policy. _CLF_

Please note that if you are not asking us to file insurance, you do not
have to give us the information below. If we are filing insurance for you,
we are obligated to have your information on file. Please note that we
comply with all HIPAA laws and that your privacy and personal information are always protected by our staff members.

Your SS# _000-00-0000_ Your employer _Captain Jack's Seafood Packers_
If your spouse is the cardholder, their SS# _000-00-0000_
Spouses's DOB _12/19/1953_ Spouse's employer _Energy Concepts Inc_
Spouse's work phone _219-876-5555_

Signature _Cathy Lynn Festus_   Date _01/15/2010_

FIGURE 5-3   A properly filled-in intake form.

3. If your statement of **informed consent** is not included on the intake form, have him sign the separate statement. Figure 5-4 is an example of a properly signed informed consent statement.

4. Have him sign the HICF, and fill out the pertinent information that goes on the form (policy number, group number, whether he is the actual insured or a dependent, etc.). If you are filing a claim electronically, you still need a written copy of the client's signature. Remember that for worker's compensation cases, the claim forms vary from state to state and should be obtained from the website for your particular state.

5. Have him sign an **assignment of benefits form**, which goes to the insurance company to let them know they should be paying you directly instead of reimbursing the policy holder. An example of the assignment of benefits form appears in Figure 5-5.

Statement of Informed Consent

I, _Tamara Oppenheimer_ , hereby acknowledge that I have requested to receive massage therapy and bodywork from _Grady Johnson_ , Licensed Massage Therapist of Johnson Therapeutic Massage, Inc. I acknowledge that I have been informed of the privacy and confidentiality policies of Johnson Therapeutic Massage.

I hereby attest that I have informed my therapist of all medications that I am taking, and listed them on the intake form. I hereby attest that I have informed my therapist of any medical conditions that I have been diagnosed with, and affirm that I am not suffering from any contagious illness or skin condition, and that I do not have any of the conditions listed below:

- Blood clots
- Cancer
- Edema
- Epilepsy or other seizure disorder
- Fever
- Hemorrhage or hemophilia
- Phlebitis or deep vein thrombosis
- Uncontrolled high blood pressure or other circulatory problems
- Under the influence of drugs or alcohol

I acknowledge that my therapist has thoroughly discussed my treatment with me, and I understand that I may verbally modify or withdraw my consent to treatment at any time during the session.

Client Signature _Tamara Oppenheimer_ Date _12/20/2009_
Therapist Signature _Grady Johnson, LMT_ Date _12/20/2009_

FIGURE 5-4   A properly signed informed consent statement.

Assignment of Benefits

I,_____Scott Ferris_____, hereby authorize the direct payment to _____Main Street Medical Massage_____, of any sum I now or hereafter owe you by my attorney, out of the proceeds of any settlement of my case, and/or by any insurance company obligated to make payment to me or you based in whole or in part on the charges made for services I have received. I understand that every attempt will be made to collect said funds from the insurance company contractually obligated, but that any amounts that are not collected after reasonable attempt to collect, be it part or all of what is due, is my personal obligation. I further acknowledge that there is no statute of limitations on my debt to you, and understand that this agreement and assignment is irrevocable until such time as all monies that are owed are paid in full.

Signature____Scott Ferris_____Date _06/20/2010_____

Therapist Signature___Janet Cordell, LMT___Date _06/20/2010_____

FIGURE 5-5 A properly filled-in assignment of benefits form.

6. Have him sign a practitioner's lien, which basically states that if for any reason the insurance company refuses the claim, the client is responsible for paying you himself (see Fig. 5-2).
7. Have him sign an **authorization to release personal information**. An example form appears in Figure 5-6.

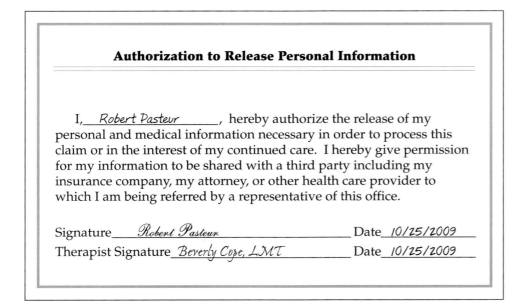

Authorization to Release Personal Information

I,___Robert Pasteur_____, hereby authorize the release of my personal and medical information necessary in order to process this claim or in the interest of my continued care. I hereby give permission for my information to be shared with a third party including my insurance company, my attorney, or other health care provider to which I am being referred by a representative of this office.

Signature____Robert Pasteur_____Date_10/25/2009____

Therapist Signature_Beverly Cope, LMT_____Date_10/25/2009____

FIGURE 5-6 A properly filled-in authorization to release personal information.

BOX 5-1   SOAP Notes: Acceptable and Unacceptable

Professional SOAP Notes

S: 20-year-old female client, initial visit. Client states feeling generally tense and having neck and shoulder pain at the level of 8 on a scale of 1 to 10; is a factory production worker, and is aware of postural problems and pain caused by bending over machinery and possible repetitive motion injury (RMI).

O: Taut bands in trapezius and rhomboids, bilateral. Active trigger points in SCM and scalenes very tender on left side. Shoulders appear rotated anteriorly. Client seems to be tense overall and stated during the session that she tends to hold her stress and tension in her neck and shoulders.

A: 30 minutes of neuromuscular therapy focused on neck and shoulders effected good releases. Client states pain level was 1 to 2 at end of session.

P: Suggested that client do neck stretches three times a day, that she stand up every hour at work, and do general stretches and 1 or 2 minutes of movement exercise. Also suggested warm Epsom baths for soreness, ice if needed for pain, increasing her water intake in order to hydrate muscles, and return for continued treatment within 1 week.

Unprofessional SOAP Notes

S: Pain in the neck.
O: A few muscles were tight.
A: Did some work on her.
P: Come back soon.

8. Keep one copy of all these forms in the client's file; send the other copy to the insurance company.
9. Keeping good progress notes is imperative. Some insurance companies require them to be sent in with every claim; others may not require it but expect you to have them on hand in case they audit a client's file or you as the health care practitioner. Box 5-1 shows examples of SOAP notes that are professionally written and SOAP notes that are not acceptable. (See Chapter 6 for a full discussion of SOAP notes.)
10. File claims in a timely manner. Many companies expect you to file within 60 to 90 days of the date of service, and of course, the quicker you file, the quicker you'll get paid.
11. Inform the client that you observe the HIPAA laws governing his right to privacy. It may be a statement on your intake form, or you can purchase HIPAA brochures from any medical supply company.

The first time you file a claim with an insurance company, you must provide a copy of your license to practice massage, a Form W-9 from the IRS, and proof of liability insurance. Some insurance companies will request photographs of your business, including the entrance, the bathrooms, and the treatment rooms so that they can verify your compliance with the Americans with Disabilities Act in having handicapped accessibility.

Controlling Growth

For the purpose of growing your business, accepting health insurance is definitely a double-edged sword. You may get more business and simultaneously more paperwork than you can handle. Therefore, you might decide to expand and hire some staff members, or to limit the amount of insurance clients you are willing to take, such as 30% of your total clientele. Keeping a higher percentage of cash-paying customers will keep your cash flowing in the right direction.

Think of your business like a garden, and plant some new seeds. If you get the ground ready, plant it, nurture it, pull the weeds, and get rid of the pests; it will not only grow but also thrive. If you don't nurture it, a few things will still pop up, but the harvest won't be nearly as abundant, and the weeds and bugs will take over. Instead, with a little extra care, you'll be like the anonymous neighbor who goes around piling excess zucchini on people's porches—you'll have more than enough.

POSTCARDS from the HIGHWAY   Linda Roisum

I had a successful career in training, development, and management for a financial data firm before coming to massage therapy as a second career. In 2006, I sold my private practice in order to focus on education and consulting. My strategies for success are simple.

You need to create a vision. If your vision isn't clear to you, it can't really be clear to anyone else. In order to be successful you have to know where you are going because if you don't, how will you know when you get there?

There are three elements to creating a clear vision. First, define a significant purpose. Purpose is what we are here for, why we exist. It means understanding what business we are really in so that we all can focus our efforts in support of that purpose. It answers the question "Why?" rather than just explaining what you do. It clarifies—from your customer's viewpoint—what business you are really in.

Second, define clear values. Values are more than just beliefs—they are deeply held beliefs. People care passionately about their values, and we all feel good when we act on our values. With that in mind, values are deeply held beliefs that certain qualities are desirable. They define what is right or fundamentally important to each of us. They provide guidelines for our choices and actions. Purpose is important because it explains "why." Values are important because they explain "how." They answer the question "How will you behave on a day-to-day basis as you fulfill your purpose?"

Third, have a picture of the future. Purpose and values alone don't explain where you're going. Vision is about going somewhere. There needs to be a sense of destination or direction. A picture of the future is a key element of vision. Spend time during the planning stages of your business envisioning what you want it to look like 5 years from now. Really get emotional about it—see it, feel it. If you've already started your business, it's not too late to create a vision. Start today! Remember your thoughts today are your experience tomorrow.

I would also advise you to learn, learn, learn. If you truly want to succeed, you must work on yourself, study business, and continually improve your skills.

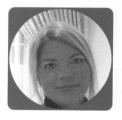

Linda Roisum is President/CEO of MassageWorks, Inc. in Falls Church, Virginia. A graduate of Marymount University with a degree in International Business, Linda retired from practicing massage and focuses full-time on being an educator, personal coach, and consultant to the massage profession. She is the author of *Creating a Prosperous Practice Spending Little or No Money Marketing*, self-published in 2004. Visit her website at www. massagetherapisttraininginstitute.com.

SUGGESTED READINGS

Association of Bodywork & Massage Professionals. *Massage Therapy Fast Facts.* http://www.massagetherapy.com/_content/images/Media/Factsheet1.pdf. Accessed 10/04/2009.

Internal Revenue Service. Department of the Treasury. *EIN Assistant.* https://sa1.www4.irs.gov/modiein/individual/index.jsp. Accessed 10/04/2009.

Jolley W. How to survive and thrive through a business setback. http://www.allbusiness.com/sales/957811–1.html. Accessed 10/04/2009.

Luther D, Callahan M. The Medical Massage Office Manual for Insurance Billing. 4th ed. Callahan/Luther Partnership, Catlett, VA, 2005.

Madison-Mahoney V. Massage Insurance Billing. http://massageinsurancebilling.com/ Accessed 10/04/2009.

National Plan & Provider Enumeration System. https://nppes.cms.hhs.gov/NPPES/Welcome.do. Accessed 10/04/2009.

Thompson DL. *Hands Heal: Communication, Documentation, and Insurance Billing for Manual Therapists.* 3rd ed. Philadelphia, PA: Lippincott Williams & Wilkins, 2005.

United States Department of the Treasury. *All About HSAs.* http://www.ustreas.gov/offices/public-affairs/hsa/pdf/all-about-HSAs_072208.pdf. Accessed 10/04/2009.

Woolsey B, Schultz M. *Credit Card Industry Facts, Debt Statistics 2006–2008.* http://www.creditcards.com/credit-card-news/credit-card-industry-facts-personal-debt-statistics-1276.php. Accessed 10/04/2009.

Worker's Compensation—The Worker's Comp Service Center. http://www.workerscompensation.com/ Accessed 10/04/2009.

My Personal Journey

In this chapter, we've discussed the obstacles a business owner might face and explored suggestions for surviving and thriving when you're facing a hurdle. Write a worst-case scenario of a crisis, financial or otherwise, occurring in your business, and then formulate a contingency plan for how you would deal with such an event.

My goals _____

_____

_____

What's in my way? _____

_____

_____

What action can I take to remedy the situation? _____

_____

_____

One-year progress update _____

_____

_____

PART III

Staying on Course

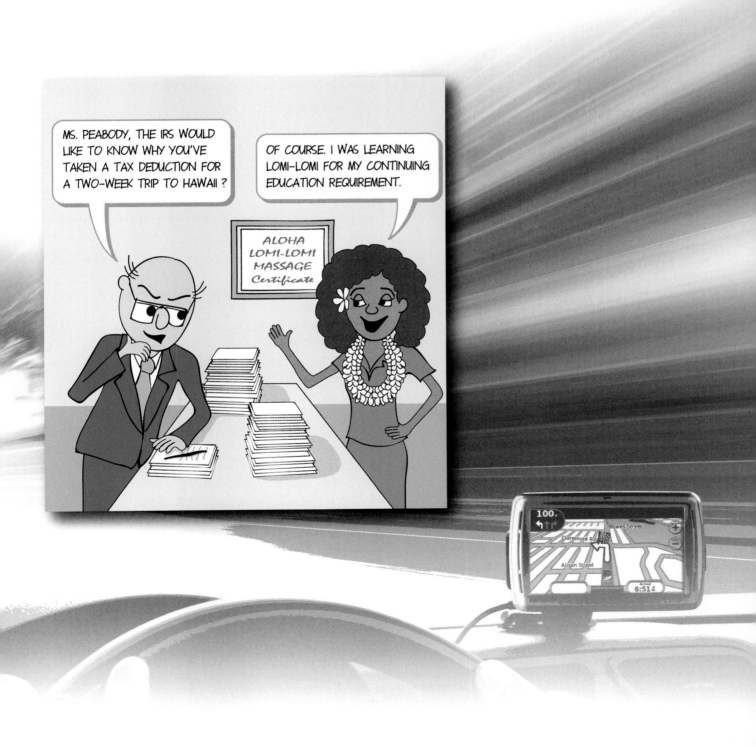

CHAPTER 6

Record Keeping

*W*hat we hope ever to do with ease we must first learn
to do with diligence.

SAMUEL JOHNSON

KEY CONCEPTS

- Keeping records is one of the obligations of owning a business.
- Office technology is useful for facilitating all kinds of record keeping and business communications, and inexpensive training is available.
- The technology products you purchase, including telephones, fax machines, and computers, are tangible assets for your business.
- Software programs are available for every office function, including financial record keeping, maintaining mailing lists, and client records and communications.
- A therapist who does outcalls has different technology needs than an office-bound therapist but is still obligated to keep records.
- There are many office systems and aids available from office suppliers to help keep records well organized.
- Electronic records should be backed up and stored in a secure location for privacy and protection.
- The office paper trail includes business records, financial records, client records, employment records, and other documents, such as warranties, corporate papers, and stock certificates.
- Keeping good business records is necessary for helping business owners stay informed about their financial status and comply with tax laws.
- Vital records, such as property deeds and insurance policies, should be stored off-site in a safety deposit box.

One of the most important obligations of a business owner is maintaining accurate, current, and complete records. Keeping good business records enables you to track your progress and to satisfy the requirements of government agencies. In addition to financial, employment, and other business records, a professional massage therapist is expected to keep records of each therapeutic relationship, and in states that regulate massage therapy, client documentation is required by law. Next to technical ability as a massage therapist, your ability to communicate effectively is the most important quality to cultivate in order to make your business a success. Technology can simplify your everyday record keeping and communication responsibilities.

MANAGING TECHNOLOGY

The word "technology" can strike fear in the hearts of some people, and there are those who don't know how to operate a computer or use the Internet, or who don't own a cell phone or any other electronic devices. If this sounds like you, the technology in your office might be a telephone (the kind that plugs into the wall), an appointment book, a checkbook, and a pen. If you're a lone practitioner, with no aspirations beyond seeing a few clients a week and no plans for future expansion, that might work fine for you, but if you want to earnestly grow a business, you'll need to jump on the technology bandwagon.

Some people avoid technology because they view themselves as technically challenged—not confident about their ability to use a computer, change the ink cartridge in a fax machine, or fix a jam in a copy machine. If that describes you, help is available. All community colleges offer inexpensive continuing education classes in computer technology and using office machines. Most computer and other office machine manufacturers provide free tutorials on CD or on the Internet for using their products, and people purchasing new products can sometimes get on-the-spot training at no extra charge at the time of purchase. The Small Business Administration also offers classes on using computer technology to help your business.

If you're the parent of a high school or college student, it's a sure bet that either your child or one of his or her friends is a bona fide computer nerd, and students are always in need of money. Ask one to tutor you. Don't be afraid of learning something new!

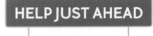

Words of Wisdom
Learning new skills empowers me to succeed.

The Well-Equipped Office

Brand-name comparisons and specific recommendations for equipment are purposely omitted from this book due to the fact that technology grows and changes so quickly. Newer products are always becoming available, so we'll just cover the basics of office equipment.

Bear in mind that different types of businesses will have different needs; a practitioner who wants to run a busy spa will have different technology requirements than a lone practitioner who makes a living doing outcalls. There are several things to consider when deciding what type of technology to purchase for your business. Ask yourself if it will save you time and/or money, make it easier for you to perform a task, or enhance your ability to communicate.

Technology products for your office do not have to cost a fortune, but remember that you get what you pay for. If you choose to buy a computer or other piece of equipment that's been previously used, the warranty will probably have expired, leaving you responsible for the full cost of repair or replacement if something goes wrong. If you do choose to buy second-hand, you're better off purchasing from a well-established computer repair person who's selling refurbished computers than from an unknown individual; you don't want to buy one that's infected with a virus or otherwise defective. Equipping your office means you are purchasing assets for your business. Get the best that you can afford, and it should last you a long time.

The Telephone

You can't operate a service-based business without a telephone. Your phone should come equipped with either an answering machine or voicemail capability; otherwise, you might miss out on appointments. Telephones are available with so many options: headsets, earphones, multiple lines, call waiting, call forwarding, call blocking, automatic redialing, voicemail, conference calling, and all sorts of other bells and whistles. The cost can vary widely depending on what kind of calling package and maintenance plan you choose, and how many options you want. If you don't hold conference calls, why pay for that capability? Choose only the options that you'll realistically use in order to hold your costs down. Your telephone company will usually give you the best rate if you purchase Internet service, cell phone, and stationary phone services together.

ROADSIDE ASSISTANCE

I answer my business phone the same way every time, and I've trained my staff to do the same: "Thank you for calling THERA-SSAGE. This is Laura. Can I help you?" It sounds friendlier than just picking up the phone and saying "THERA-SSAGE." I've also tried to make the message on our voicemail informative without being overly long: "Thanks for calling THERA-SSAGE. Please leave a message and we'll call you back as soon as possible. You can visit our website at www.thera-ssage.com for information and online gift certificates." Directing callers to our website saves me a lot of time I would otherwise be spending on the phone.

The Fax Machine

A fax machine is handy for sending and receiving communications. Many businesses, such as office supply stores and shipping stores, will send and receive faxes for you, but the fees can be as high as several dollars per page, and if you have to go some distance, that's time spent away from your business. It's better to have your own fax machine. An "all-in-one" is a machine that can phone, fax, scan, copy, print, and e-mail documents, making it a good investment for your office.

Faxing is sometimes viewed as obsolete compared to e-mail, but it might actually take more time to scan a large document, so you can e-mail it, than it does to send it by fax. A fax machine is a worthwhile piece of equipment for your office.

The Computer

A computer may not be a necessity, but it can certainly make your work easier. The computer, printer, and any accompanying devices are referred to as **hardware**.

Whether you're typing client progress notes, preparing an advertisement, or balancing your checking account—a computer can do all these things. The Internet has made it possible to do banking and bill paying online, which gives you the use of your money right up until the last minute; no more mailing checks off a week or 10 days ahead of the due date so that they'll arrive on time.

The public almost expects that anyone who is in business has a website. You can even sell gift certificates and set appointments online. We'll discuss the different ways you can use your telephone, computer, and other office technology as tools to market your business in Chapter 13.

The Credit Card Terminal

A credit card terminal enables you to accept credit and debit cards from clients. You should not have to pay for this machine; your bank or other merchant account provider should give you the use of a terminal as part of your contract. Avoid dealing with companies who want to sell or lease you a terminal.

Accepting credit cards and debit cards is a convenience to your customers. The processing fees are tax deductible as part of the cost of doing business.

Going with the Flow

Sometimes we have to unite and take matters into our own hands, so to speak, when it comes to getting rid of a tired old trend. There is a long-standing tendency among banks and other credit card processors to classify any massage business as a massage parlor, in the numerical occupational classification system the federal government obligates them to use. The North American Industry Classification System (NAICS) code for therapeutic massage is 621399, while the code for a massage parlor is 812199. Many people now have debit cards tied to a Health Savings Account (see Chapter 5). If your credit card processor has your business classified as a massage parlor, those debit cards would be turned down. Check with your bank or credit card processor to see how your business is currently listed and insist that it is coded as therapeutic massage.

Office Software

A computer is useless until it's loaded with **software** or application programs. Programs may be purchased on a CD or downloaded from the Internet.

When buying a computer for your office, bear in mind that most come preloaded with software, such as e-mail programs, word processing programs, database programs, and graphics programs, and these vary from one manufacturer to the next. You can purchase any additional software you want and feel comfortable using them; if you're spending a substantial amount of money in a computer store, they may even throw in extra software if you ask.

There's a saying in the computer world: GIGO—"garbage in, garbage out." In order for a computer to be useful to your business, you have to enter the correct information into it. For instance, a financial software program will let you check your status at the touch of a button. This type of program will keep a continual record from the first day you're in business, as long as you enter your sales and expenses daily, weekly, or whatever works best for you.

You can generate the necessary forms for filing your taxes, and compare the figures from the first year you were in business at each year's end to see how much your business has grown. You can instantly find out where you're over budget in expenses, get reports showing the breakdown of the income different services you offer are bringing in, what retail items are selling, and so forth. Again, the key to successfully using such a program is diligent input. Each transaction at your office should be recorded carefully—whether on paper or in the computer, or some combination of the two.

Using a database program to keep your client list and client contact information makes sending mailings to your clients a simple task. A database of names and addresses can easily be imported into your e-mail program, allowing you to send mass mailings of newsletters or other communications to your clients.

A desktop publishing program lets you create your own business cards, brochures, flyers, and other advertising or informational materials. Such programs are usually easy to use. (For full discussions of promotion and advertising, see Chapters 13 and 14.)

There is software created specifically for massage therapy offices. It consists of a word processing program with templates for progress notes, schedule and calendar features, and a database program for your clients. Most of the currently available products sell for $200 to $300. As mentioned in Chapter 5, more sophisticated medical office software is also available for those who intend to build their business by accepting health insurance, but it's much more expensive ($1000 minimum) and not worth the investment unless you have a medically oriented business and are filing a substantial amount of insurance claims.

All software programs contain instructions and help functions to assist you in learning how to use them. Practice makes perfect!

Equipment for the Mobile Massage Therapist

If you make your living doing outcalls, you still have to maintain records, and you may own some or all of the office technology equipment and products described above. A therapist who's constantly on the go also needs a cell phone. You may choose to carry a regular appointment book, or get a **personal digital assistant (PDA)**, which is basically a hand-held computer that can be used to send e-mails, keep track of appointments, keep client files, and many of the other tasks a full-size computer can do. More and more people are using smart phones—cell phones that have all the same features as a PDA, along with the ability to take pictures, record and send videos, download and share music, and other fun activities.

Tips for the Organizationally Challenged

Maybe you're the type of person who has a filing cabinet in your home, and your bills are paid and bank statements filed the day they arrive. Or maybe you use the shoebox method, throwing everything into one place. While that's definitely better than doing nothing at all, it is not the recommended method for running an efficient office. Setting up a proper filing system is a must. Organization is a skill that can be learned; it just requires discipline.

You'll want to have an in-box and a file labeled "Bills to Pay" for things that haven't been taken care of yet. An inexpensive expanding portfolio organizer that's labeled with the dates of the month is helpful. When a bill arrives, file it in the slot for the appropriate date of payment so that you won't forget to take care of it on time.

The simplest filing system for general office paperwork is an alphabetical system. Label file folders with the names of vendors and services—electricity, rent, water, and so forth—and file them alphabetically. Once you've paid the bill, staple the check stub to the invoice and file it. Use a cardboard file box or a plastic file holder with a secure lid; at the end of each year, take the year's records out of the filing cabinet and store them. Label the box with the year: "Financial Records 20xx." It's very simple—as long as you take the time to do it.

Suze Orman, a well-known financial advisor and author, has this piece of advice: "Clutter in your home and office is a sign of clutter in your financial life." That makes good sense. How can you know where you stand financially if you can't find your last bank statement or keep your checkbook balanced? You can't. Professional organizers exist in almost every locale. If you need to, hire one to set up your office filing system, so you'll start out on the right foot.

Words of Wisdom
Resolve to be organized!

ELECTRONIC RECORDS

Running a paperless office is something many people aspire to in the interest of saving trees and cutting down on waste. If you're really organized and computer-savvy, you may already be paying your bills online and receiving online bank statements. You can keep almost any record electronically. Any document not created on your own computer can be scanned and saved on a hard drive or CD.

It's very important to have a backup of all your documents. If everything pertaining to your business is saved on your hard drive, and your computer crashes, you'd be lost. Back everything up regularly on an external drive or disk, and store it away from your office. Many Internet companies offer secure web-based storage. Off-site data storage is becoming a popular business; there may be one in your town.

Words of Wisdom

Whether it's your financial records, address book, or other business documentation, you wouldn't want to lose it due to a crash or an office fire. Back it up.

Just like paper files, electronic records are also easier to maintain when they're well organized. You can create folders in "My Documents" and "My Databases" and label them accordingly, such as "Employees," "Gift Certificates," and "Advertisements." When you create a new document, save it in the correct folder. If you organize things at the outset of setting up your office, it will save time later.

The Paper Trail

Maintaining a careful paper trail will make your life easier in the long run, and particularly if you are ever audited by the Internal Revenue Service (IRS). Even if you have the majority of your records stored electronically, you still need to keep paper receipts for purchases you have made, and they should be filed by category. Paper records, both printed and handwritten, are often referred to as **hard copy**.

Health care businesses are one of the most frequently audited types of business. According to the IRS, the reason is the filing of fraudulent tax returns—not by those in the holistic sector, but mainly by unscrupulous physicians and hospitals who abuse the Medicare and Medicaid systems.

Small businesses, incredibly, come under more scrutiny by the IRS than billion-dollar corporations. The IRS assumes that small business people, especially those in service-based businesses, are apt to be the recipients of cash payments that might go unrecorded, or they might be getting unreported tips. Because of the profession we're in and the fact that we're entrepreneurs, it's essential to keep a careful paper trail. Then, if the IRS ever calls on you, you'll be ready.

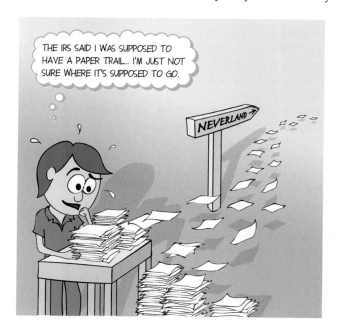

BUSINESS RECORDS

Business records are all pieces of documentation related to operating your massage business, paper and electronic: financial records, client records, employment records, and any other records that contain pertinent information. There are many things a business owner must document in order to comply with tax laws.

Specific laws govern how long you should maintain records. According to the IRS, the length of time you should keep a document depends upon the action, expense, or event the document records. Generally, you must keep your records that support an item of income or deductions on a tax return until the period of limitations for that return runs out. This is the time period in which you can amend your tax return to claim a credit or refund, or that the IRS can assess additional tax. As of November 2008, the rule was 3 years for personal tax records; 4 years for employment tax records, and 7 years if you have taken a deduction for a bad debt. Documentation relating to property should be held onto until the period of limitations expires for the period in which you disposed of the property. If you have ever been convicted of filing a fraudulent tax return, or have ever failed to file a return, you are obligated to keep your records indefinitely.

Financial Records

If you're a lone practitioner, you may think your checkbook register is the only financial record you need to keep. While no one wants to be bogged down in paperwork, as a business owner, you must be familiar with—and must maintain—certain financial documents.

We discussed the preliminary budget in Chapter 2 as part of your business plan. Keeping an ongoing budget, and adjusting it as needed based on cash flow, is smart business. Maintaining a profit and loss sheet will keep you current on exactly where you stand. You need to be aware of the amount of equity you've invested in your business; it's important to your tax return, and if you ever decide to sell, it's important when setting the asking price.

Since this is the age of online banking, get in the habit of frequently comparing your bank account as it appears on your financial software, or in your written journal, to what's appearing in the online statement. During the Christmas season, and on Valentine's Day and Mother's Day, when the sales of gift certificates are high and your office is very busy, it's easy to let things pile up. You may find there are transactions that haven't been entered. Performing frequent audits of your bank account is a great idea.

If you accept credit cards, remember to check your settlement tape against what you have recorded every day, or however often your batches are settled. The credit card processor can make a mistake just like you can, and you don't want to be cheated out of any money.

If you choose not to join the computer age, you'll need to keep a financial journal, a handwritten daily record of incoming and outgoing cash. Business journals, available in office supply stores, are acceptable to the IRS and the Department of Revenue in any state. Purchase one that is self-explanatory, with preprinted categories to help you keep track of expenses that are tax deductible and those that are not.

REALITY CHECKPOINT

If you're incapable of keeping careful financial records or so busy that you don't have the time, hire someone to do that for you. A bookkeeper's services are usually less expensive than a Certified Public Accountant or Certified Financial Planner because the duties of a bookkeeper are limited to record keeping and do not include giving financial advice. Ask other business owners for a referral to someone who is competent and honest. Some banks have bookkeeping services available for their small business accounts. You might even be able to offer massage to a qualified person in exchange for bookkeeping services. (For a discussion of bartering, see Chapter 7.)

Client Records

When clients come into your office for the first time, have them fill out an intake form, listing their contact information and their medical history (see Fig. 5-3). Intake forms should be updated regularly. When you see clients who come in sporadically, always ask if their contact information has changed, and if they have developed any medical conditions since their last visit.

Written **SOAP notes** for every session are an essential part of client records. SOAP notes, also referred to as progress notes, are a form of documenting client progress during massage sessions and are also widely used by other health care practitioners.

- *S* stands for *Subjective*: What the client said. Example: "I think I hurt my back yesterday while I was doing yard work."
- *O* stands for *Objective*: What the therapist observed, through a combination of interviewing, posture assessments, and palpation. Example: "Client appears to be tense in general. Active trigger points in quadratus lumborum, bilateral. Client is very tender in lumbar erectors."
- *A* stands for *Assessment*: What the therapist did to help the client, and outcome of those actions. Example: "Applied alternating hot and cold packs for 15 minutes, following by NMT (neuromuscular therapy) focused on lower back. Noted good trigger point releases. Client stated pain level dropped from 8 to 2 on a scale of 1 to 10."
- *P* stands for *Plan*: What the therapist suggests as self-care for the client. Example: "Soak in a warm tub, drink extra water, and use ice for pain." The care plan is a mutual agreement between practitioner and client that includes a discussion of the benefits of future massage therapy appointments.

Writing SOAP notes takes a certain amount of self-discipline if you work alone; there's no one to remind you, and you may think you can just keep it all in your head. What if a client who has been seeing you for several years comes in one day and says she's moving out of state and asks for her records so that she can give them to her new therapist? It would be unprofessional—and embarrassing—to have to tell her you don't have any records. You are presenting yourself as a professional massage therapist, and therefore, people should be able to expect you to keep progress notes. If you hope to have mutual referral relationships with other health care practitioners, or if you intend to file health insurance claims, maintaining SOAP notes is a necessity. Figure 6-1 is an example of a professional SOAP note form, illustrating several correctly documented massage therapy sessions.

In addition to the intake form and progress notes, client records include documentation on any incidents pertaining to the client. For instance, if a client made a sexual overture, it must be recorded. If an accident happened, such as a client slipping and falling in your office, even if she said she wasn't hurt at the time, make sure you have it all written down. If you're filing an insurance claim, the releases and other forms mentioned in Chapter 5 are part of that documentation. (For further discussion on policy and procedure documentation, see Chapter 9.)

If you are practicing in a state that currently has no licensure laws and a license to practice does become required, keeping client records might be the deciding factor in whether you can be "grandfathered in" as a licensee. As more and more states regulate massage, licensure boards have been making education requirement exceptions for therapists who have been operating a business for a certain number of years, and/or who have documented a certain number of client sessions.

You may choose to keep your client files on the computer, have actual paper files, or a combination of the two. Failing to maintain regular client records that are complete and accurate is inexcusable. You must find a system that works for you and for your business structure and style.

ROADSIDE ASSISTANCE

I maintain two sets of client files: one paper and one electronic. Each client is entered into my electronic database, for the convenience of doing mailings. Each client is numbered in the electronic database, and the paper file is labeled with the corresponding number on an end-tab file folder. A separate paper card file is arranged alphabetically by the client's last name, and the file number is noted in the upper right-hand corner of the card. When a client comes in, I look in the card file to find the file number and pull the paper file. This step could be eliminated by keeping the online database open all the time, but in the event of a computer crash, or more than one person looking for a file at the same time, the card file is conveniently located beside the paper client files and serves as a backup to the electronic database. SOAP notes are entered into the computer and a paper copy is printed for the client's paper file, so the notes are accessible to a practitioner conducting an interview or having a follow-up conversation with a client in the privacy of the treatment room. This also serves as a backup measure.

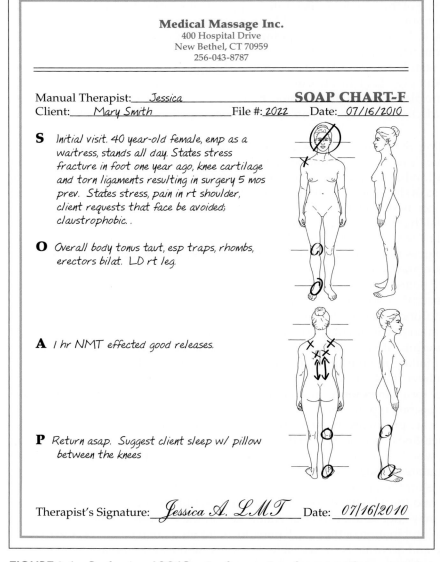

Medical Massage Inc.
400 Hospital Drive
New Bethel, CT 70959
256-043-8787

Manual Therapist: _Jessica_　　　**SOAP CHART-F**
Client: _Mary Smith_　　File #: _2022_　Date: _07/16/2010_

S Initial visit. 40 year-old female, emp as a waitress, stands all day. States stress fracture in foot one year ago, knee cartilage and torn ligaments resulting in surgery 5 mos prev. States stress, pain in rt shoulder, client requests that face be avoided; claustrophobic. .

O Overall body tonus taut, esp traps, rhombs, erectors bilat. LD rt leg.

A 1 hr NMT effected good releases.

P Return asap. Suggest client sleep w/ pillow between the knees

Therapist's Signature: _Jessica A. LMT_　Date: _07/16/2010_

FIGURE 6-1　Professional SOAP notes for a series of massage therapy sessions.

Medical Massage Inc.
400 Hospital Drive
New Bethel, CT 70959
256-043-8787

Manual Therapist:___Jessica_____   **SOAP CHART-F**
Client:____Mary Smith_____   File #:_2022___   Date:__09/27/2010__

S *Client states pain in shoulders; just had second knee surgery, so avoid lower rt ext.*

O *Taut bands traps and rhombs bilat.*

A *30 mins focused upper body session, good releases w/NMT.*

P *Increase water to hydrate muscles, shoulder rolls and stretches, return 1-2 weeks.*

Therapist's Signature:___*Jessica A. LMT*___ Date:__09/27/2010__

FIGURE 6-1   *(Continued)*

EXPLORATIONS

The next time you're at the doctor's or dentist's office, ask to see your file (you have the legal right to do so; by law, patient files are the property of the patient). Observe the documentation: the intake form, releases you've signed, insurance information, progress notes, and medical reports. Notice that the papers are in chronological order and that correct medical terminology is used in the notes. Aspire to keep your client records in the same professional manner as those you find in a medical or dental office.

Medical Massage Inc.
400 Hospital Drive
New Bethel, CT 70959
256-043-8787

Manual Therapist:___Jessica___   **SOAP CHART-F**
Client:___Mary Smith_____ File #:_2022___ Date:__09/29/2010__

S   Client states stress and tension in shoulders.
       Still need to avoid rt knee.

O   Taut traps, rhombs, erector sp taut bands
       bilat.

A   1 hr NMT effected good releases.

P   Stretch, soaking baths for soreness, return
       as needed.

Therapist's Signature:___Jessica A. LMT___ Date:__09/29/2010__

FIGURE 6-1   *(Continued)*

Employment Records

If you have employees or independent contractors in your office, you are bound by law to keep employment records. Keep a file on each individual who works in your office, regardless of the person's status. In addition to the job application, you would keep either an employment contract or an independent contractor agreement, and the appropriate tax forms, as part of the employment record for every member of your staff. (A discussion of the differences between employees and independent contractors, including the tax forms that apply, and examples of employment agreements appear in Chapter 8.)

Medical Massage Inc.
400 Hospital Drive
New Bethel, CT 70959
256-043-8787

Manual Therapist:___*Jessica*_____   **SOAP CHART-F**
Client:___*Mary Smith*_____File #:_*2022*___Date:_*10/24/2010*___

S   *Client overall tense and says she feels "out of balance"; rt knee that was recently op on is not healing well and giving her problems. MD has told her to "baby it".*

O   *Traps, delts, levs, erect sp taut bands bilat. Rt knee is swollen and hot.*

A   *1 hr session; Swedish massage for tension w/NMT on neck and shoulders. Elevated knee and applied ice pack during session. Client reported very relaxed after session.*

P   *Warned her to keep MD constantly informed about the knee problem.*

Manual Signature:___*Jessica A. LMT*___Date:_*10/24/2010*___

FIGURE 6-1   *(Continued)*

Any incidents related to staff members should also be kept on file. If a client makes a complaint about a staff member, it should be documented; if a staff member reports a client for doing something inappropriate, that should be documented in the client's file, as mentioned above, and a copy placed in the staff member's file as well. Be sure to document any injuries that occur on the job.

As your business grows, you may decide to implement a staff evaluation process. Informally, however, you should just note any problems, such as excessive absenteeism or failure to observe cleanliness standards, in the staff member's file, including what actions you have taken to rectify the situation. (See also Chapter 9.)

Medical Massage Inc.
400 Hospital Drive
New Bethel, CT 70959
256-043-8787

Manual Therapist: _Jessica_   **SOAP CHART-F**
Client: _Mary Smith_   File #: _2022_   Date: _10/30/2010_

S Stressed out about knee, which is still hot and swollen. Carries her tension in her shoulders.

O Traps, levs, rhombs taut bands bilat.

A 1/2 hr NMT focused upper body. Good releases. Kept rt knee elevated and iced during massage.

P Recommended client keep knee elevated as much as poss and see MD again asap due to the condition of it and how much pain it is causing her. Suggested ice if needed at home. Return 1-2 weeks.

Therapist's Signature: _Jessica A. LMT_   Date: _10/30/2010_

FIGURE 6-1   *(Continued)*

ALTERNATE ROUTES

Employees and Independent Contractors

Keep copies of any employment contracts, insurance policies, tax forms, and so forth in a safe place away from your workplace. SOAP notes and other client records should *not* be removed from the office. However, if you ever have to document anything that could result in legal action, such as sexual harassment, or a client claiming injury due to your negligence, keep careful records of that as well, away from the office in a secure location.

Business Partners

Be sure that both partners know the location of all important papers. All partners should have their own copy of any partnership agreements and access to any off-site record storage, such as safety deposit boxes, where insurance policies and other important papers are stored.

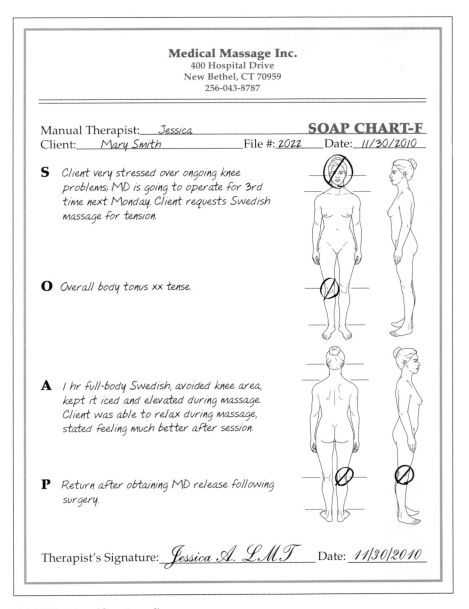

Medical Massage Inc.
400 Hospital Drive
New Bethel, CT 70959
256-043-8787

Manual Therapist: _Jessica_   **SOAP CHART-F**
Client: _Mary Smith_   File #: _2022_   Date: _11/30/2010_

S *Client very stressed over ongoing knee problems; MD is going to operate for 3rd time next Monday. Client requests Swedish massage for tension.*

O *Overall body tonus xx tense.*

A *1 hr full-body Swedish, avoided knee area, kept it iced and elevated during massage. Client was able to relax during massage, stated feeling much better after session.*

P *Return after obtaining MD release following surgery.*

Therapist's Signature: _Jessica A. LMT_   Date: _11/30/2010_

FIGURE 6-1 *(Continued).*

OTHER DOCUMENTATION

In addition to financial and tax records, client records, and employment documents, your paper trail should include any corporate or partnership records; licenses and permits; copies of insurance policies; and, if you're in a state or professional association that obligates you to receive it, continuing education records. Save the warranties on any equipment purchased for your business; stapling a copy of the receipt to the warranty is a good practice.

Important paper documents, such as insurance policies, your lease agreement, or the deed to your property, or corporate papers or stock certificates, should be kept in a fireproof cabinet or a safety deposit box at the bank. Remember, if it's your business, everything in it and everything that happens in it is personally important to you in one way or another. The paper trail is a long one, but the purpose of it is primarily to protect you as the business owner.

POSTCARDS from the HIGHWAY

Felicia Brown

I graduated from massage school in 1994, and a few years later started Balance Day Spa on my own. Eight years later when I sold the business, it had grown to over 50 employees and annual revenues in excess of $1.6 million. In my 16 years as a massage therapist, spa owner, and consultant to the spa and bodywork industry, I've learned some important lessons for success along the way:

1. *Follow your heart.* Be passionate about your life, love what you do.
2. Live your dreams.
3. *Listen to your instincts.* Follow your hunches and impulses, and "tune in" to your inner voice. You know what is best for you.
4. *Give thanks.* Be grateful for everything in your life, good and bad, and look for the hidden gifts in each problem or crisis you encounter.
5. *Be positive.* Believe in yourself, allow yourself to succeed, and be ready to do what it takes to achieve your dreams.
6. *Set an example for others.* Give back to your community, live a healthy life, and always take the high road.
7. *Help others succeed.* Assist clients and colleagues, refer business to others, and be available as a mentor.
8. *Always be willing to learn.* Learn to accept feedback and criticism, read constantly, and find new ways to expand your horizons.
9. *Do what is important.* Know your priorities, take care of yourself, and enjoy your life.
10. *Pay yourself first.* Invest in your retirement, education, and self-development every single month.
11. *Get lots of massage.* This last step will help you achieve everything else on the list, and to remember exactly why you joined this profession in the first place.

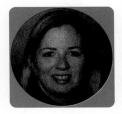

Felicia Brown, LMBT is a licensed massage therapist and the owner of Spalutions, a firm that provides continuing education, business consulting, and marketing coaching to spa and wellness professionals. She has received numerous business awards including 2009 Spa Person of the Year from the Day Spa Association and 2005 Small Business Person of the Year from the Greensboro, NC Chamber of Commerce. Felicia is also an approved NCBTMB provider and Certified Guerrilla Marketing Coach. She may be reached at Felicia@spalutions.com or www.spalutions.com.

SUGGESTED READINGS

American Massage Therapy Association. *Credit Card Processors May Code Your Practice Wrong.* http://www.amtamassage.org/member/credit_card_processors_codes.html. Accessed 09/03/2008.

Gegak T, Bolsta P. *The Big Book of Small Business: You Don't Have to Run Your Business by the Seat of Your Pants.* New York, NY: Harper Collins, 2007.

Isidro I. *Commonsense Tips on Keeping Business Records.* http://www.powerhomebiz.com/vol4/commonsense.htm. Accessed 08/18/2008.

Island Software Company. *Software Downloads.* http://www.islandsoftwareco.com/ecommerce/catalog/software_downloads.php?osCsid=o29ic8tts2ppg4e8os6orbgkd7. Accessed 08/16/2008.

Kendall S. *The Technology Coach.* http://thetechnologycoach.blogspot.com/2008/08/online-backup-good-small-officehome.html. Accessed 08/16/2008.

Orman S. *The 9 Steps to Financial Freedom: Practical and Spiritual Steps So You Can Stop Worrying.* New York, NY: Three Rivers Press, 2006.

QuickBooks. *Professional Service Solutions.* http://quickbooks.intuit.com/product/accounting-software/professional-services-industry/business-software/. Accessed 08/16/2008.

Sylvester J. *401 Questions Every Entrepreneur Should Ask.* Franklin Lakes, NJ: Career Press, 2006.

Managing technology. Inc.com: The Daily Resource for Entrepreneurs. http://www.inc.com/resources/technology/. Accessed 04/26/2010.

U.S. Census Bureau. North American Industry Classification System (search results for: massage). http://www.census.gov/cgi-bin/sssd/naics/naicsrch?code=621399&search=2007. Accessed 04/26/2010.

My Personal Journey

In this chapter, we've discussed managing office technology. Make a list of the technology products you want to obtain for your office, and do comparison shopping in order to find the best products for your business at the most reasonable price.

My goals _____

_____

_____

What's in my way? _____

_____

_____

What action can I take to remedy the situation? _____

_____

_____

One-year progress update _____

_____

_____

CHAPTER 7

Managing Your Finances

The safest way to double your money is to fold it over and put it in your pocket.

KIN HUBBARD

KEY CONCEPTS

- By tracking your personal spending habits and answering some honest questions about your finances, you will gain insight about your attitudes toward money.

- Making a household budget before attempting to construct a business budget gives a realistic picture of how much money you need to meet your obligations.

- The break-even point is reached when income exceeds expenses.

- The balance sheet, profit and loss sheet, and statement of cash flow are useful documents for tracking business finances.

- The most common budget busters are procrastination and expenses that are allowed to spiral out of control.

- Reconciling bank statements and scrutinizing bills for mistakes should be done monthly.

- Variable expenses should be proportionate to income.

- Managing inventory involves keeping a modest amount of product on hand for a minimum investment.

- There are certain tax obligations for self-employed people.

- Failing to pay the income tax you owe is illegal, but legitimate tax deductions can help you minimize your tax obligation.

- Small businesses are exempt from certain tax laws until a threshold number of employees is met.

- Bartering for goods and services can save you a lot of money, but it still incurs a tax obligation.

- Planning for retirement should be factored into your goal setting, and it's never too early to get started.

- Preparing to sell a business requires research, paperwork, and strategizing.

How you manage your finances directly relates to your business success. The importance of preparing yourself financially to open your business has been reinforced throughout this book, but there's more to learn, especially regarding your *attitude* about money and the effect that has on how you handle your finances. Getting your personal finances in order before going into business is a must. Learning to avoid budget busters, educating yourself about the various taxes for which you are responsible, and planning for the future are needed at the outset and will improve over time as you evolve into a more experienced businessperson.

ATTITUDES ABOUT MONEY

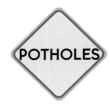

Your attitude concerning money has a lot to do with the way you were raised. If you are from a family of hardworking, frugal people who have a simple lifestyle and save for the future, you might have a much different attitude toward money than a person who was raised in an affluent household with no worry about saving for tomorrow. Everyone comes from different circumstances.

Have you ever thought—or said out loud—"I'm broke?" That implies you need fixing! And if you find yourself saying it with any frequency, maybe you do. If you have bad financial habits at home (the kind that leave you broke), they will carry right over to your business. Having a healthy attitude toward money is not about things that are beyond your control, such as an unexpected expense when your car breaks down or a medical emergency; it's about those things you *can* control.

Don't fool yourself into thinking that owning your own business is miraculously going to straighten out your life and your finances. Get a handle on your financial situation before taking the plunge—whatever that entails. You want to stack the deck in favor of your business succeeding, and it's hard to do that when a financial mess at home is hanging over your head. Clean it up first.

Tracking Your Personal Spending

REALITY CHECKPOINT

If you carried around a notepad for a week and wrote down every dollar you spent, do you think you'd have a rude awakening? A cappuccino here, a magazine there, a lottery ticket every day, and another eye shadow when you already have a dozen at home—these are all small expenses that really add up over time.

Eating fast-food breakfast on the way to work and lunch out every day can easily add up to more than some people earn in a week (not to mention compromising your health). I did this as an experiment and discovered I was spending $100 a week on things I didn't need. That's $400 a month or $5200 a year—the cost of a nice vacation.

The thing about "spending money" is that we spend it without thinking about it. Bear in mind that you're about to be self-employed, with no guarantee of turning a profit within a certain amount of time, and resolve to save more money. You might need it for necessities until your business is operating in the black. To get an honest picture of how you really handle your finances, in addition to writing down every dollar you spend for a week, answer the questions in Box 7-1 truthfully. This exercise will have a lot more impact if you actually write the answers instead of just thinking about them.

If your answers to the questions in Box 7-1 are less than satisfactory, take a good hard look at where you're going wrong. Better yet, find an impartial credit counselor to get some advice. If you can't handle your finances at home, how are you going to handle them in a business? You might need real help and an attitude adjustment about money.

BOX 7-1   The Money Test

1. Do I live from paycheck to paycheck?
2. How much money do I have in savings?
3. Do I save regularly?
4. Have I ever written a bad check? If so, was it a one-time mistake in my checkbook, or has it happened repeatedly?
5. Do I use my credit cards for living expenses?
6. Do I use my credit cards for things I don't have the cash to pay for? Are they things that are necessities or just things I want?
7. Can I take a vacation or buy a new wardrobe without putting it on a credit card?
8. Have I been forced to borrow money to make ends meet?
9. Have I consolidated debt and then gotten right back into it?
10. Do I only make the minimum payments on my debts?

ALTERNATE ROUTES

Independent Contractors and Employees

Your employer may expect you to collect the money for your sessions, or there may be a designated person who handles the cash. Be sure you're clear on the employer's policies; for example, if more than one person is using the cash register, who will be held responsible if there is a shortage?

Business Partners

If all partners are active participants in the business and not just silent investors, it's wise to keep abreast of cash flow on a daily or at least weekly basis. If one person is accountable for handling the cash, the other partners should have the expectation of being informed immediately of any potential problems or discrepancies.

Words of Wisdom

Money should serve you; you shouldn't be a slave to money.

Most businesses that fail do so because of money—not because the entrepreneur doesn't have the desire or the work ethic or the good intentions. Losing money in the first year or two after opening a business is a real possibility, not necessarily because of financial mismanagement. It's a given that you're going to invest sweat equity in your business, but unfortunately, sweat equity won't repay your bank loan or make your car payment; that takes cold cash.

HELP JUST AHEAD

Meeting with a credit counselor can help you get back on track with your finances if you feel overwhelmed by debt. The Consumer Credit Counseling Service is a nonprofit organization, founded in 1964, that provides reliable and confidential budget counseling and money management education. Avoid any for-profit credit counseling company that makes unrealistic claims about wiping out your debt or that charges you a fee for a consultation.

Your Household Budget and Massage Pricing

Your household budget is not part of your actual business plan. However, you should construct it first, so you can be realistic about how much money you require in order to meet basic expenses before you go into business for yourself.

Your wish list in Chapter 1 indicated you want to be debt-free by age 50 and have enough money to send your kids to college (see Fig. 1-1). Let's say you have a mortgage of $135,000 with monthly payments of $800 and $8000 in credit card debt you incurred training for your new career that you're trying to pay off at $500 per month. Your other household expenses, including utilities and groceries, run to another $1500 a month, and you have a $300 monthly car payment. That's $3100 per month just to get by, not counting any extras such as going out to eat, buying clothes, paying for haircuts, and taking vacations. In addition, health insurance for self-employed people tends to cost quite a bit more than for employees who get group rates. All this amounts to about $3600 per month to live on in the style you're accustomed to.

The median price of a massage in the United States is $65 an hour, according to *Massage Therapy Fast Facts* on ABMP's public education website. For research purposes, I asked therapists across the country who are members of my social and business Internet networks to provide me with the average charge for an hour of massage in their locale. The price varies widely from one area to another, as shown in Table 7-1. In addition to geographic location, the price is determined by the workplace. The cost of an hour of massage in a gym or home office was consistently stated as being less than in a day spa or medical setting.

If you are charging $65 per session for massage—fulfilling your objective to offer affordable treatments—you would have to do 56 sessions a month in order to support yourself. Bear in mind we haven't gotten to any of your office expenses yet; we're just talking about your household budget and what you need to make ends meet.

TABLE 7-1	Average Price Ranges for One Hour of Massage
Location	**Hourly Cost**
Albuquerque, New Mexico	$45–80
Atlanta, Georgia	$75–85
Bristol, Virginia	$40–60
Charlotte, North Carolina	$45–90
Denver, Colorado	$55–75
Florence, Alabama	$65–80
Minneapolis, Minnesota	$50–125
Nashville, Tennessee	$75–120
New York, New York	$90–120
Olympia, Washington	$55–60
Palm Beach, Florida	$65–90
Portland, Oregon	$50–60
Rochester, Minnesota	$55–65
San Francisco, California	$65–80
Tucson, Arizona	$55–75
Tulsa, Oklahoma	$55–85
Washington, District of Columbia	$85–100
Williamsville, New York	$50–75

One of your objectives was to work 5 days a week with weekends off. Divide the 56 treatments by 20 days, and you have to see 3 clients a day to support yourself. The mortgage will be paid off in 17 years (before you're 50, one of the goals). That $800 per month can then go into the college fund. Allowing for inflation, that won't be nearly enough to pay for college, but one of life's great lessons for your child is to earn money to help pay her own expenses and to take out student loans she can pay off when she gets that nice job for which she's been educated.

If you pay off your credit card debt as quickly as possible, you can apply that money toward extra payments against the principal on your home loan. Removing that debt faster will enable you to save more for future college expenses and other things.

EXPRESS LANE AHEAD

The Break-Even Point

Remember, unless you're only doing outcalls or working at home, office expenses have to be factored in to determine your **break-even point**—the point at which your business income exceeds your expenses. For instance, at my office, it takes 52 massages in a month to meet my break-even point. So if you need 56 massages a month in order to pay your personal bills, and it takes 56 massages to pay the bills at your office, that realistically means you need to perform 112 massages a month or 5.6 massages a day during a 5-day workweek. That's pretty hard work for one person, especially if you're the business owner with other duties, such as laundry, cleaning, and record keeping.

This brings us to the last objective: to have others working with you. Wouldn't it be easier for you to personally do only three sessions per day and to get the rest of your income from those who are working with you, either by collecting rent or by receiving a percentage of what they earn? Of course it would. That doesn't mean you'd get to relax for the rest of the day. There's always plenty for you to do, if you're running a business.

The Balance Sheet

A **balance sheet** is a document that shows the financial state of your business. It has three categories:

- Assets: everything your business owns and money that is due to your business, also referred to as **accounts receivable**
- Liabilities: everything your business owes, also referred to as **accounts payable**
- Equity: the monetary value remaining when total liabilities are subtracted from total assets

When a balance sheet is prepared correctly, the amount of total liabilities and the amount of the owner's equity will equal the assets. While a basic balance sheet is a simple document, particularly at the outset of a business, bear in mind that some of your assets, such as furnishings and equipment, will depreciate over time. Your financial software may calculate depreciation for you; you can also find instructions for calculating depreciation on the IRS website or seek the help of an accountant. A sample balance sheet appears in Figure 7-1.

Naturally you want the balance to be in your favor, and that may not be the case when you first start out. As time goes by, your accounts receivable should increase, your accounts payable should decrease, and the amount of equity will increase.

BALANCE SHEET

ASSETS	AMOUNT
Cash in checking account	$10, 486.00
Accounts receivable	$720.00
Inventory on hand (retail items)	$960.00
Supplies	$1, 126.00
Equipment and furnishings	$4,905.00
Total assets:	**$18, 197.00**

LIABILITIES	
Accounts payable	$7, 006.00
Owner's equity	$11,191.00
Total liabilities and owner's equity:	**$18, 197.00**

FIGURE 7-1   A balance sheet.

Tracking Profit and Loss

A **profit and loss sheet**, sometimes referred to as an income statement, indicates whether or not a business is operating at a profit. You'll want to prepare a profit and loss sheet, for your own information, that tracks revenues and expenses monthly or quarterly, as you choose. An example appears in Figure 7-2. Again, you may be showing a loss initially, but that's one of the purposes of preparing this document. The number representing the loss should grow progressively smaller until a balance begins to appear as profit.

Many new small business owners struggle with not having enough cash for their daily operations. A **cash flow statement** compares money coming in

PROFIT AND LOSS SHEET

From: _____ (date) to: _____ (date)

REVENUES	AMOUNT
Revenues from massage	$32, 060.00
Revenues from retail sales	$9, 344.00
Total revenues:	**$41, 404.00**

EXPENSES	
Rent	$9, 000.00
Products purchased for resale	$1, 000.00
Laundry service	$2, 400.00
Utilities	$2, 400.00
Marketing	$1, 800.00
Supplies	$1, 000.00
Membership dues for professional associations	$500.00
Continuing education	$500.00
Total expenses:	**$18, 600.00**

Net profit (revenues minus expenses)	**$22, 804.00**
Less income tax	$3, 450.00
Net profit after taxes	**$19, 354.00**

FIGURE 7-2   A profit and loss sheet.

with money going out. You can also use a cash flow statement to project your revenues and expenses. In addition, a cash flow statement lists any draws taken by the owner and money used to purchase new assets. (A **draw** is money taken out by the owner until such time as the amount invested in the business has been returned. For example, if you've spent $10,000 in getting your practice opened, any money you take out of the business up to $10,000 is considered a draw. After you've earned back the $10,000 investment, money taken out of

CASH FLOW STATEMENT

Cash flow from: _____ (date)   to: _____ (date)

	AMOUNT
Cash receipts from revenues	$41, 404.00
Cash payments for expenses	($21, 850.00)
Net cash for operating:	**$19,554.00**
Capital expenditures for equipment	($3, 500.00)
Draws by owner	($12, 000.00)
Total expenditures and draws:	**($15, 500.00)**
Cash on hand at beginning of period	$1, 650.00
Net increase or decrease in cash	$4, 054.00
Cash at the end of the period:	**$5, 704.00**

FIGURE 7-3   A cash flow statement.

the business is your salary.) If you've prepared a projected budget as a preliminary to opening your business, a monthly cash flow statement can show you where adjustments are needed. An example of a cash flow statement appears in Figure 7-3.

ROADSIDE ASSISTANCE

When I was a kid, I received the princely sum of 50¢ a week for my allowance, and I had to do a lot of chores to earn it. I used to save that money until I had $50 or more so I could spend it on something big! I didn't blow it at the candy store; I wanted something to show for it. That's still what I want for the money I earn today: *something to show for it.* Being diligent about managing your personal and business finances will ensure you'll have something to show for it, whether that's your dream vacation, a retirement fund, a new home, the ability to increase your charitable giving, or all of the above.

Words of Wisdom
I spend wisely so I can reap the fruits of my labor.

BUDGET BUSTERS

J. Paul Getty said if you can count your money, you aren't a billionaire. Let's assume for argument's sake that applies to you. You should be consulting your budget and counting your money frequently. The purpose of a budget is to plan how much money you're going to spend and then to track how much you actually do spend. It's incredibly easy for things to get out of hand if you don't stay on top of them at all times. Let's take a look at some real budget busters.

Procrastination Versus Paperwork

The most serious offense that can cause your budget to go haywire is simply dropping the ball on paperwork. If revenues coming in and expenses going out are not recorded in a timely manner, it's easy for things to be overlooked. Keeping a **daily ledger**, whether on paper or on the computer, works best and requires just a few minutes of attention every day. If you wait until the end of the month to record your transactions, it'll seem like drudgery instead of a simple task. The purpose of a ledger is to keep track of who you paid and who paid you, the date of each transaction, what category the income or expense is attributed to, and the form of payment. A sample ledger appears in Figure 7-4.

Reconciling your bank statement is an essential task that should be performed every month without fail. It's a simple process of ensuring that the bank statement balance matches the balance you have recorded in your checkbook or tracked online using financial software. A sample reconciled bank statement is shown in Figure 7-5.

Out-of-Control Advertising

Advertising is a business expense that can easily spiral out of control. Your rent and your utilities usually aren't going to be the problem areas, because they're more or less fixed amounts. Say you've budgeted $5000 for your first year's advertising. Your Yellow Pages ad is $100 a month, or $1200 for the year, leaving you with $3800. The newspaper ads you'll schedule for reminders to buy gift certificates around the major holidays account for another $2000, leaving you with $1800. A year's worth of business cards and brochures costs another $500, leaving you $1300. Your website costs $25 per month, leaving you $85 per month to spend elsewhere on advertising for the year. You can't get a whole lot for that price, so shop around carefully to get the most exposure for the least amount of money. (For more on advertising, see Chapter 14.)

Be aware that when the ad salesperson says, "it's a great ad and it's only $100 a month," that may be so, but spend it and you're already $15 over your monthly budget. It can get away from you quickly. Don't ever pay for advertising by putting it on a credit card, unless it's a charge card you pay off in full every month. You don't want to be paying for the ad in last Sunday's newspaper a year from now.

ROADSIDE ASSISTANCE

One month I noticed an extra $45 service charge on my bank statement. When I called the bank to find out what it was for, they told me it was because I had made too many deposits. In my most incredulous tone of voice, I asked the customer service rep if I was really being penalized for putting my money in his bank. He removed the charge and upgraded my checking services to handle the increased volume of business. If you don't know what it is you're being charged for, call and question it. Just as in my scenario, the bank will sometimes forgive a charge in the interest of maintaining good customer relations.

DAILY LEDGER

Revenues
Type: Income from retail sales

DATE PAYMENT RECEIVED	RECEIVED FROM	ITEMS	INVOICE #	AMOUNT	TYPE OF PAYMENT	YEAR-TO-DATE
01/02/10	Tim Mott	Neck pillow	6181	$25.00	Cash	$25.00
01/03/10	Jo Kerns	Essential oils	6182	$178.10	Check # 5100	$203.10
01/03/10	Alice Catt	Biofreeze	6183	$14.95	Cash	$218.05
01/03/10	Bob Nitze	Biofreeze	6184	$14.95	Cash	$233.00

Expenses
Type: Office supplies

DATE PAID	PAID TO	PURCHASES	AMOUNT	TYPE OF PAYMENT	YEAR-TO-DATE
01/02/10	Office Depot	Paper, calendar, ink	$78.15	Check # 2301	$78.15
01/03/10	Bubba's	File storage boxes	$27.70	Check # 2302	$105.85
01/03/10	Amazon.com	Tax software	$129.00	Debit card	$134.85

FIGURE 7-4   A daily ledger.

Scrutinizing Your Bills

Scrutinize all your bills every month. Utility bills can be simplified by your agreeing to pay a flat rate every month and make up any difference from actual usage at the end of the year. Check those bills anyway. If your water bill is supposed to be $35 and it suddenly goes up to $50, you should be calling the water company to ask the reason.

Check your phone bill. Most of the businesses you'll deal with probably have a toll-free customer service number, so be sure you have those numbers and use them. Look for any unusual long-distance calls that aren't to a toll-free number, and question any charges you can't identify.

Check your other bills: laundry, office supplies, advertising bills, and everything else. You want to pay what you owe, and no more.

BANK RECONCILIATION

Enter balance for this statement: $ 8749.10

Add: Outstanding Deposits (recent deposits that do not appear on this statement)

Date	Amount
10/11/10	$444.00
10/13/10	$231.00
Total	**$675.00**

Subtract: Outstanding Checks (checks that have not yet cleared the bank)

Check #	Amount
1321	($124.60)
1322	($178.00)
1323	($29.25)
1324	($147.15)
Total	**($479.00)**

Checkbook balance: $ 8945.10

Subtract service charge: $ (20.00)

Actual current balance: $ **8925.10**

FIGURE 7-5   A reconciled bank statement.

Expenses Proportionate to Income

In addition to checking your expenditures, keep track of how you're doing in terms of income projections. If you're not getting as much business as you planned, you need to cut back on expenses wherever possible. But if you have exceeded your revenue projections, there are variables you may need to spend more on, such as massage supplies and sheets from the linen service. It's a good thing when your business grows enough to warrant an increase in your expenses.

Managing Inventory

If you are planning to sell retail items in your office, it's important to manage your inventory carefully. Be careful not to invest hundreds of dollars in retailing when you're just starting out. If selling on consignment is an option—you get the product and pay as you sell—that's one good way to keep your money in your pocket. If you're tempted to purchase outright goods to sell, start with very small amounts. If you sell out, you can always reorder, and if you don't, it's much better to have an inventory consisting of a small amount of product than a large amount of product.

A friendly reminder: Retailing places you in the position of assuming dual roles with clients. As long as you aren't prescribing or telling people that they *need* something you're selling, you'll be okay.

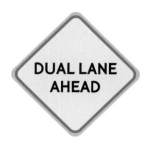

> ### ROADSIDE ASSISTANCE
>
> My personal experience has been that the retail items that sell well in my office are the things we actually use with our clients. The first item I ever retailed and still sell today are the gel packs that can be heated or frozen. They're inexpensive to buy and sell well, for $3 to $5 each. Buckwheat neck warmers are another item that works for us, as are the essential oils and topical ointments we use with clients. When people experience the products directly during a massage session, they're more likely to want to buy them for use at home.

TAXES

Due to the fact that all tax forms are subject to change from year to year, the actual forms are not included in this book. Federal tax forms are available on the IRS website, as is a schedule for business owners detailing the filing deadline for each type of tax. State tax forms and filing schedules are available on your state's Department of Revenue website.

Taxes are a fact of life. Nobody enjoys paying them, but the country couldn't run without them. We all contribute a portion of our income so the government and its thousands of agencies and projects can keep going. It sometimes seems we're taxed every way we turn: federal income tax, state income tax, county tax, city tax, sales tax, gasoline tax, lodging tax, property tax, capital gains tax, estate tax, and so on. We don't have to like it; we just have to pay it.

It is illegal to evade paying income tax, but you can reduce the amount of tax you have to pay by taking advantage of all the legal deductions at your disposal. According to the IRS, in order for an expense to be deductible, it must be incurred in connection with your business, it must be ordinary and necessary to the running of the business, and it must be based on precedence and the reasonable belief that you're entitled to it. A list of tax deductions appears in Box 7-2.

You don't have to be an accountant in order to understand taxes, but if you're mathematically challenged, or you're lacking in the self-discipline necessary to keep good records and adhere to the due dates for filing, you'd be wise to hire one. An accountant or tax professional is likely to find deductions for you to which you may not realize you're entitled. An additional benefit to seeking professional tax preparation help is that if you're ever audited, the tax preparer can represent your interests and defend the tax returns he prepared on your behalf.

Social Security Tax

A practitioner who works as an employee is subject to having Social Security taxes withheld from her paycheck; the employee pays half and the employer contributes half. FICA, the Federal Insurance Contribution Act, was created in 1935 as a social insurance for the elderly, disabled, and survivors.

BOX 7-2   Tax Deductions

- General office supplies (e.g., paper, pens, printer ink)
- Office equipment (e.g., computer, copier, fax machine)
- Office furnishings and decor
- Massage supplies (e.g., creams, oils, lotions, CDs, etc.)
- Massage equipment (e.g., massage tables, table warmers, hand tools)
- Home office expenses
- Bank service charges
- Credit card fees (on your business credit cards)
- Credit card processing charges (cards accepted at your business)
- Rent or mortgage payments
- Utilities at the office
- Telephone charges
- Internet service
- License and permit fees
- Insurance
- Membership fees for professional and business associations
- Attendance at professional and business conferences
- Continuing education expenses
- Subscriptions to trade journals
- Subscriptions to magazines for the waiting room
- Books, DVDs, and other media related to the profession
- Laundry service
- Cleaning service
- Property tax
- Sales tax
- Business taxes
- Fees to professionals, such as attorneys and accountants
- Printing and reproduction for office and promotional literature
- Postage and delivery costs
- Travel and mileage costs related to business. (The trip from your home to your office is not deductible; if you do outcalls from your home office, the first and last trips of the day are not deductible.)
- Gifts to clients ($25 limit per gift)
- Repairs
- Cost of goods purchased for resale
- Business-related meals (50% deductible)
- Uniforms (if required for the job)
- Bottled water for clients
- Wages paid to employees and fees paid to independent contractors
- Charitable contributions
- Your salary (applies only if your business is a corporation instead of a sole proprietorship)

Social Security is a retirement benefit, and the amount you're entitled to receive is based on the amount of money earned, as well as Social Security taxes you paid during your working life. You become eligible for retirement benefits at age 62, and the longer you continue to work, the more your retirement benefit will be.

Social Security taxes are sometimes referred to as FICA taxes. As of the end of 2009, Social Security tax was 12.4%. Those who are self-employed have to contribute the entire amount of the tax to their own Social Security account.

Self-Employment Tax

According to the IRS definition, self-employment tax (SE tax) is a combined Social Security and Medicare tax for individuals who work for themselves. You can calculate your tax liability yourself using Schedule SE; Social Security and Medicare taxes of wage earners are usually calculated by their employers. You can deduct half of your SE tax in figuring your adjusted gross income. Employees cannot deduct Social Security and Medicare taxes. The self-employment tax rate as of 2009 was 15.3%. The rate consists of two parts: 12.4% for Social Security (old age, survivors, and disability insurance) and 2.9% for Medicare (hospital insurance). The income subject to self-employment tax was capped at $94,200 as of 2008. The specifics of tax obligations pertaining to employees and independent contractors are discussed in Chapter 8.

Federal Income Tax

According to the IRS, any self-employed person with an income over $400 should file a tax return and pay income tax. There are literally hundreds of IRS forms, and your individual circumstances will dictate which ones you file. Form 1040 is the standard personal federal income tax form, and this long version lets you itemize your tax deductions, such as interest on a mortgage, medical expenses, charitable contributions, and contributions to a retirement account.

Form 1040A is a shorter form that allows you to take standard deductions. Form 1040EZ is an even shorter form whose use is limited to taxpayers who have an income of less than $100,000 and no dependents.

In order to get every dollar you're entitled to, you or your tax preparer should use the long 1040 form and itemize your deductions. In some circumstances, when you don't have enough deductions to make a difference, you may be better off taking a standard deduction and filing one of the shorter forms. Your tax professional should know which way of filing will best fit your situation and save you the most money.

State Income Tax

As of 2010, there were seven states that have no income tax: Alaska, Florida, Nevada, South Dakota, Texas, Washington, and Wyoming. Two other states, Tennessee and New Hampshire, only collect income tax on dividends and interest earnings. The rest of the citizenry pays state tax in rates that range from less than 1% in Iowa and Oklahoma to a flat 25% of the taxpayer's federal tax liability in Rhode Island. State income taxes fund government programs just like federal taxes do, except they're state programs instead of federal ones.

Retailing and Taxes

If you are going to sell retail items in your business, check with your state Department of Revenue to see if you need to obtain a retail license. The license will include an account number for paying retail tax on the items you sell, and it will also allow you to purchase things from suppliers at wholesale prices that you can sell at retail prices. Most states require you to pay your retail taxes quarterly and then to file a simple year-end summary. Your town or county may also require a retail license, so be sure to check with your local offices.

Bartering and Taxes

Bartering is trading goods and/or services for goods and/or services, without a cash exchange taking place. Barter dollars or trade dollars are identical to real dollars for the purpose of tax reporting. If you conduct any direct barter—barter for another's products or services—the IRS expects you to report the fair market value of the products or services you received on your tax return. For example, let's say that during the course of a year, you have given $1000 worth of massage in exchange for goods and services for which you bartered. However, the cash value of the goods and services you received was $2000. That means the extra $1000 is taxable income and should be reported as such when you file your tax return.

Bartering can get you a lot of things you need but can't afford to pay for. Just remember, though, when you're bartering with someone, your main commodity as a practitioner is your *time*. Assuming that you need a certain amount of actual cash to be able to pay your bills, you have to be careful not to go so overboard on bartering that you don't have enough time left for cash-paying customers. You might be glad to perform a massage in exchange for a bushel of organic apples, but you can't use them to make your car payment.

Bartering possibilities are endless. Every client is a potential barter partner, even if he or she isn't a businessperson. Maybe he or she's a great babysitter, part-time cleaner, or talented artist. I've bartered in the past for carpet cleaning, furniture refinishing, music lessons, artwork for my office, graphic design services, and home-cooked meals delivered to my door by a client who's a professional chef. A colleague who lives near a university tells me that students are constantly posting messages online and on community bulletin boards offering all kinds of goods and services in exchange for massage, and she has done many such exchanges, including babysitting services, custom-made clothing made by a design student, and Spanish lessons. Bartering is a mutually beneficial proposition. Both parties get something they want, and their money stays in their pockets.

EXPLORATIONS

Make a list of people you could potentially exchange with for massage, and contact them.

PLANNING FOR YOUR RETIREMENT

Maybe you're a young practitioner who hasn't thought about retirement yet, but don't think you have to wait until you're middle aged to start making those plans. One of your goals for being self-employed is to make a comfortable living; another goal should be to make enough money to be able to put some aside for retirement. Even if you're only 21, planning ahead for retirement can save you money on your income taxes right now. The only restriction on eligibility to contribute to an Individual Retirement Account (IRA) is that you must have earned taxable income and you must not be older than 70.5 by the end of the year in which you are contributing.

There is more than one type of IRA, and the amount you can contribute varies based on your age, your marital status, and the particular kind of retirement account you have. As of 2010, the maximum amount that most people could contribute per year to their basic IRA is $5000 for those under the age of 50 and $6000 for those over 50. One type of IRA, known as a SEP IRA or Simplified Employee Pension, is for those in a higher income and tax bracket, and you may contribute as much as $49,000 per year. Contributions to your IRA are tax deferred, meaning you won't pay any tax on the money until you retire and actually start withdrawing. (There are heavy penalties for early withdrawal of retirement funds, to discourage spending the money ahead of time.)

A banker or a certified financial planner can advise you about the options available for saving for retirement. It's never too early to start planning your retirement strategy, particularly if one of your goals is to retire by a certain age.

Going with the Flow

According to the Society for Human Resource Management, there is a trend among women to be substantially less prepared for retirement than men. Statistics compiled by Associated Massage & Bodywork Professionals indicate that almost 83% of massage therapists are women and 64% of massage therapists are self-employed. That's a lot of people who should be planning more diligently for their retirement.

SELLING YOUR BUSINESS

You just got started; why would you want to sell? Perhaps you're ready to retire. Sometimes there's a need to relocate, a divorce, the dissolving of a partnership, or any number of other reasons for selling a business. Maybe someone just made you an offer you can't refuse!

One of the first things to consider when preparing to sell your business is whether or not it includes real estate. It is possible to sell a business without any real estate changing hands. For instance, you might lease your office instead of owning the property. That doesn't mean you can't sell your business. If it doesn't include real estate, a potential buyer would be getting **tangible assets**, such as office furnishings and equipment with a monetary value, along with linens and a lot of other supplies conducive to running a massage therapy practice; plus **intangible assets**, including your business name and client files.

Setting the Price

If you have any intention of selling, be prepared to produce profit and loss sheets for the past few years for the potential buyer to see. A potential buyer will want to see a list of tangible assets, as well as intangible assets, so he knows exactly what he's getting for his money. Detail any financing options, if you're prepared to offer any. Intangible assets are difficult to place a value on. How would you value the well-known name of your business, or the years of customer goodwill you've built up? If you want to be really nice, you could offer to write a letter of introduction to your clients urging them to continue to patronize the business once it changes ownership. That's an intangible asset that could be worth a lot of money. Another value-added strategy is to offer to remain on the job for a period of time in order to ease the transition for the new owner. Price and value aren't always the same thing.

Some formulas for selling a business suggest multiplying the gross annual sales three to five times and starting from there. Another thing to consider is the selling price of similar businesses in your area. Consulting a broker who specializes in selling health care practices is probably your best bet for getting a realistic picture of what your business is actually worth when you're ready to put it on the market.

Finding a Buyer

Ideally, if you are ready to retire or to sell for some other reason, the best person to sell to may be one of your employees or independent contractors. They're already established with your business, and chances are they know at least something about how the office runs; their presence would provide a sense of continuity for the existing clientele. Otherwise, you might do best by seeking a broker to sell your business for you. Brokers are in business to make money, too, and they'll immediately tell you what your strong and weak selling points are and what you can do to address the weak ones.

Another possibility is to sell to the competition. If you own a successful day spa, for instance, and you're ready to sell, consider approaching the day spa across town and asking the owner if she'd be interested in a second location. If you are a member of professional organizations, many of them offer free online classified ads where you can list your business for sale. If your business is still continuing to increase every year, and if the talented practitioners who work there now and who have a clientele built up agreed to stay for a new owner—these would be benefits for the buyer.

POSTCARDS from the **HIGHWAY**   **Ruth Werner**

It's always in the back of my mind to get one of those books specifically for women in business to see how my gender role is limiting or empowering me. . . but then, I'd rather do other things with my spare time. And I guess that's what success is, isn't it, being able to choose what to do with one's spare time? Here are a few of my guiding principles for success:

- You learn a lot more with your mouth closed than with your mouth open.
- The time to speak is when you're sure you have something important to say.
- Humility is strength: the ability to admit not knowing everything means you still have the capacity to grow.
- Life is an open-book test.
- Be the same person and make the same choices, regardless of whether anyone is watching.
- Ask for help when you need it.
- Identify people you respect, analyze what they do, and try to emulate those qualities.
- Have an idea of what you want, so you can recognize it when it falls into your lap.

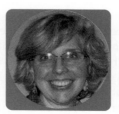 Ruth Werner is the author of *A Massage Therapist's Guide to Pathology*, now in its 4th edition, published by Lippincott Williams & Wilkins. Ruth graduated from Reed College in Portland, Oregon, with a degree in theater and literature in 1982. A massage therapist since 1985, she discovered her passion for anatomy while a student at the Brian Utting School of Massage in Seattle, Washington. Ruth has been an educator since 1991, teaching in a number of massage schools and offering continuing education all over the United States. Since 2006, she has served on the Board of Trustees of the Massage Therapy Foundation as the Educational Chair and is currently serving as the president of the Foundation. Ruth has recently moved to the Oregon coast. Visit her website at www.ruthwerner.com.

SUGGESTED READINGS

Alternative Health Business for Sale. http://us.businessesforsale.com/us/search/Alternative-Health-Businesses-For-Sale. Accessed 10/29/2009.

Brunner N. *Massage Profession Metrics.* http://www.massagetherapy.com/media/metricscharacteristics.php. Accessed 10/29/2009.

Consumer Credit Counseling Service. *What We Do.* http://www.cccsatl.org/whatWeDo/index.jsp. Accessed 10/29/2009.

Internal Revenue Service. *Operating a Business.* http://www.irs.gov/businesses/small/article/0,id=99930,00.html. Accessed 10/29/2009.

Massage Therapy Fast Facts http://www.massagetherapy.com/_content/images/Media/Factsheet1.pdf. Accessed 10/24/2009.

Massage Today.com eclassifieds. *Practices for sale.* http://eclassifieds.massagetoday.com/eclassified/view.php?mc_categoryid=2&MERCURYSID=a7f69f58d610625acf6f2467c33551e0. Accessed 10/29/2009.

Siegel P. *Business Formula Valuation: Learn More Here.* http://www.usabizmart.com/articles/26-article.php. Accessed 10/20/2008.

Society for Human Resource Management. *Women's Retirement Income Substantially Trails Men's.* http://www.shrm.org/rewards/retirement/rt.asp. Accessed 10/22/2008.

My Personal Journey

In this chapter, we've discussed your personal attitudes about managing your money. Based on your answers to the Money Test in Box 7-1, state your concrete goals for getting your personal finances in order, and brainstorm about the positive actions you can take in order to make that happen before you open your business.

My goals _____

_____

_____

What's in my way? _____

_____

_____

What action can I take to remedy the situation? _____

_____

_____

One-year progress update _____

_____

_____

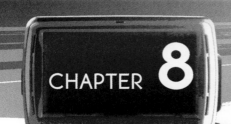

The People in Your Business

Hard work spotlights the character of people: some turn up their sleeves, some turn up their noses, and some don't turn up at all.

KEY CONCEPTS

- Practitioners who choose to work alone must make an extra effort not to become too isolated.
- Supervising student interns can be a good way to experiment with having another person in your office; it benefits the student, the school, your clientele, and you.
- The benefits of sharing a work space include having help meeting expenses and being able to offer expanded hours and/or services to clients.
- Practitioners who are expanding their business have a choice between renting space to another practitioner, hiring an employee, or entering into an agreement with an independent contractor.
- It's important to define in writing what qualities you are looking for in the people you wish to add to your business.
- For tax purposes, it's vital to understand the difference between employees and independent contractors.
- Having a written contract for the employee or contractor protects the employer by detailing exactly what is expected of the worker.
- Depending on the number of people in the business, a business owner who employs others may be obligated to pay worker's compensation and unemployment insurance.
- Providing employee benefits makes your business a more attractive place to work for people who are seeking a job.
- Interviewing potential staff members should serve the purpose of gathering the information the employer is seeking without being discriminatory in any way.
- Firing a staff member is sometimes necessary, and never pleasant.

Some practitioners prefer to work independently, coming and going as they please with no one else to worry about, while some would rather work with others. If working with other people was one of your goals and part of your business plan, think it through very carefully before making any final decisions. There are many considerations involved in choosing others to work with you. You want the people in your business to be talented, to coexist in joyous harmony and cultivate the atmosphere of wellness and serenity in your healing space. You obviously don't want trauma and drama, people who bring negativity into the workplace, or unprofessional or unreliable staff members.

THE LONE PRACTITIONER

People choose to work alone for a variety of reasons. Some people are just solitary types who prefer being on their own. In a rural area or small town, one massage therapist might be the only practitioner around. Home practitioners usually work alone; some people work at home in order to save on office overhead expenses, or to be home with children or someone who needs caretaking. Therapists who specialize in outcalls or chair massage usually work alone; the equipment and overhead are minimal, and having a change of scenery every day can be fun.

We've talked a lot about growing your business, but realistically, not everyone aspires to that. Many therapists love the freedom of working alone and wouldn't have it any other way.

Words of Wisdom
Success is relative; it's whatever it means to you.

Being Aware of Isolation

If working alone is what you want to do, you should certainly do it. Be careful, though, when it comes to isolation. Make it a point to regularly get out of the office, especially if you work at home. (Therapists who do outcalls are exempt from this part.) You don't want to fall into the trap of feeling like you're at work every minute because your practice is at home or of becoming a totally unsociable person because the only people you see are your clients. Have lunch with a friend, get out of the office to network with other therapists, go to the gym or the park for some exercise, go out into the community to introduce yourself and publicize your business, and you won't suffer from isolation.

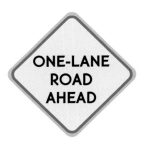

The Ups and Downs of Working Alone

The upside of being a lone practitioner is that you have no one but yourself to worry about, no one to pay, no one to generate extra paperwork, no one to cause you any scheduling or other problems. Deciding to take a day off, or a vacation, is as simple as locking the door.

The downside is that you can only do so much by yourself, and eventually you'll get to the point where your business can't grow. When you work alone, with no receptionist or support staff of any kind, it's easy to become overwhelmed by the amount of work you have to do that goes along with running a business, over and above performing massage. Whether you're in an office or practicing at home, you have to clean, you have to do laundry, and you must keep up with your record keeping.

Furthermore, if you've got the "Closed" sign on the door and the answering machine is picking up calls because you are with a client, you're going to miss out on a certain amount of business. People who stop by to purchase gift certificates may be put off at finding the office closed and decide to go elsewhere to make the purchase. If a prospective client calls and gets an answering machine, she might hang up instead of leaving a message. These are some of the pitfalls of working alone.

OPPORTUNITIES
AHEAD

If you are doing all the massage you can personally provide, plus all the accompanying chores, and you're happy with the amount of income you're making, that's great. But if you still aren't earning enough, the decision to include others in your business can be your ticket to making that goal a reality.

Supervising Interns

If you're not yet sure that you want to have other people as a permanent part of your business, one solution is to host student interns in your office. Many massage schools require their students to do internships, working in the office of experienced therapists who can supervise and mentor them for a certain number of practice hours.

In most states with licensure requirements, students are prohibited from being compensated; their internship hours are considered part of their training to become a professional therapist. While the students might not be allowed to be paid, it is usually acceptable for the supervising therapist to charge something for the student's services. You might offer your regular clients the opportunity to receive a student massage at half your going rate, for instance, or at the same fee the school charges for a massage in the student clinic (if there is one). The student can also help you with tasks around the office; the purpose of an internship is not only to get practice in massage but also to gain practical work experience.

HELP JUST
AHEAD

If there's a massage school within driving distance, make an appointment to see the director and offer your services as a practicum supervisor. You'll be helping the school, helping the student, helping your clients, and helping yourself.

The Benefits of Sharing Work Space

There are benefits to sharing space, whether you're renting to someone else or hiring staff. You don't have to start out on a grand scale. Depending on the amount of space in your massage setting, you might want to have just one other practitioner—perhaps a therapist who provides a different modality than yours—or who has a different skill altogether, such as an acupuncturist or a naturopath, or even a person who is willing to work different hours and different days than you do. Offering increased hours and having different services available are both great benefits for your clients.

If you're paying rent or the mortgage on an office and you're there only 4 days a week, you're letting 3 days go by while you could be earning money. If you're only working during the day while your children are in school, someone could be using the space in the evenings and helping pay the rent. Think it over, and weigh the benefits to your clients and to you as a businessperson.

> ### ROADSIDE ASSISTANCE
>
> I live in a small town, and when I started my business, I knew people who were driving an hour or more out of town to get services that weren't available in our area. I contacted a Rolfer, an acupuncturist, and a therapist who practices manual lymphatic drainage and arranged for them to work in my office one day a week. I pay them a higher percentage than usual to make it worth their while to come to my place, and it's been a win-win situation for everyone.

Renting Space to Others

If you have the space but you're not ready to take personal responsibility for staff members, one option is to rent space to another practitioner. When you rent to someone, he is neither your employee nor an independent contractor; he's the tenant, and you're the landlord.

If you enter into a rental agreement with anyone, put it in writing, and spell out the details:

- The amount of rent.
- The amount of a security deposit, if you decide to require one.
- The date the rent is due, and whether you will charge any added fees for paying late.
- The duration of the lease, such as month-to-month, or otherwise.
- The exact space the person will be entitled to use, including the use of common areas such as the lobby, the break room, the laundry room, or a storage area.
- The tenant's responsibility in terms of cleaning and maintenance.
- The amount of notice expected if the tenant decides to move out.
- Any prohibitions you are imposing, such as no access to your telephone, cash register, or linens.
- The reasons for you to terminate the rental agreement
- Proof of renter's insurance, if you require the tenant to have it.

You could consider trading part of the rent in exchange for office support, such as cleaning or doing laundry, but again, spell out the expectations so that both parties are clear. Ask your tax professional about how to handle the financial exchange. Remember that bartering is subject to income tax, as explained in Chapter 7.

A Good Impression

Bear in mind that although the person is just renting space from you, people could easily have the impression that he is a part of your business, and thus a reflection on you. If you rent to a massage therapist or other person who is subject to licensure in your state, you should insist on proof of a current license. In addition, you should ask for character references and also insist on a criminal record check. You don't want to find out after the fact that you're the landlord to America's Most Wanted, or someone who is violating the state's practice act.

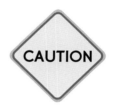

If a person is renting from you, a lot of things are beyond your control—such as the way he dresses. If you make it a point to dress professionally yourself and your tenant comes strolling through the lobby barefoot in cut-off jeans and a shabby T-shirt, that's going to drive you crazy, not to mention making a bad impression on your clients. Screen a renter just as carefully as you would screen an employee. Let him know up front what kind of professional image it's important to you to project, and explain that as a tenant in your work space, he is a part of that image. If the potential renter is not willing to uphold the same standards you require, keep looking. (For more discussion on professionalism, see Chapter 10.)

ASSEMBLING A STAFF

If you are in the market for a staff member, make a wish list just like you did in the context of Chapter 1, but make it about the person you're looking for. Say you want a practitioner to come into your office part-time. Here's a possible wish list for a massage therapist:

- An independent contractor.
- Will work 2 to 3 d/wk, including every other Saturday.
- Willing to work an afternoon shift from approximately 2 to 6 p.m.

- Has good references.
- Dresses and acts professionally.
- Willing to do outcalls

Where are you going to find this person? You can try placing a classified ad. You can list the opening on your website, if you have one. If you are located near a massage school or a school of the healing arts, place an ad on the bulletin board. Look on your state licensure board's website to see if practitioners are listed, peruse the web listings of the professional massage associations, or search general job matching websites where people have posted their resumes.

Be very specific about what you want in a member of your staff, and you will be a lot better off in the long run. Keep refining your wish list. If it is important to you that the person wear scrubs and white shoes to work every day, write that down. If he needs to use a certain greeting every time he answers the office telephone, say so. If you want someone who is computer savvy, put it on the list. Writing down your wish list will give you notes to refer to when you conduct job interviews. Thoroughly laying out your expectations before beginning any business relationship is much better than being disappointed and trying to change someone later.

EXPLORATIONS

If you're looking for nonlicensed personnel, such as a receptionist, post a notice on the bulletin board in the business department of your local community college, or attend a school career day as a potential employer. If you're seeking a part-time person, the local senior citizens' center could be a great place to find one. Retired people often have a wealth of experience to bring to a job; they appreciate the opportunity to keep busy and are limited in how much money they can make in addition to drawing Social Security. You just might find someone there who'd love to have a part-time job.

Employees

Let's examine some of the differences between employees and independent contractors.

If you want a staff member to work specified hours that you set up, and you want to have control over her activities as well—such as having her do cleaning, filing, or other tasks when she's not attending to clients—you are looking for an employee.

When you have an **employee**, you pay her an agreed-upon wage for her services.

As mentioned in Chapter 7, you are also obligated to pay half of her Social Security tax and to withhold federal and state tax amounts from her wages, which you then submit to the IRS and the state Department of Revenue on her behalf. You're required to have each employee fill out Form W-4, an Employee's Withholding Allowance Certificate, stating her filing status as married or single, and number of dependents, for the purpose of determining how much to withhold from her paycheck. At the end of the year, you furnish her with a Form W-2, officially referred to as a Wage and Tax Statement, that shows how much she has earned and how much tax has been withheld. All tax forms are available on the IRS website.

Spelling out exactly what you expect from an employee, in writing, protects you as the employer and leaves no room for doubt in the employee's mind. Figure 8-1 is a sample employment agreement for an employee.

ROADSIDE ASSISTANCE

I'm proud of the staff I have assembled. They're a mixture of people who have been practicing their art for a long time, and people who are relatively fresh out of school. With me, attitude counts more than expertise. I can teach someone how to give a massage or do paperwork; I can't teach anyone how to have a great personality. I've deliberately chosen cheerful, outgoing people who are positive in their outlook on life and who are service oriented. If you're thinking of adding a staff member to your business, seek out someone who has those qualities. I've made a point of cultivating staff who are skilled in a wide variety of modalities. If we don't offer a modality someone requests, we promise our clients that we'll make an effort to find them a therapist who does, and we follow through on that promise. It's an extra little bit of service that people truly appreciate.

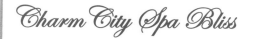 *Charm City Spa Bliss*

2700 Palmetto Boulevard
Tidal Creek, Texas 20202
950-230-4444

Employment Agreement for Massage Therapist (Employee)

Charm City Spa Bliss, Inc. expects the following duties and observation of the following rules from the massage therapists we employ:

1. The massage therapist shall arrive at work 10 minutes prior to opening at 9 a.m. in order to check your treatment room and gather any needed supplies for the first client.
2. The massage therapist shall wear and launder the scrubs we provide with the Charm City Spa Bliss logo on them when on duty.
3. No high-heels or bare feet are permitted at the office. Shoe soles must be made of rubber or other quiet material.
4. The massage therapist shall greet the client in the lobby and take her to the treatment room to conduct the intake interview in private. The massage therapist shall inform each client of her right to privacy by giving her a HIPAA brochure. Any aftercare instructions should be given to the client while she is still in the privacy of the treatment room.
5. The massage therapist shall pull the client's file prior to the client's arrival and write complete SOAP notes as soon as the client departs. Insurance client files are given to the receptionist at the end of the session. Non-insurance files should be refiled by the therapist.
6. The massage therapist shall ask each client if she would care for water before the massage, and give a bottle of water to each departing client.
7. The massage therapist shall ask each client if she would like to schedule her next appointment before she departs.
8. If the receptionist is busy assisting other clients, the therapist shall collect payment from the client and record it on the log sheet.
9. The massage therapist shall assist with answering the phone, filing, cleaning, or other duties as needed, in her spare time.
10. The massage therapist shall replace tissue, toilet paper, soap, or other supplies in the restroom when necessary.
11. The massage therapist shall take soiled laundry to the laundry room after changing the table and start the washer anytime there is a full load. She should check the laundry room during slow periods to see if sheets need folding or laundry needs transferring from the washer to the dryer.
12. The massage therapist is expected to see a maximum of five clients per day, unless prior arrangements have been made with the manager.

FIGURE 8-1 **An employment agreement for an employee.**

13. The massage therapist shall spend one full hour in the treatment room performing work on the client, unless a shorter session has been booked by mutual agreement.
14. The massage therapist is entitled to 30 minutes in between clients to change the linens, use the bathroom, and so forth.
15. The massage therapist is entitled to a one-hour lunch break, which will be scheduled by the receptionist to accommodate the daily flow of clients.
16. The massage therapist shall keep her own treatment room clean and uncluttered, and the trash emptied; the room is to be dusted and vacuumed at 5 p.m. after the last client leaves.
17. The massage therapist shall clean up after herself in the break room. Food should not be left in the refrigerator overnight.
18. The massage therapist shall assist clients with gift certificate, package, and retail purchases. No high-pressure selling is allowed.
19. The massage therapist shall display her framed license and certificate of liability insurance in the room she is working in at all times. A therapist going on an outcall should carry a photocopy of her license with her.
20. The massage therapist shall immediately report any sexual behavior by a client, any sexual behavior by any other therapist on the premises, or any injury to a client or other staff member, to the manager.
21. The massage therapist shall agree to give a notice of 14 days in the event she decides to leave the employment of Charm City Spa Bliss.
22. The massage therapist acknowledges that she is to punch the time clock when coming and going from the job, and to sign the time card by the close of business on Thursday in order to be paid at the close of business on Friday. Failure to sign the time card will result in payment being delayed until the following Friday.

I, _Billie Jean Smith_ , acknowledge that the management of Charm City Spa Bliss has thoroughly discussed this employment agreement with me, and verify that any questions I have about the conditions of this agreement have been answered. I hereby enter into this employment agreement with Charm City Spa Bliss effective date <u>12/10/10</u> for the pay rate of <u>$25</u> per hour for <u>30</u> hours per week.

Employee's Signature   *Billie Jean Smith*

Manager's Signature   *Monty P. Dickerson*

FIGURE 8-1 (*Continued*).

Paying for Worker's Compensation

Depending on the number of people you employ, you may have other financial obligations in addition to paying salaries. Worker's compensation is a type of insurance intended to cover your workers in case of job-related injury, illness, or occupational disease. In 2009, Texas became the last of the 50 states in which covering worker's compensation payments is required by law. Each state has an employee threshold; you may have a certain number of employees before you are obligated as the employer to purchase the insurance, and in some states, that number is as low as three. Check with your state Employment Security Commission to find out the obligation that applies to you.

Going with the Flow

According to the U.S. Department of Labor, the demand for massage therapists is expected to increase 20% by the year 2016, growing faster than the average of all other occupations.

Paying for Unemployment Compensation

During the Great Depression (1929–1939), the federal government implemented the Federal Unemployment Tax, an insurance plan employers pay into that is intended to help workers who through no fault of their own have lost their jobs. Even though it is a federally mandated program, each state has its own rules and schedules of unemployment payments concerning displaced workers, including the employee threshold at which employers must start paying the tax. If you hire only one employee, chances are you don't have to pay it, but if you grow to the point of having several employees, check with your state Employment Security Commission to find out if you are obligated to pay unemployment compensation tax.

In order to qualify to receive the insurance payments, a worker must have worked a certain number of weeks during the year and must also be out actively looking for employment. Being fired for reasons such as using drugs on the job or chronic absenteeism and lateness will cause an unemployment claim to be denied. Employers who don't have any claims filed against them for unemployment receive credits in their account.

As a self-employed business owner, you are not entitled to receive unemployment benefits if you go out of business, unless you have incorporated and made yourself an employee of the business. Check with your tax professional. Independent contractors are not eligible for unemployment benefits either because they are considered to be self-employed.

Providing Employee Benefits

If you have employees, you are not obligated to provide employee benefits, but you may wish to. Benefits can give your company the status of being a better place to work, thereby attracting dedicated workers. Here are some examples of benefits an employer could provide:

- Health insurance, with the company paying at least part of the monthly premiums
- Uniforms
- Employee meals
- Paid vacations
- Paid holidays
- Sick days
- Maternity leave
- Day care for worker's children
- Funeral leave
- Tuition for continuing education
- Paying for membership at a gym or health club
- A profit sharing plan, matching employee contributions to an Individual Retirement Account (IRA), or other type of retirement benefits

When you're first starting out in business, you probably won't be able to offer many, or any, employee benefits. However, it's something to keep in mind and work toward in the future.

Independent Contractors

Independent contractors are self-employed individuals who conduct their work in your place of business. The IRS code states that people who follow an independent trade, business, or profession, in which they offer their services to the public, are generally not employees. However, whether someone is an employee or an independent contractor depends on the facts in each case. The earnings of an independent contractor are subject to self-employment tax, as mentioned in Chapter 7.

An independent contractor may be paid an hourly rate, a commission, or percentage of the price of the work she performs, or a certain flat rate per client, regardless of the type of massage or spa treatment. Independent contractors are not entitled to receive any benefits. Guidelines set forth by the IRS determine whether a worker is an employee or an independent contractor. They are as follows:

- Behavioral: Does the company have the right to control what the worker does, and how the worker does his job?
- Financial: Does the payer determine how the worker is paid, whether or not he is reimbursed for expenses, and whether he provides his own equipment and supplies?
- Relationship: Are there written contracts? Does the worker receive any benefits? Is the work vital to the business?

The IRS states that these guidelines are not black and white, and that there may be overlap in the conditions determining whether one is an employee or an independent contractor. If there is any doubt, you can submit Form SS-8 to the IRS, and they will make a decision about the worker's status, based on your answers to a questionnaire.

If you use an independent contractor, you do not withhold any taxes from her pay. You are obligated to have her complete Form W-9, Request for Taxpayer Identification Number and Certification, when she begins working in your establishment. At the end of the year, you should provide her with Form 1099-Misc, Miscellaneous Income. You are also obligated, as the business owner, to furnish copies of these forms to the IRS. It helps them keep track of freelance workers.

Many employers choose to have independent contractors because it relieves them of a lot of responsibility in the tax and paperwork departments. Just bear in mind that an independent contractor is a self-employed individual who practices massage therapy on your premises. You can't have her wash the windows or scrub the toilet. You can, of course, require her to clean up after herself and change her own linens, but you can't make her mop the lobby or take over desk duty without crossing the line between independent contractor and employee. You don't have to provide her equipment, massage cream, or other supplies. A sample employment agreement for an independent contractor appears in Figure 8-2. Notice the differences with the employee contract (see Fig. 8-1).

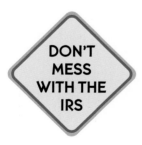

Be particularly careful in determining that a worker is an independent contractor. If the IRS were to audit you and deem that the worker was in fact an employee, you would be liable for the tax that should have been withheld from the worker's pay, including any penalties and interest imposed by the IRS.

INTERVIEWING, HIRING, AND FIRING

It's essential to be thorough and conscientious when interviewing potential candidates to work in your business. You don't want any surprises after someone has already been accepted into your company, especially something that might have been a deal-breaker, had you discovered it during the interview process. Part of that process includes checking the employment and character references of any

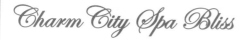

2700 Palmetto Boulevard
Tidal Creek, Texas 20202
950-230-4444

Job Description for Massage Therapist (Independent Contractor)

Charm City Spa Bliss, Inc. expects the following duties and observation of the following rules from the massage therapists we utilize as independent contractors:

1. The massage therapist shall put circles in the appointment book under her name when she is available to work and draw a line through the column on the days and hours she will not be available.
2. The massage therapist shall wear the scrubs we provide with the Charm City Spa Bliss logo on them at all times when on duty. The scrubs will be left here at the end of the shift to be laundered.
3. No high-heels or bare feet are permitted at the office. Shoe soles must be made of rubber or other quiet material.
4. The massage therapist shall greet the client in the lobby and take her to the treatment room to conduct the intake interview in private. The massage therapist shall inform each client of her right to privacy by giving her a HIPAA brochure. Any aftercare instructions should be given to the client while she is still in the privacy of the treatment room.
5. The massage therapist shall pull the client's file prior to her arrival and write complete SOAP notes as soon as the client departs. All client files are given to the receptionist at the end of the session.
6. The massage therapist shall ask each client if she would care for water before the massage, and should give a bottle of water to each departing client.
7. The massage therapist shall collect payment for the treatment and record it on the log sheet.
8. The massage therapist shall take her own soiled laundry to the laundry room after changing the table.
9. The massage therapist shall display her framed license and her liability insurance certificate in the room she is working in at all times, and if doing outcalls, should carry a photocopy with her.
10. The massage therapist is expected to see a maximum of five clients per day, unless prior arrangements have been made with the manager.
11. The massage therapist shall immediately report any sexual behavior by a client, or any injury to a client, to the manager.
12. The massage therapist shall turn in her invoice by the end of business on Thursday for payment each Friday by 12 p.m.

I, _Bobbie Jo Smith_, acknowledge that the management of Charm City Spa Bliss has thoroughly discussed this independent contractor agreement with me, and verify that any questions I have about the conditions of this agreement have been answered. I hereby enter into this independent contractor agreement with Charm City Spa Bliss effective date _12/10/10_ for the pay rate of _50% commission_ for the massage services I perform.

Employee's Signature   *Bobbie Jo Smith*

Manager's Signature   *Monty P. Dickerson*

FIGURE 8-2   **An employment agreement for an independent contractor.**

candidate. When you check someone's job references, chances are you won't get the information you're looking for in much detail. In accordance with privacy laws, basically the only thing an employer can tell you about a former employee is whether or not the person is eligible to be rehired.

Of course, you're taking a chance with anybody you don't know—or, for that matter, anybody you do know. If you've never worked with your best friend, for instance, and she came into your business, you might find that she has an entirely different persona at work than the one you're used to. The same goes for family members. A family-owned business works out well for some people, while others couldn't imagine going to work with relatives all day, every day. When you interview someone, naturally you want to find out what she'll bring to the table in terms of skills and experience. But the real purpose of an interview is to get a feel for the person, in order to tell whether or not she will be a good fit for your business.

Avoiding Discrimination

CAUTION

Be sure to keep in mind that when interviewing a candidate, you should never ask any questions that are discriminatory. Sometimes it's hard to avoid because it can happen unintentionally. Nevertheless, it can still set you up for a lawsuit to do so. Federal and state regulations prohibit questions being asked about the following:

- Race or ethnic background
- Color of skin
- National origin
- Gender
- Sexual orientation
- Religion
- Age
- Disability
- Marital or family status

There are many examples of potentially troublesome opportunities for discrimination. For instance, as massage therapists, we've all seen people who suffer from fibromyalgia, and we know that some days they just can't get out of bed, or if they do, they're not at their best. Would you want to hire a therapist knowing she has fibromyalgia? If that would keep you from hiring her, you would be discriminating against someone who has a disability, even though she may not have what most people think of as a visible handicap. Would you hire a blind massage therapist? A blind person's touch can often be more sensitive because it's used in place of his eyes; in fact, in some areas of the world, the blind are the only ones allowed to do massage.

The caveat to all this is that the Americans with Disabilities Act, intended to protect handicapped workers from discrimination, exempts businesses with fewer than 15 employees from compliance with the law. However, from a humanitarian standpoint, you wouldn't want to be guilty of that type of discrimination, even if the law doesn't apply to you.

A person's religion or sexual orientation isn't any of your business. But if you are a fundamentalist Christian, would you be willing to employ a pagan, a Muslim, or a gay person? If you had it in mind to employ someone young and fashionable, and a grandmotherly type showed up to apply, would you consider her for the job or automatically discount her, regardless of the skills she has, because of her appearance? What about overweight people? Would you refuse to hire someone who doesn't fit your idea of health and beauty?

REALITY CHECKPOINT

I have visited spas where the staff members look as if they were cloned: all under 30, all perfectly tanned, all beautiful, and all skinny to the point where I wanted to hand them a sandwich. Such places are missing out on a wealth of talent by practicing staff profiling.

What You Can and Should Ask

Refer again to your wish list, and ask the candidate if she's willing to work the days and hours you have in mind. Here are some other basic questions you should ask to determine suitability:

- What is your educational background?
- Describe your previous experience in massage therapy.
- Are you licensed or nationally certified? (Explain your state requirements, or whatever is important to you or your business. You may want someone who is nationally certified, even if there is no licensure law in your state.)
- Do you have your own liability insurance, and if not, are you willing to obtain it before coming to work here?
- If I needed someone to cover during different days or hours than what we agree upon, would you be able to accommodate that?
- What type of compensation are you seeking?
- Do you want an employee position or an independent contractor position?
- Why did you leave your last position?
- Would they rehire you there?
- Are you willing to obtain a copy of your criminal record and turn it over to me as part of your employment process?
- Are you looking for a long-term position, or is this temporary?

It is perfectly within your right as an employer to ask for a criminal record check, and you should. There are predators out there, and some of them infiltrate our profession. Some state massage boards require a criminal record check as a prelude to licensure, so if you operate in such a state, a license can be accepted as proof that the person had nothing on his record that was serious enough to prevent him from getting one. Some employers also test potential employees for illegal drug use, and that's usually done at the employer's expense.

ROADSIDE ASSISTANCE

The fact that someone wants to work in my massage business for a year or two before striking out on his own is not a deal-breaker for me, although it might be for you. I welcome the chance to mentor someone who's new to the business, and there are enough aching bodies to go around. If he eventually leaves and some of his clients follow him to his new setting, more will come along to take their place. I've found that asking the question about permanent or temporary employment sometimes takes candidates by surprise, but I let them know that it's not going to prevent me from hiring them if they eventually plan to be on their own. I just like to know what I'm getting into when I agree to take someone on.

Noncompete Agreement

It is a common practice for employers in the massage profession and spa industry to get workers to sign what's known as a noncompete agreement, stating that they will not open up a business nearby, or go to work for a local competitor, for a certain time period after leaving their employment. Having such a contract is an option for you if you are concerned that one of your therapists leaving and opening up a competing business could shut you down. However, attorneys warn that none but the most iron-clad agreements will stand up in court; the most common reasons such agreements are ruled invalid are because they demand too much time, cover too wide a geographic area, and/or place too many limitations on the type of business that can be conducted. An example of a noncompete agreement

Charm City Spa Bliss

2700 Palmetto Boulevard
Tidal Creek, Texas 20202
950-230-4444

Non-Compete Agreement

I, Billie Jean Smith, hereby agree that for a period of six months, commencing on the last day of my employment at Charm City Spa Bliss, I will not work as a massage therapist, either on my own or for someone else, within a 10-mile radius of Charm City Spa Bliss. I further acknowledge that I am prohibited from removing any client files or records of any kind from the premises of Charm City Spa Bliss. I further acknowledge that my violation of this agreement will result in suit being brought against me for breach of contract.

Employee's Signature Billie Jean Smith Date 10/11/2011

Manager's Signature Monty P. Dickerson Date 10/11/2011

FIGURE 8-3 A noncompete agreement.

appears in Figure 8-3. It can also be contained within the employment or independent contractor agreement, and in that case is referred to as a noncompete clause.

Noncompete agreements are not legal in every state. The safest thing to do is to have an attorney look over the document before you commit yourself to an employer who is insisting that you sign a noncompete agreement.

ALTERNATE ROUTES

Employees and Independent Contractors

If you live in a rural area or small town, you may want to think twice before signing a contract that contains a noncompete agreement. If the job doesn't work out, would it be a burden on you to travel farther out of your way to work? If you plan to work somewhere else for awhile as a prelude to opening your own business, a noncompete agreement could ruin those plans, if you were thinking about setting up shop in the same town. Even though such agreements are often ruled invalid, it could still cost you time and attorney fees to prove your case. Weigh your options.

Business Partners

A noncompete agreement is much more likely to be enforceable by law on a business partner than on an employee. The more senior the position one has in a company, or the extent of his access to company secrets, the more likely the agreement could be ruled valid by the court.

The Art of Firing

Sometimes it's necessary to let a staff member go. If you discover an employee has committed a blatant offense, such as an ethics violation that could cause you to be the subject of a lawsuit, or stealing from the cash register, feeling upset and angry is natural, and you're well within your rights to fire the offender on the spot.

Most of the time, firing someone without prior warning is not recommended. If a staff member has violated the rules of your business, or if her performance isn't up to standard, giving her a verbal warning, followed by a written warning, protects you, the employer. Documenting any problems in writing, conducting an evaluation session with the person, and giving her a definite timeframe in which to turn things around—all of this is proof that you treated the worker fairly in the event of a lawsuit.

In spite of being competent, reliable and punctual, neatly dressed, and courteous to clients, for some intangible reason the person might not be the right fit for your business. That makes it more difficult to let him go, but even though he isn't right for your company, he may be exactly what someone else is looking for. In a case like this, you could offer the person assistance in finding another job, or give him a letter of reference.

Firing someone is never pleasant, regardless of the reason. Be prepared for a reaction. It might be anger and cursing, or grief, or tears and begging to keep the job. You have to stand your ground and say that your mind is made up. The experience will probably be just as emotional for you as it is for the departing staff member.

Firing should always take place in private, out of earshot of other staff members. However, you might decide to have one trusted colleague in attendance as a witness to the proceedings. Avoid embarrassing the person; being fired in itself is humiliating enough.

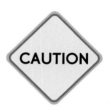

POSTCARDS from the HIGHWAY   Ann Catlin

In 1979, I began my career as an occupational therapist. For the next 30 years, I witnessed how people of all ages cope when faced with serious disease, injury, or disability. The reactions of those dealing with these life-changing circumstances are as individual as the people themselves. But no matter what the person's age, condition, or the impact on his or her life, I noticed something that affected them all—that human connection holds the power to heal.

I can remember one time when I was in a therapy session with a woman who had suffered a severe stroke. As an OT, my job was to teach her how to dress herself using one hand because the stroke had left her left arm paralyzed. She was so frustrated by this task that she began to cry. I stopped what I was "supposed" to be doing and just sat with her, holding her arm while she cried. At that moment, just being present while I touched her was what she needed. Her tears and my acceptance and support allowed her to move past her grief just a little bit. This woman was one of my early teachers about how touch heals. I've never forgotten that lesson.

My career took a turn in 1998 when I entered massage school. It was while I was a massage student that I discovered Compassionate Touch, an approach specifically designed for people dealing with the effects of aging, disease, or disability. It was then I realized that I could serve the same population I had known all those years—only this time, I'll offer the gift of my touch!

I decided to specialize in serving elders in facility care and those in hospice care. That was the best decision I could have made. Working with this special population is a personally rewarding experience. The gift of touch for those in eldercare and hospice uplifts individual lives and reclaims the human touch in caregiving.

(continued)

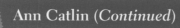

Ann Catlin (*Continued*)

I have been blessed with the privilege of teaching Compassionate Touch to others who feel drawn to serve those in later life stages. This offers a viable and growing scope of practice for massage therapists. Long-term care and hospice settings are seeing the value of massage for frail elders, those with dementia, and the dying. It is my privilege to be a leader in the effort to bring massage into eldercare and hospice settings.

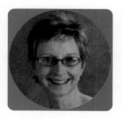

Ann Catlin, LMT, OTR, has 30 years' experience with elders in facility care, persons with disabilities, and the dying, using her skills as both a massage therapist and an occupational therapist. She is the owner/director of the Center for Compassionate Touch LLC, an organization that provides Compassionate Touch training for health professionals across the nation. She is the author of numerous articles in massage publications and the creator of an instructional massage DVD. Her vision is a world where a healing presence in the form of touch is commonplace and every elder, every ill and dying person, has access to the benefits of Compassionate Touch. Visit her website at www.compassionate-touch.org.

SUGGESTED READINGS

Hamlet C. *How to Fire Someone.* http://www.ehow.com/how_4500247_fire-someone. html?ref=fuel&utm_source=yahoo&utm_medium=ssp&utm_campaign=yssp_art. Accessed 11/08/2009.

Internal Revenue Service. *Independent Contractor or Employee?* http://www.irs.gov/ businesses/small/article/0,id=99921,00.html. Accessed 11/08/2009.

MassageTherapy.com. Massage Profession Metrics. http://www.massagetherapy.com/ media/metricsgrowth.php#income. Accessed 11/08/2009.

U.S. Department of Labor. *Disability Resources: Employer Responsibilities.* http://www.dol. gov/dol/topic/disability/employersresponsibilities.htm. Accessed 11/08/2009.

U.S. Department of Labor. *Occupational Projections and Training Data.* Feb. 2008. http:// www.bls.gov/emp/optd/optd.pdf. Accessed 11/08/2009.

My Personal Journey

In this chapter, we've discussed working with other people in your business. Based on what you've learned about the differences between employees and independent contractors, and the options of having a student intern or a renter, write down your wish list of what type of person you would like to hire or work with, and which situation you think would suit you the best.

My goals _____
_____
_____

What's in my way? _____
_____
_____

What action can I take to remedy the situation? _____
_____
_____

One-year progress update _____
_____
_____

CHAPTER 9

Policies and Procedures

*I*ncidents should not govern policy; but, policy incidents.

NAPOLEON BONAPARTE

KEY CONCEPTS

Policies and procedures protect the business owner and serve as guidelines for operating a safe and efficient workplace.

- Established ethics codes and practice standards serve as a starting point for building your policies and procedures.

- Creating a convenient and easily accessible manual that you and your staff members can refer to is a necessity.

- Clarity, conciseness, and coherence are the hallmarks of effective policies and procedures.

- Some policies may be mandated by federal, state, or local laws.

- Policies and procedures for clients and staff members ensure that everyone is treated fairly and consistently.

- Policy issues should be documented, whether they concern clients, staff, or both.

- The policies and procedures manual is a work in progress that can evolve as you discover new problems or new options for dealing with situations.

Policies and procedures are guidelines for operating a safe and orderly workplace. They serve the purpose of making sure that people who patronize your business and the people who work for you, are treated fairly and consistently, and that everyone in the company has the same approach when it comes to handling different situations. Policies reflect the rules of a business; procedures reflect the implementation of those policies. Having, and adhering to, written policies and procedures can save your business if legal action is ever brought against you by a disgruntled employee or client.

BUILDING A POLICIES AND PROCEDURES MANUAL

I suggest you purchase a three-ring binder for your policies and procedures manual and keep it in a convenient, easily accessible place. Divide your manual into sections: one section for policies concerning clients and another for policies concerning personnel, if you already have or plan to have staff members. Include a table of contents and section tabs to make it easy to use. Including the policy statement within the procedure document will make your policy manual easier to write and more user-friendly.

Begin by stating the purpose of the policy: what issue or problem the policy addresses. Then write the policy itself, followed by the procedure that should be followed to resolve it.

It is also helpful to write a script to use as a guideline. You and your staff member will be holding a conversation with each other, or with someone else about the matter. That conversation should be as courteous, neutral, and nonjudgmental as possible, while at the same time addressing the problem in a direct manner. An example is shown in Figure 9-1, which includes a sample script and a blank template appears in Appendix A.

Let the Code of Ethics Be Your Guide

When you are considering policies and procedures, let the AMTA's code of ethics, as well as the NCBTMB's Standards of Practice, serve as the barometer for writing your guidelines (see Chapter 3). You are not borrowing the actual policies from the code, but you are following their *spirit*.

The primary purpose of ethics codes and practice standards is to make massage safe and effective for the public. Take those same principles and apply them to the important task of creating the policies and procedures for your business. Bear in mind that your objective is to make conducting business safe and effective for *you*, the business owner. Following ethical principles will help you develop policies and procedures that are in keeping with the highest standards of the massage and bodywork profession.

The Three Cs: Clarity, Conciseness, and Coherence

The three Cs are qualities to keep in mind when writing policies and procedures.

- *Clarity*: The policies and procedures are written in a way that is clear and straightforward.
- *Conciseness*: Each policy and every procedure is exact and brief; anyone consulting the manual shouldn't have any doubt about what action to take for the issue at hand.
- *Coherence*: There is a logical flow of information and consistency from one thought to another.

Ask several people to read the text of the manual for you. Ask for feedback on whether the policies and instructions for following procedures are clearly stated and easy to understand.

HELP JUST AHEAD

Legal Obligations

The policies and procedures of your business must be in line with federal, state, and local statutes. There are numerous laws that concern businesses, and many apply only to businesses with a minimum number of employees. Some of these obligations include compliance with the Equal Employment Opportunity Act, the Americans with Disabilities Act, the Immigration Reform Act, the Family Medical Leave Act, and

Main Street Massage: Policies and Procedures Manual

Situation:
A client has missed an appointment without calling to cancel.

Policy:
Clients are allowed one missed appointment without penalty. After the one allowance, a bill is sent for a missed appointment.

Procedure:
At the time of the missed appointment, the therapist the appointment was scheduled with should call the client. Politely inform the client that he or she missed a scheduled appointment, and try to reschedule. Inform the client that the cancellation policy of Main Street Massage is that unless we receive 24-hour notice of cancellation, he or she will be billed for the appointment, but that we are allowing one missed appointment without penalty. A sample script is below. Staff members should not argue with a client at any time and should always remain professional and courteous, regardless of what the client says. If a client is rude and argumentative, inform management immediately.

Sample Script:

Therapist:
Mrs. Johnson, this is Sally calling from Main Street Massage. You were scheduled for a 2:00 appointment today, and we are concerned that you didn't show up and didn't call to cancel.

Client:
Sorry, I got busy and forgot all about it.

Therapist:
We all do things like that from time to time. Would you like to reschedule the appointment?

Client:
Yes.

Therapist:
(Handle the rescheduling first, and thank her for rescheduling.) Mrs. Johnson, we do make one allowance for everyone, but I need to remind you that we have a 24-hour cancellation policy. In the future, if you miss an appointment without calling to cancel, we'll have to send you a bill. Do you need a reminder call the day before your appointment next time so that won't happen?

Client:
Yes, that would be a big help.

Therapist:
Thank you, Mrs. Johnson. Your appointment is set for _____ at _____, so I'll give you a call the day before. Have a nice day.

FIGURE 9-1   A sample page from a policies and procedures manual.

other federal mandates. If your business grows beyond a couple of employees, it's wise to obtain legal advice to make sure you are in compliance. Who knows—you just might become the next entrepreneur to give Massage Envy a run for their money!

Action Versus Reaction

Your policies and procedures will not be written the same as mine or the practitioner's across town, because different people have different reactions to situations.

You have to decide what policies suit you as a business owner and an individual, based on your own reaction to a given issue. One therapist may be very casual about no-shows; her reaction might be, "Oh, I guess it just wasn't meant to be for me to see that client today," and she might head out to go shopping or take a nap during the downtime. Another therapist might get upset about no-shows and bill for every missed appointment, because he has a strict budget and a waiting list of potential clients who are hoping for a cancellation.

You do not want to say or do something to a client or staff member that you will regret later. Having a written procedure in place for handling situations can keep you from reacting inappropriately in a moment of anger or confusion. When setting your policies, ask yourself a few questions:

- Am I comfortable with the policy?
- Is the policy discriminatory in any way?
- If the tables were turned and I was subject to this policy, would I think it was fair, or would I leave this business and never come back?

REALITY CHECKPOINT

Strive to create policies that are fair, and follow them.

Words of Wisdom
A positive action is always better than a negative reaction.

An Exception to (Almost) Every Rule

Policies and procedures are always written with the intent that they be respected and observed. However, common sense and/or compassion will sometimes override the policy manual.

If a client missed an appointment because of an unexpected death in the family, you would understand how he could forget an appointment at such an upsetting time, and you would not send him a bill. You might temporarily overlook the forgetfulness of an employee going through a family tragedy, or make allowances for a staff member who is grieving because she had to put her pet down yesterday. Rules are made to be broken—*sometimes.*

When Not to Make an Exception

Most times, the rules must be enforced. The only reasonable excuse for a staff member missing work without calling in is that she is in labor, in a coma, or something equally serious. There is never sufficient reason to tolerate sexual molestation, physical abuse, threats, or theft, for instance, from a client or a staff member. Such incidents must be dealt with swiftly and firmly.

Remember, policies and procedures are there to protect you, as the business owner, and to make your business run more safely and efficiently. Do not allow anyone to get away with behavior that could cause harm to you or your business.

A POLICY FOR EVERY PURPOSE

You would be surprised at how many circumstances there are that warrant having a written policy and procedure. If you are a lone practitioner with no intention of future expansion, you may think you do not have the need for written policies, but it will still serve you to have them. You may not need personnel policies, but you will still need policies for issues that arise with clients. Taking the time to create policies and procedures at the beginning of your business means you will have the tools in place to handle a difficult situation when it presents itself, instead of wondering what to do and second-guessing yourself after the fact.

A policies and procedures manual is usually a work in progress. A new situation will arise that you have not previously thought of, or through trial and error, advances in technology, or suggestion from a staff member, and you might learn a new way to handle a problem. Update and revise your manual as often as needed. Date each revision, and document the reason why it was made. If a policy is accidentally violated, or a procedure is handled in the wrong way, do your best to minimize the damage, document what happened, and vow to do better the next time.

Going with the Flow

A write-in survey in *Massage Magazine* asked therapists to share how they handle no-shows and last-minute cancellations. Not surprisingly, the majority of therapists do not do anything about it; one responded that he gives the client a lecture; very few stated that they had clear, written cancellation policies. One therapist commented, "We are teaching people how to treat us by not having clear policies and procedures. How can we expect anyone to respect us if we don't respect ourselves and ask for respect in return?"

Policies and Procedures for Client Relations

Many client-related issues require clear policies and procedures. Consider these situations, and start thinking about how you might handle each one:

- A client shows up late for her appointment.
- A client does not show up at all and does not call to cancel his appointment.
- A client cancels an appointment without giving ample notice.
- A client writes a bad check to your business.
- A client says or does something inappropriately sexual.
- A client trips on the rug and gets injured at your workplace.
- A client claims that you or a staff member injured him during a bodywork session.
- A client (or a stranger) solicits you to support a charity or other cause by giving gift certificates or free services.
- A client brings a child along with her who is loud and unruly enough to disturb other clients.
- A client brings a pet to an appointment.
- A client appears to be under the influence of drugs or alcohol.
- A client has insurance that will pay for massage.
- A client is involved in a workers' compensation case.
- A client is involved in a personal injury case.
- A client is a minor.
- A client has a contraindication that requires a doctor's release to receive massage but does not have the release.
- A client leaves his cell phone on in the building or even during the session.
- A client claims to have lost or misplaced something valuable in your workplace.
- A client wants to bring another person into the treatment room during the massage.
- A client makes a complaint (the massage was not what she expected, the room was too cold, or something else she did not mention until after the session was over).
- A client accuses you or a staff member of sexual impropriety or another ethics violation.
- A client shows up for her appointment and is obviously sick.
- A client has a skin condition or other contraindication that was observed after the session started, but he did not mention it on the intake form or during the interview.

- A client shows up dirty and/or smelly for her appointment.
- A client wants to redeem a gift certificate that has expired.
- A client wants a refund.
- A client wants to transfer a gift certificate or package deal to someone else.
- A client asks for a discount.

Consider a couple of the possibilities. For example, your cancellation policy might look something like this:

> Clients who give less than 24 hours notice in the event of a cancellation will be billed in full for the missed appointment.

The procedure is to send the client a bill and a friendly reminder of your cancellation policy. Here is another version:

> Clients who give less than 12 hours notice of a cancellation will be billed at half-price for the missed appointment and will be required to guarantee all future appointments with a credit card.

The procedure is to send the client a bill, along with a friendly reminder of your cancellation policy and a notice about guaranteeing future appointments with a credit card.

A sample form letter for billing for a missed appointment is shown in Figure 9-2. A blank template appears in Appendix A.

ROADSIDE ASSISTANCE

In my state, due to the fact that my staff members are all independent contractors, it is against the law for my business to bill anyone for a missed appointment, unless the appointment was personally with me. The contractors may send the client a bill if they choose to; it is at their discretion. I have provided the independent contractors a form letter asking for payment that they can send to repeat offenders. The law may be different in your state, and you can check that out before setting your policy.

Informing Clients

You cannot expect people to adhere to your policies unless they know what they are. You are actually doing yourself and others a favor when you inform them up front about your expectations. Remember: Successful relationships are built on clear and direct communication.

Obviously, you cannot give a copy of your policies and procedures manual to everyone who comes in the door. However, there are a number of ways to inform clients about your policies:

- Include policy statements about cancellations, no-shows, and late arrivals on your intake form; reiterate them verbally to clients on their first visit, and have them initial the paragraphs to acknowledge their understanding.
- Include the same information on your brochures.
- Put nicely lettered signs in the waiting area, at the front desk, and in the treatment rooms stating your cancellation and late arrival policies.
- Add your cancellation policy to the message on your answering machine or voice mail.
- Include the policies on your website.
- State your policies in every issue of your newsletter.

Main Street Massage
101 Main St.
Big Creek, NC 28012

Maddy Tempo
800 Pippin St.
Big Creek, NC 28012

October 9, 2010

Dear Ms. Tempo,

Please submit payment of $75.00 for the appointment you missed without notice of cancellation on Friday, October 6.

It is our policy to collect payment for missed appointments after the first offense, as stated on our intake form and on your appointment card.

While we value your business, and regret having to collect money for a session you didn't receive, we must do so in order to protect the income of our staff members. We have a waiting list of clients who want to get an appointment in the event of a cancellation, and if we have the required 24-hour notice, we can fill the appointment with someone else. Please note that future appointments must be guaranteed with a credit card. You are also welcome, in the future, to send a friend or family member to take your scheduled appointment.

Thank you for understanding that we must enforce this policy.

Regards,

Cameron Jobe

Cameron Jobe, Owner

FIGURE 9-2 A sample form letter for billing for a missed appointment.

- Each time a person calls for an appointment, especially if it is a new client, be sure to state your cancellation policy.
- If you use appointment cards, or have business cards with appointment space printed on the back, have the cancellation policy printed on the card.
- Gift certificates should include this kind of statement: "Canceling appointments with less than 24 hours notice will result in this certificate being forfeited."

You know the old saying about reading the fine print. Do not print your policies in a font so small that people cannot read it.

Enforcing Client Policies

Practitioners sometimes feel hesitant about enforcing a policy, especially when it comes to money and especially when they are just starting out in business. If that sounds like you, get over it! You need to protect your income, and that of your staff. Starting your business with policies in place, and upholding them from the beginning, will make your business run smoothly. Do not let things slide, and try hard to avoid enforcing policies after the fact with people who have already been allowed to take advantage of you.

The key to enforcing your policies is to be polite but firm. Let us say a client asks something like this: "Do I really have to pay the full amount even though I was twenty minutes late?" The correct answer is a polite version of this: "Yes, because I had the whole hour reserved just for you. I could have taken another half-hour appointment had I known you weren't going to be here until 12:30."

Be consistent with policy enforcement. If you allow one client to extend the expiration date on her gift certificate, you must allow the next client who asks for the same courtesy. Avoid playing favorites. There will be the occasional client who gets mad and does not come back; let her go. You will be better off with clients who will respect you and abide by your policies.

INFORMATION AHEAD

ROADSIDE ASSISTANCE

My policy concerning no-shows is to give everyone the benefit of the doubt—one time. After that, I insist on getting paid. I am not rude about it. I call the person and say, "Fred, you missed your massage appointment with me today, and I didn't get a cancellation call. I'll let you off the hook this time, but if that happens again, I'll have to bill you for the appointment." Fred apologizes and says it will not happen again. After a polite reminder, I have found people generally comply.

We keep a "must-pay-up-front" list of clients who have to guarantee their appointments with a credit card due to their past failure to observe our cancellation policy. When one of them calls, I politely say, "Carolyn, you have missed two appointments in the past couple of months without giving us a cancellation notice. I'm sorry, but we can't save that spot for you unless you guarantee it with a credit card. It's a policy we have in order to protect our business from losing income. Your card will not be charged unless you fail to give us a 24-hour notice." In the years I have had this policy, the majority of clients comply.

EXPLORATIONS

Thousands of massage therapists have websites, and many list their late arrival and cancellation policies online. Spend some time browsing websites, to see how other professionals are handling cancellations, lateness, and no-shows in their place of business.

Documenting Client Issues

Documentation concerning a client is kept in the client's file. Whether someone is chronically late, or had an accident on the property, or has acted inappropriately sexual, should be noted in the file, along with a written record of the steps you or a staff member took in attempting to address the problem. Print these incident reports on brightly colored paper, to distinguish them from the rest of the file. When you document something concerning a client that other staff should be aware of, such as an accident or a complaint, the colored paper will make it visible and easy to find. A sample incident report is shown in Figure 9-3, and a blank template appears in Appendix A.

Centennial Sports Massage
243 Oakland St.
Davidson, MS 45098

Incident Report

Persons involved: **Date:** December 18, 2010

_____James Earwood_____client

____Amber Smith, Will Byers_____staff member(s)

Place where the incident occurred: The front porch steps of Centennial Sports Massage.

When the incident occurred: 1:45 p.m.

Description of the incident: Mr. Earwood was leaving the office after his session with me (Amber Smith) when I heard him yelling for help. Mr. Earwood was on the concrete at the bottom of the stairs in front of the building, holding onto his ankle. He stated he had missed a step and feared he had broken his ankle. I asked him if he felt he could stand with assistance and he said he could. He was in obvious pain. Will Byers, another therapist who was about to leave for the day, offered to take Mr. Earwood to the emergency room. Will drove his car up onto the sidewalk and he and I assisted Mr. Earwood into the car. Will took Mr. Earwood to Memorial Hospital and stayed with him until his wife arrived. Mrs. Earwood called the office several hours later to report that the ankle was in fact broken, and that Mr. Earwood had been discharged from the hospital and was resting at home. Since Monica Allgood, the owner of the business, was out of town, I informed Mrs. Earwood that Monica would be in touch with her when she returned the following day.

Signature:_____Amber Smith,_____Date: 12/18/2011

Addendum: Amber Smith informed me of the accident Mr. Earwood had at our office yesterday. I first spoke with Bill Moore, the insurance agent, who assured me that my policy would cover Mr. Earwood's medical bills and his time missed from work due to the accident. I called Mr. Earwood and assured him that he would be taken care of. I told him that Bill Moore would be calling him in the next couple of days about our insurance coverage and he said that was fine. Bill will follow up with me within a week.

Signature: _Monica Allgood_ Date: 12/19/2011

FIGURE 9-3   A sample client incident report.

Policies and Procedures for Staff Relations

The employment agreements for employees and independent contractors in Chapter 8 can be used as the jumping-off point for writing your personnel policies. However, you need to expand on them and write policies that spell out exactly what behavior you expect of the people working in your office. Here are some common staff issues that require a policy:

- A staff member commits a violation of the code of ethics.
- A staff member fails to observe HIPAA protocols, such as privacy precautions during intake and exit interviews.
- A staff member chronically arrives late for work or leaves early.
- A staff member has excessive absences.
- A staff member fails to maintain licensure and/or liability insurance.
- A staff member does not follow the protocol for greeting clients and assisting departing clients.
- A staff member is rude, either on the phone or in person.
- A staff member gets injured on the job.

Other issues affecting staff members that should be part of the policies and procedures manual include

- Performance evaluations
- Payment procedures
- Tipping
- Dress code
- Personal items in the workplace
- Bringing children to the office
- Service expectations
- Housekeeping expectations
- Record-keeping expectations
- Marketing expectations, such as whether independent contractors are allowed to, or required to, advertise themselves
- Moonlighting
- Using the office phone or other equipment for personal use
- Discounting services
- Performing community service
- Giving free massage to friends or family members on the premises

If someone other than you will have authority to hire and fire, be sure the procedures for doing so are in the policy manual.

ROADSIDE ASSISTANCE

I have more than a dozen practitioners on staff, some of whom share rooms because of the different shifts they work. I ask them to observe a limit of one or two personal items in the treatment rooms, in addition to their lotions and potions. There is nothing wrong with having a picture or two, or a couple of personal mementoes, but a treatment room should not look like a booth at a flea market. A cluttered space is not conducive to a calming experience.

Informing Staff Members

If you have staff members, you want to feel secure that they can handle things in the right manner when you are away from the office. The policies and procedures manual should not be hidden on a back shelf in the storage closet; it should be easily accessible at all times. It is even better to provide all staff members with their own copy.

Avoid having your manual sound like a broken record of "don't, don't, don't." Instead of using negatives like "don't do this, don't do that," state *positively* what action is expected.

When new persons join your business, they should be expected to read the manual. Have them sign a statement acknowledging that they have read it and understand the policies and procedures of the workplace and your business.

Enforcing Staff Policies

As the owner of the business, your responsibilities are to effectively communicate your expectations to staff members and to lead by example. If your policy manual states that staff members are not allowed to go around the office in their bare feet, do not go around in yours.

Remember that one of the main purposes of having policies and procedures is for ensuring that everyone is treated fairly and consistently. We are emotional human beings, and of course we like some people more than others. However, as a business owner, you have to keep in mind the importance of treating everyone the same, regardless of your personal feelings.

For instance, if you discipline an employee for failing to follow the dress code, you must discipline every employee who fails to follow the dress code in the same way. If you fire a staff member for coming into work late three times in a month, you must fire the next one who comes into work late three times in a month. Failure to do so is an invitation to legal action by an employee who might feel he or she was singled out and treated unfairly.

Documenting Staff Issues

Documenting policy issues with a staff member is just as important as documenting an incident involving a client. If a staff member has committed an offense you consider serious enough to discuss with her, record the details of your discussion and put that report in her personnel file; have the person sign an acknowledgment that she has received a verbal warning about the situation. Doing so can protect you from legal action down the road, if the circumstances warrant firing the person sometime in the future. You may want to have a third person present when you are discussing a disciplinary matter with a staff member. Lawsuits are sometimes a "he-said/she-said" situation, and having a witness provides you, the business owner, with additional protection.

SECURITY CHECKPOINT AHEAD

Personnel files should be kept in a secure location. They should not be available to other staff members, unless you have a designated secretary or office manager who should be allowed to access them.

James Waslaski

People need to set powerful goals to tap into their spiritual blueprint for success in life as well as business. Successful people find great mentors and align themselves with capable people. They maintain a balance in life in terms of spirituality, family, employment, and giving, as well as in physical, emotional, social, learning, and financial areas. Successful people turn challenges into opportunities.

I strongly believe in the *be/do/have* theory of life. *Be* committed to *doing* what it takes to *have* what you want. Be grateful, and strive to be increasingly more humble. Learn to create or find value in all things.

I recommend getting involved in personal growth seminars and taking an active role in helping others.

We all play certain tapes in our mind all day long. I live by the fact that the thoughts we give energy to, and pay attention to, will always become our reality. Based on the law of attraction, we draw into our life what we consistently think about.

Finally, do not measure success in terms of money and material things, because financial freedom will actually be a manifestation of tapping into what we are passionate about. I believe that strong intuition will guide each person to his or her spiritual blueprint for success. Pay attention to your heart and to the powerful intuitive message inside, and you will discover "true" success. Enjoy the journey to making a positive difference in the world. That is what success is really all about.

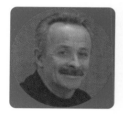

James Waslaski is an internationally respected lecturer and author in the fields of chronic pain and sports injuries. Prior to becoming a massage therapist, James spent 20 years working as a paramedic and in trauma centers, while teaching emergency medical courses. His unique structural and multidisciplinary bodywork approach has been taught all over the world, and he is consistently one of the most popular presenters at state, national, and international conventions. He is the author of numerous articles, books, manuals, and a series of DVDs. In 2008, James was inducted into the Massage Therapy Hall of Fame. Visit his website at www.orthomassage.net.

SUGGESTED READINGS

Gegax T, Bolsta P. *The Big Book of Small Business: You Don't Have to Run Your Business by the Seat of Your Pants.* New York, NY: Harper Collins, 2007.

Heet L. Guide to Company Policies. http://www.work.com/company-policies-2269/. Accessed 11/11/2008.

Institute for Therapeutic Massage, Inc. Industry Trends: Massage Therapy. http://www.massageprogram.com/goto/1/5/34/29/. Accessed 11/11/2009.

Onofrio J. Cancellation Policies for Massage Therapists. http://thebodyworker.com/massage_blog/cancellation-policies/. Accessed 12/03/2008.

Weltman B, Silberman J. *Small Business Survival Book: 12 Surefire Ways for Your Business to Survive and Thrive.* New York, NY: John Wiley & Sons, 2006.

Write Express. How to Write a Policy Manual. http://www.writeexpress.com/or/employee-manual/Employee-Manual-eBook.pdf. Accessed 11/11/2009.

My Personal Journey

In this chapter, we have discussed developing policies and procedures for your business. Based on the lists of potential issues with clients and staff, start creating your policy manual. If you are still in school, or not prepared to go into business yet, start creating it anyway—so you will have your manual ready on opening day.

My goals _____

_____

_____

What is in my way? _____

_____

_____

What action can I take to remedy the situation? _____

_____

_____

One-year progress update _____

_____

_____

PART IV

Traffic Signals

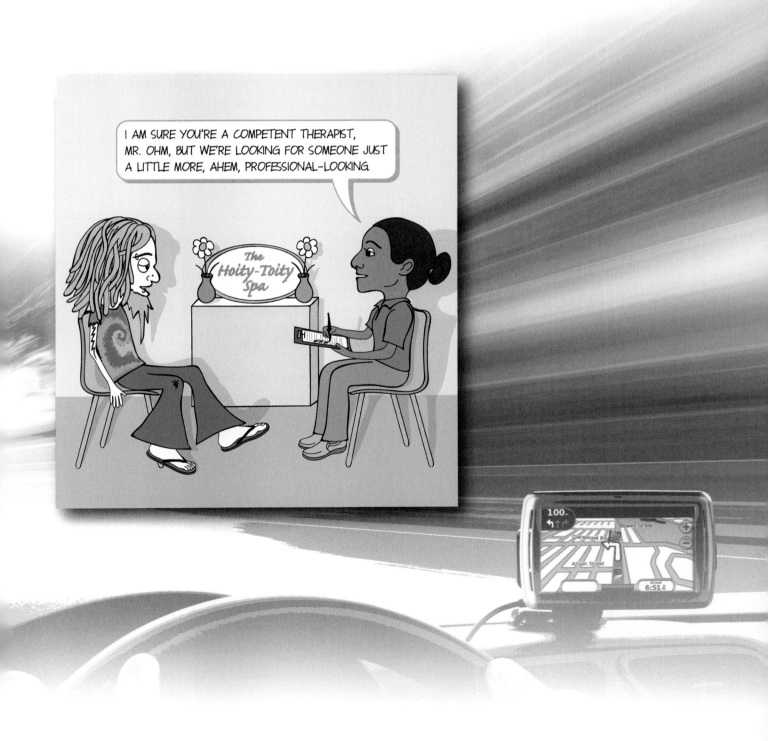

Projecting Professionalism

> *A professional is a person who can do his best at a time when he doesn't particularly feel like it.*
>
> ALISTAIR COOKE

KEY CONCEPTS

- Projecting professionalism depends on a combination of professional training and acquired skills that anyone can learn.

- A practitioner who obtains massage therapy education and credentials, even though her state does not require any, sets herself apart as a professional massage therapist.

- An untrained therapist might be uninformed about the contraindications for massage.

- Projecting a professional image inspires client confidence, as well as the confidence of peers and other practitioners in the health care community; it can help you get referrals.

- Dressing like a businessperson is part of projecting professionalism.

- Communicating in a professional manner involves the correct use of grammar and medical terminology when speaking, as well as cultivating listening skills.

- Practicing social and business etiquette means using good manners in all situations.

- When you assume professional and personal responsibility, you gain respect from your community.

- A professional is constantly striving for self-improvement through continuing education and personal development.

- Roadblocks to professionalism are behaviors that one can choose to avoid.

OPPORTUNITIES AHEAD

There are many qualities that contribute to whether or not a person projects professionalism. The way a therapist dresses, his speech and other communication skills, his manners, and the decor and cleanliness of his treatment room—everything affects the way he's perceived by the public and, just as importantly, by other professionals. People constantly judge our character, our competence, and our commitment based on the way we present ourselves. As with any service-based business, public perception is a major factor in whether or not your massage therapy business is going to succeed.

STANDARDS OF PROFESSIONAL BEHAVIOR

Professionalism was touched on briefly in Chapter 2 as a component of your business plan and in Chapter 3 pertaining to the Standards of Practice. In this chapter, we'll examine more closely what it means. We aren't born knowing how to act like professionals; it's a process that's influenced by our environment, our upbringing, our socialization, our education, our self-perception, and our aspirations. Projecting professionalism involves a commitment to upholding certain standards, and it involves behavioral skills that anyone can learn.

Inspiring Client Confidence

The nature of our work as massage therapists demands that we inspire confidence in our clients. A client wants to feel safe and secure; she wants to feel that she's in a place where she'll be treated with courtesy and compassion, where professional ethics are respected, and where the highest levels of technical skill and professional behavior are observed.

There are so many facets of a client's experience within the therapeutic relationship, starting with the first contact. You only get one time to make a first impression, and that impression is usually the deciding factor in whether or not there's going to be a continued relationship. Try to see things from the client's point of view. If your new client was the official undercover Professionalism Inspector, see how you would score if you were being evaluated on the following criteria:

- The first telephone contact was courteous and professional.
- I was greeted warmly and taken into the treatment room on time.
- The therapist conducted a thorough intake interview and took the time to answer all my questions.
- The treatment room was serene, uncluttered, and comfortable.
- The therapist was skillful, and checked in with me several times to ask if the pressure was okay.
- I had to go to the bathroom during the massage, and the therapist had a robe for me to wear so I wouldn't have to put my clothes back on.
- The entire facility was spotlessly clean.
- After the massage, the therapist brought me some water and took time to explain to me about aftercare, such as stretching, soaking in an Epsom salts bath, and using ice if I needed it to help ease my pain.
- The therapist thanked me for my business and talked to me about rescheduling but didn't pressure me.
- I was satisfied with the entire experience, and I felt I had chosen a massage therapist who is a true professional.

Would you make the grade? Bear in mind that most clients will not tell *you* that they think you were dressed unprofessionally or that your office was messy or your restroom is dirty, but they will tell other people, and they just won't come back.

REALITY CHECKPOINT

Your Professional Credentials

Displaying your massage school diploma, other educational credentials, and your license in your office is a good idea. If you're in a state where massage is regulated, displaying your license is probably a legal requirement. A massage therapist who performs outcalls should carry a copy of her license at all times. Clients appreciate knowing that they're being treated by a person who's well trained and abides by the law.

If you have gained other forms of professional recognition, such as being named Volunteer of the Year, being voted the best massage therapist in your town, receiving a community service award, or other similar accolades, display those, too. If you don't toot your own horn, who will? Those types of things impress clients.

If you practice in a state with no regulations, or if you were grandfathered in when licensure became required in your state, you may be practicing without any training in massage therapy at all. Obtaining a professional credential, such as one of the credentials from the National Certification Board or the Asian Bodywork Therapy Certification from the National Certifying Commission on Acupuncture and Oriental Medicine, is a sign to the public that you are a professional massage therapist, who has expended the time and money to get an education and passed an examination to prove competence, even though it isn't a legal requirement. It's never too late to get an education—even if you already have plenty of clients who think you're great. Massage school is not just a learning experience; it's a personal growth experience as well.

A professional massage therapist has training in anatomy, physiology, kinesiology, pathology, body mechanics, ergonomics, the history and development of massage therapy, contraindications for massage, proper draping methods, professional ethics, business, and marketing and has passed an examination that proves competency in all those areas.

The Untrained Therapist

There are many talented and caring massage therapists and business owners who have been practicing for years and don't have any education or professional training. However, there's a big difference between being able to give a good backrub and possessing the same knowledge as a professionally trained therapist. Anyone who holds herself out as a massage therapist should have at least done enough exploring on her own to know when massage is contraindicated. The potential for serious consequences exists for the therapist (not to mention the client) who lacks that knowledge.

Just as for any health care professional, your obligation as a therapist is to *first do no harm*. The general public is uneducated about contraindications for massage. There have been a number of times over the years when I had to send a client away without giving him the massage he was looking forward to, because he had a health condition that is a contraindication, but he didn't know any better.

An untrained therapist can rub the tension out of a muscle, but she might unintentionally do harm. If she doesn't know the places of origin and insertion, and the action the muscle performs, she would be blindly groping around hoping to get the right one, merely from hearing the client say "It hurts when I do *this*." In order to restore lost motion, you have to know which muscle causes that motion, and a trained professional has that knowledge.

Inspiring the Confidence of the Professional Community

Mutual referral relationships were discussed briefly in Chapter 2 as part of the business plan, and business communications with others will be discussed in Chapter 11. We'll discuss those relationships here as they are affected by your projection of professionalism. While clients may be the people you care about impressing the most, they are not the only ones you want to have to think of you as a professional. The way you are viewed by your peers, and the other health care practitioners in your community, can have a very real effect on your business, and obviously you want that effect to be positive. Your ability to inspire the confidence of the professional health care community depends on your own projection of professionalism.

Your Peers

You may not think of a therapist across town that you've never met as a peer—but you should. People usually become massage therapists because they're caretakers, because they understand that the awesome power of touch can be used to heal and restore, and because they've found something they can do that blesses other people and themselves at the same time. Being able to make a good living while doing something we love is the icing on the cake. We all want to give the gift of touch, and we all need to support ourselves and our families.

It's important to cultivate relationships with the other massage therapists in your community and to have them think well of you. You want your peers to regard you as a professional colleague, not a rival. That therapist across town may take time off to have a baby, or she might have a family emergency that interferes with her work; at some point she might move away. She'll refer her clientele to someone she thinks of as a fellow professional. She wouldn't want to refer them to a therapist she's heard about acting unprofessionally, and word travels fast.

There may be therapists in your community who perform other modalities that would benefit your clients or who maintain schedules different from yours. Or you may be the one who takes time off to have a baby or who moves away. You want to be able to refer your clients to people who are as professional as you are. You wouldn't want to send someone to an office that's dirty or to a therapist who is rude.

Networking with other therapists in your community serves a couple of different purposes. It's a marketing opportunity, but over and above that, it lets other therapists see that you project a professional image. Behaving as if you're superior, or acting stand-offish to other therapists, won't get you anything except a reputation as being aloof or conceited. If you're so competitive that you act badly toward other therapists, or say something negative about another therapist to a client, it will backfire. Treating other therapists, including those you think of as your competitors, with courtesy and respect will leave them with the impression that you treat clients with courtesy and respect. It's the way a professional conducts herself.

Other Health Care Professionals

Within the health care professions, massage therapy is being used more increasingly to supplement conventional medical techniques to address muscle problems, certain illnesses and diseases, and stress-related health conditions. The growing acceptance of massage as a therapeutic tool by medical practitioners and insurance companies is having a strong impact on employment opportunities for massage therapists. According to the AMTA, as of 2008, 63% of massage therapists already reported receiving referrals from other health care providers, and that number will surely rise as massage becomes more mainstream.

The other health care professionals in your community are potential sources of referrals—if they perceive you to be a credible member of the health care team. Projecting professionalism is the only route to take, if you intend to be taken seriously by physicians, physical therapists, occupational therapists, nurse practitioners, and others who could potentially help your career. Effective communication with other health care professionals will be discussed in Chapter 11.

Going with the Flow

According to the Bureau of Labor Statistics, demand for massage therapy should grow among older age groups because they increasingly enjoy longer, more active lives. People who are 55 and older are projected to be the most rapidly growing segment of the U.S. population over the next decade (2010–2020). However, as of this writing, the demand for massage therapy is greatest among young adults, and they are likely to continue to enjoy the benefits of massage therapy as they age. Offering family package deals is a good way to reach across generations and an opportunity to gain new clients.

Your Professional Image

Cultivating a strong professional image as a massage therapist is something you should be practicing all the time. In addition to dressing professionally, speaking professionally, and following the rules of social and business etiquette, it's also important to maintain an attitude of self-confidence and to be committed to an ongoing process of self-improvement.

REALITY CHECKPOINT

People who are impressed by your professional image will refer you to others. As for those who aren't impressed—they'll spread the word, too. Obviously, it's much better for business to have people talking about you in a positive manner, so keep your professional image in mind—always.

Dressing Professionally

It might not be fair to judge people based on the way they're dressed, but it happens all the time. If you were going to have brain surgery, and the surgeon met you sporting a lime green Mohawk, flip-flops, and a T-shirt with a picture of a marijuana leaf on it, you'd probably cancel that appointment and go to someone who presents an image of a medical professional. You want to be treated by someone who inspires confidence, and the same is true for your clients in your own profession. If you met the same surgeon under different circumstances and he was wearing scrubs or nice street clothing, you'd form an entirely different opinion of him.

Many vendors of massage equipment and supplies sell scrubs and clothing with massage-related logos on them, or you can have your own logo printed on a T-shirt or polo shirt. If your work attire is something you would wear to a job interview if you were trying to impress the management, you're on the right track.

ROADSIDE ASSISTANCE

A young woman came into my office the other day to apply for a job. She was very personable and friendly, but she was wearing cut-off jeans and a T-shirt bearing the slogan, "Dip me in chocolate and throw me to the lesbians." I don't have a homophobic bone in my body, and her sexual orientation is none of my business. But the fact that she would come for a job interview dressed that way was a deal-breaker for me; it showed a lack of professionalism. I don't require the therapists in my practice to wear a uniform, but I do stipulate that they should not wear any clothing that's revealing or anything that advertises alcohol, tobacco, or illegal drugs, and nothing that anyone would find racially, spiritually, politically, sexually, or otherwise offensive. In other words, no slogans are allowed, unless related to the profession, such as "Have You Had Your Massage Today?"

Polishing Your Professional Speech

Speaking like a professional businessperson depends on the correct use of language. For many people, language has become filled with slang, colloquialisms, and jargon; the rules of grammar and syntax often fall by the wayside, if they were ever learned at all. While some might think, "Hey, whassup?" is an okay alternative to "Hello, how are you?" on the street, it isn't acceptable in a business environment.

People appreciate speech that is clear and succinct. Banish such "filler" words as *um, huh,* and *like* (as in, "Like, I saw a client today, and like, he had a bad knee).

When speaking to the client and when writing your progress notes, use correct medical terminology. Be conscious, however, of not talking over the client's head. Most people know where the pectorals and hamstrings are located, but if you use a term such as *latissimus dorsi,* point out its location on the client's body.

EXPLORATIONS

Record a video of yourself having a half-hour conversation with a friend, and see how your image projects and how your speech sounds when you play it back. You really aren't aware of how you look and sound until you see and hear it for yourself.

Practicing Social and Business Etiquette

Practicing proper etiquette is more than knowing which fork to use at a fancy dinner. Following social and business etiquette translates to using good manners—treating people with courtesy, consideration, and respect. Manners are learned behavior from the time we're born. If good manners are something you weren't taught at home and didn't learn in school, assume the responsibility and learn them for yourself.

Saying "please," "thank you," and "excuse me" should become automatic. Always remember to thank people for their business and thank anyone for sending you a referral. In addition to thanking people in person, sending handwritten thank you notes is even better, particularly for referrals from physicians or other health care professionals. Opening a door for someone, inviting her to have a seat, offering a glass of water—these are basic tenets of polite behavior.

One of the most important rules of etiquette—social or business—is to be punctual. Be on time for your appointments. If you are running late, and have to keep a client waiting, even for a few minutes, apologize sincerely. Failing to do so will leave the client with the impression that you think your time is more valuable than hers.

When it comes to business etiquette, there are other rules to be observed. Use "Mr." and "Ms." until you're given permission to do otherwise. With the intention of being polite, you might say, for example, "I'm Mary Richards and I'm going to be your therapist today. Is it okay if I call you Elizabeth?" But that could make the client uncomfortable; you might be putting her on the spot. It would be better to ask, "What would you like me to call you? Being overly friendly and calling people by their first name at the initial session might seem presumptuous to some people, especially if they are much older than you.

The appropriate manner of address can be a matter of regional variation, too. For instance, in the southern United States, it's customary to address older adult clients as Mr. or Mrs., whereas in other regions, addressing clients by their first name at the initial encounter is the norm.

EXPLORATIONS

Professional coaching has exploded in popularity. A coach will help you define the areas of business etiquette in which you need improvement. She can either help you herself or give you a referral. Many coaches work by telephone, and it's easy to locate one on the Internet. Alternatively, ask someone whose professional persona you admire to mentor you. She doesn't have to be a professional coach to give you help and guidance. There are also plenty of etiquette tips available on the Internet, numerous books on the subject, and classes offered in many places.

Words of Wisdom
Treating people with respect and kindness is the most important etiquette lesson you can learn.

GROWING AS A PROFESSIONAL

There's a saying that if you're not moving forward, you're backing up. In the business world, that's very true. It doesn't mean you need to be "trendy," but you don't want to get stuck thinking that your way is the only way. Professional growth comes about through learning from your mistakes, being willing to listen and take advice from others when it makes sense to do so, and having the desire to improve yourself and your business whenever you can.

Professional growth often depends on personal growth, and that's especially true when you are the owner of a business. If a client says something critical to you about your demeanor, how long she was left sitting in the waiting room, or the cleanliness of the bathroom, would you automatically take offense, or would you see it as constructive criticism and be willing to use it as an opportunity to make a positive change?

The challenge, for any professional, is in making decisions where there aren't any right or wrong answers—only consequences. For the business owner, that challenge is magnified by trying to find a balance between your professional life and your personal life in order to avoid burnout—and keeping an eye on the ideals and goals that made you want to go into business in the first place.

Professional growth means that as time goes by, your collective personal experience as a therapist and business owner becomes a bank of wisdom from which you can draw. Having pride in yourself and your business, and confidence in your abilities, while maintaining humility, will enable you to maximize your opportunities and help you realize your highest potential.

Continuing Education

An important facet of professional growth is continuing your education. The professional associations and the National Certification Board require proof of continuing education (CE) attendance in order to maintain professional membership, and in regulated states, it might be a legal obligation as well. You might think you learned everything you need to know in massage school. Some therapists consider CE a waste of time and a financial burden they have to bear, and that's a shame. CE is really a great chance to learn something new—a technical skill or new modality you can add to your menu of services or something intended to help you grow your business. CE classes are always great networking opportunities, too.

ROADSIDE ASSISTANCE

I'm a provider of CE, and it happens often that a therapist calls and says "I need five CE hours. Do you have any classes that length?" I appreciate the business, but if I attended a class I had no interest in just because it meets the CE requirement, I'd feel like it was a waste of my hard-earned money and be snoring before the first break. When I seek CE, I am looking for a class that will excite me, teach me a new skill I can use on my clients, show me a new way to promote myself, or make me aware of something I should be doing in my office to benefit the business. I want to attend a class that causes a lightbulb to go off in my head, so I think, "I should be doing that!"

ALTERNATE ROUTES

Employees

When negotiating an employment contract, it never hurts to ask the employer if she provides CE as a benefit. It's a tax deduction for her and a benefit for you.

Independent Contractors

Your CE should include classes on taxes. Being self-employed entitles you to tax benefits, and you want to be sure to get all the available deductions.

Business Partners

If one partner is handling most of the details of running the business because that's her strength, the other partner should include business classes in her plans for CE. Don't let the business end of your partnership depend on just one person's ability.

Professional Responsibility

A professional massage therapist has many responsibilities; attending CE classes in order to build upon the entry-level technical skills and knowledge of science, ethics, and business skills you started out with is just one of them.

You have a professional responsibility to *first do no harm*, as I've repeated throughout this text. This means not only staying current with contraindications, but also not performing massage when you're sick or have an infection you might pass on—regardless of whether the rent is due and you really need the money. Giving anyone a guarantee that you are going to make him better or remove his pain is a serious violation of professional responsibility.

If you're working for someone else and you decide to leave the company, you have a professional responsibility to give a reasonable advance notice. If you have agreed to supervise interns in your workplace, it's your professional responsibility to provide adequate supervision. You have an obligation not to associate yourself with any project or practice that is dishonest or fraudulent in nature. Professional responsibility is characterized by everyday individual acts that you handle in the correct, ethical manner.

Professional responsibility can also entail being in service to the massage profession—by teaching, mentoring a less-experienced therapist, participating in your professional association, or volunteering to serve on a board, a committee, or an emergency response team. That will be as beneficial to you as it is to the person or entity you're helping. Being in service can provide networking and marketing opportunities, not to mention the self-satisfaction gained from doing something positive for the profession. As an additional bonus, the NCBTMB accepts teaching and certain volunteer activities, in lieu of CE attendance, as proof of professional development for the renewal of national certification.

Social Responsibility

Social responsibility is the theory that a business should contribute to the welfare of society, rather than being solely devoted to making a profit. With the advent of evidence-based practice and the increasing popularity of peer-reviewed research in the profession of massage therapy, continually educating ourselves for the benefit of the public is one aspect of social responsibility. Even if attending CE classes is not a legal requirement for you, it's still a service to your clients to keep up with the latest research. It also sends the message that you're a professional massage therapist who's always interested in improving herself and her ability to help others.

There are many other ways a small-business person can practice social responsibility, such as conducting business in as "green" a manner as possible. Simple acts such as recycling, conserving energy, making your office as paperless as possible, and using sustainable and biodegradable products at your office are examples.

Doing anything you can to improve the community you live and work in is a form of social responsibility. While performing community service, such as giving time to a hospice, a women's shelter, or a homeless shelter, is an act of social responsibility, and not education in the traditional classroom use of the word, there's no doubt that such pursuits are educational and sometimes life-changing as well. Organizing or joining in on a community cleanup day, and participating in local service organizations are other examples. Being involved in your community gives the public a good impression of you and your business; people like to support businesses that they perceive as giving something back. It's a win-win situation.

Removing the Roadblocks to Professionalism

Roadblocks to professionalism are usually behavioral, and removing them is generally within your control. Dealing with those roadblocks is relatively simple: First, you identify the problem; then, you remove it. That could mean an attitude adjustment on your part. For example, if you resist fulfilling your obligation to attend CE classes, adjust your attitude and start viewing that as an opportunity for growth, instead of a burden.

REALITY CHECKPOINT

Here's another example: Dressing professionally is a personal choice, but to some therapists, it's a roadblock to success. They might have the attitude that they can give massage dressed in their pajamas and fuzzy slippers, because there's no one to tell them not to. Maybe they have clients who are comfortable with that. But if you're committed to presenting yourself as a professional, getting rid of that roadblock is as simple as making the decision to dress professionally.

Other qualities of a professional, such as speaking appropriately and practicing proper etiquette, are all about choice: You can choose to behave one way, or you can decide to behave another way. You can make the effort to learn the social and business skills that you don't know, or you can decide not to.

OPPORTUNITIES AHEAD

The decisions you make have consequences, as most of us learned in childhood. Back then, you might have been punished for ignoring your mother's rules or gotten a failing grade in school for not doing your homework. The consequences in your adult professional life are more far-reaching. Following the path of professionalism in your work can mean the difference between barely getting by and having a practice that thrives.

Unethical Behavior

One of the most serious roadblocks to professionalism is failing to abide by the code of ethics. Adhering to a code of professional ethics and observing the NCBTMB's Standards of Practice are the most important obligations of the massage therapist. Conducting business in an ethical manner applies not only to clients, but to the other people with whom you do business, such as vendors and salespeople, and, if you are an employer, to your staff members, as well.

Honoring the sacredness of the therapeutic relationship by safeguarding client confidentiality, maintaining careful roles and boundaries, and staying within your scope of practice is the only acceptable route. A professional who practices unethically will be found out, and the consequences are severe, including loss of certification and/or licensure, not to mention loss of reputation. The National Certification Board, AMTA, and many state massage therapy boards consider the ongoing study of professional ethics to be so important that CE hours in ethics is required for every renewal period.

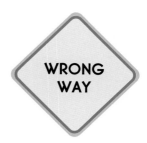

Unprofessional Behavior

Rude behavior of any kind is unprofessional. A study by the Joint Commission on Allied Health Occupations has determined that rude behavior by health care practitioners, including doctors, nurses, and other hospital personnel, undermines patient safety. As members of health care teams, massage therapists must observe the same standards. An inappropriate behavior, such as showing impatience with a client who is asking you questions or using a condescending tone when answering, can destroy client confidence. You can always improve your "people skills" by attending a communications class or an etiquette class.

You may hold the opinion that your personal life is your personal business. But if you live in a small town where gossip travels quickly, be careful how you behave outside the workplace. You wouldn't want the word to get around town that the massage therapist from Main Street Massage was seen dancing on the bar at the local saloon. A good party is fine, but within the neighborhood of your business, unprofessional behavior is not okay.

Remember, every action has a consequence. Choosing to project a professional image and behaving in a manner that will make people think well of you are part of the journey to success.

Leading by Example

If you're a therapist who is expanding your business from a sole proprietorship to being an employer, you'll be learning to delegate responsibilities as your company grows. You will constantly strive to improve your communication skills and learn to lead by example.

If you pay your staff low wages, or get a reputation for treating staff members badly, you won't attract quality people. Get a reputation as being a fair and caring employer, and you'll have therapists lined up at the door waiting to apply.

Conduct your business in the way you want your staff members to conduct business. Act the way you want your staff members to act. Dress the way you want your staff members to dress. Treat all clients the way you want your staff members to treat them, and treat your staff members the way you want to be treated. When you model professionalism and lead your staff with the highest ethical standards, as well as respect and trust, they in turn become inspired to create excellence instead of mediocrity. What a credit to you to be thought of as the leader of a top-notch staff.

John Barnes

When I was younger, as an athlete I was very aware of and interested in the mind/body connection. I attended the University of Pennsylvania and graduated as a physical therapist.

I was involved in a multitude of competitive sports, including karate and weight lifting. I seriously injured my back, falling with over 300 lb while working out, crushing the L5 disc and ripping ligaments in my lumbar area. I tried every form of massage and physical therapy known, only to be disappointed with temporary results. Nobody wanted to get better more than I did. My life had been focused on motion and competition. In one moment, everything that I loved had been taken from me!

After years of unsuccessful therapies, I was in more pain than most of my clients. There was a point when I realized nobody was going to help me but me. In my desperation, I began to experiment by treating myself on my living room floor. My attitude of "never give up" eventually led me to what is now called the "John F. Barnes Myofascial Release Approach."

I realized that myofascial release was the "missing link" in all forms of massage, bodywork, energy work, and physical therapy. Too often, without myofascial release, these approaches are blind alleys leading to the frustration of temporary results. Myofascial release enhances all other forms of therapy, elevating them to more profound and long-lasting results. In other forms of therapy, we were taught to force a system that can't be forced. This, over time, injures the therapist and leads to the frustration of temporary results. Myofascial release uses totally different principles that instead strengthen the therapist and provides the fulfillment of profound, lasting results.

Recent research has shown that trauma, surgery, and inflammatory responses create myofascial restrictions that can produce crushing pressures of approximately 2000 lb per in^2 on pain-sensitive structures. It is also important to note that myofascial restrictions do not show up on any of the standard tests, so myofascial problems have been misdiagnosed for a long time.

I wish I hadn't been injured, but as I look back, I realize it was an opportunity for me to grow and help others in pain. I believe that to be successful, one needs to be curious and not accept everything we are taught just because it is logical. I have found that just because something is logical does not mean it has any basis in reality.

Persistence is important. Never give up. Life will always present obstacles, but there is always a way. Dare to be different. Our society has tried to homogenize us. Honor your uniqueness; it is strength. Have compassion come from your heart. There is an old saying, "Your client doesn't care what you know, until they know that you care." Be confident and trust yourself! I teach that myofascial release is a process, and as we learn to trust the process, we learn to trust ourselves. And most important, have a passion for what you do and who you are. Enjoy your journey!

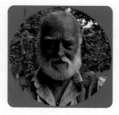

John F. Barnes, PT, LMT, NCTMB, is an author and acknowledged expert in the area of myofascial release. He has taught over 50,000 therapists and physicians worldwide who use his techniques on millions of clients per month through his Myofascial Release Seminars. You can visit his website at www.myofascialrelease.com.

SUGGESTED READINGS

American Massage Therapy Association. *Massage and Healthcare.* http://www.amtamassage.org/news/MTIndustryFactSheet.html#8. Accessed 12/27/2009.

American Medical Association. *Declaration of Professional Responsibility: Medicine's Social Contract with Humanity: Preamble.* http://www.ama-assn.org/ama/upload/mm/369/decofprofessional.pdf. Accessed 12/27/2009.

Etiquette Police. *Online Etiquette Training Program.* www.etiquettepolice.com. Accessed 12/27/2009.

Michigan State University. *Professional Behavior Expectations.* http://mdadmissions.msu.edu/main/probehavior.htm. Accessed 12/27/2009.

Quan K. *Patient Safety Threatened by Unprofessional Behavior.* http://www.ultimatenurse.com/patient-safety-threatened-by-unprofessional-behavior/. Accessed 12/27/2009.

Roberts L. *Creating a Positive Professional Image.* http://hbswk.hbs.edu/item/4860.html. Accessed 12/27/2009.

Slawski B. *Social Responsibility and the Small Business.* http://searchengineland.com/social-responsibility-and-the-small-business-14397.php. Accessed 11/16/2008.

Williams P. *More Than Just Eating with the Right Fork.* http://www.ravenwerks.com/practices/etiquette.htm. Accessed 12/27/2009.

My Personal Journey

In this chapter, we've discussed the importance of projecting professionalism and all that entails, including the use of proper etiquette. Etiquette 101 is a free online class composed of five modules pertaining to social and business etiquette. The course can be found at www.etiquettepolice.com. After completing all five modules, you can take a final exam. Whether you take the class or not, write about your goals for professional development and your goals for learning proper etiquette.

My goals _____

_____

_____

What's in my way? _____

_____

_____

What action can I take to remedy the situation? _____

_____

_____

One-year progress update _____

_____

_____

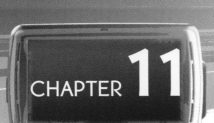

CHAPTER **11**

Effective Communications

*T*he most important thing in communication is to hear
what isn't being said.

PETE DRUCKER

KEY CONCEPTS

- Effective communications involve speaking clearly, listening actively and intently, observing body language, and cultivating writing skills.
- Business obligations include communication with clients, staff members, other professionals, and the general public.
- Communications serve the purpose of letting people know important details about you and your business and allowing you to gather important details about others.
- Word choice is less important to the listener than *how* the message is being said.
- Asking questions that have definite answers facilitates better communication.
- It's important to observe the rules of e-mail courtesy when using e-mail for business purposes.
- Handwritten notes are a personal touch that gives the impression you're making special time to communicate with someone, whether a client, a staff member, or another health care professional.
- Form letters should be letter-perfect and professionally polished.
- Conducting staff training and holding regular staff meetings are effective ways to communicate expectations to your employees.
- Mutual referrals add value to your business and benefit all concerned.
- Timely and professionally presented communication with your referral sources is a must for maintaining effective relationships with other health care practitioners.

As the owner of a massage therapy business, you want your daily contacts—clients, staff members, and other professionals—to perceive you as an effective, professional, and engaging communicator. Communicating well is a skill every businessperson should cultivate. An effective communicator is a good speaker, a good listener, and an observer of facial expressions and body language as well. In addition to speaking, listening, and observing, there are many occasions in business that call for written communications. Sometimes a neatly typed letter or a personal, handwritten note is appropriate, and producing one is a skill you'll need to master as well.

CLIENT COMMUNICATIONS

Your ability to communicate clearly with clients is equally as important as your massage technique, and your success as a therapist depends upon it. Effective client communications serve several different purposes:

- To make the client feel comfortable about receiving massage.
- To give the client an impression of you as a professional therapist.
- To convey information about your business.
- To allow you to collect the information you need about the client.
- To fill specific business needs pertaining to the client, such as billing and other notifications.

Our client communications matter the most because clients are the reason for our work; without them, we don't have a job. We discussed speaking in a professional manner in Chapter 9, and let's now look at some of the other important elements of communication.

Verbal Communications

Every encounter with a client includes verbal communication, from the first telephone contact, to the intake interview, to conversation during the massage, to the last goodbye as she is leaving.

Here's a fascinating finding about conversation. According to research, your choice of words is the least important factor in the effectiveness of verbal communication; only 7% of the effectiveness of conversation is attributed to words, while 43% is attributed to tone of voice, and the remaining 50% is attributed to nonverbal clues, including body language, facial expression, and the emotions of the speaker and the listener.

Words of Wisdom
What you say is not nearly as important as how you say it.

Making eye contact with the person you're speaking with is perceived by many people to be the key to whether the speaker is honest and trustworthy. In addition, people pay more attention when they think you are speaking from the heart; there's a fine line between sounding confident and sounding condescending, and it's the tone of voice that makes the difference.

Enthusiasm should be tempered with an attitude of calmness. Not all massage therapists are born talkers—there are shy therapists, too. Appearing interested and concerned to the client is much more important than being thought of as a witty conversationalist.

Honoring the Client's Comfort Zone

As massage therapists, we get very intimate with people in a short amount of time. A new client goes from the first hello to allowing a perfect stranger to lay hands on her unclothed body in less than 15 minutes. That requires faith and trust. Making someone feel comfortable at the first contact is often the deciding factor in whether or not any further contact will occur.

When greeting people, you want to respect their need for personal space, but on the first meeting, you don't yet know what that is. Try this technique to make the person feel more comfortable. Introduce yourself: "Hi, I'm Laura Allen and I'll be your therapist today." Then extend your hand and take a step or two toward them, and stop. Let the client be the one to enter *your* personal space. It's a small thing, and yet it can set someone at ease who might be nervous about receiving a massage from a total stranger.

ROADSIDE ASSISTANCE

In an extensive course about body structure and function, I learned that you can tell a lot about a person by his or her facial structures. For instance, a person with extremely high eyebrows prefers a more formal approach, while a low-browed person will barge right into your space and hug you the first time you meet. People with wide-set eyes are "looking at the big picture" and want a lot of information, while those with narrow-set eyes are very focused and appreciate it when any conversation gets directly to the point. I base my approach when meeting someone for the first time on those two theories and have had years of success.

Proactive Conversation

Proactive conversation is different from social conversation in that there is an intent to produce definite results. In the case of a therapist-client interaction, the desired results are for you to gather the information you need about the client and for you to gain the client's trust. You do that by *listening*. You'll need to ask some questions, but the most important role you play during a conversation with a client is being an engaged, active listener.

Maintaining eye contact, lean in a bit toward the client and nod affirmatively; answer her questions, but don't interrupt. Taking notes will reinforce the client's perception that you're interested in what she is saying. Avoid distractions and unnecessary interruptions, such as taking phone calls while you're speaking to a client; you don't want her to feel as if other things are infringing on her time. Another technique that's useful is repeating back what the client says to you; it reinforces for her that you are listening attentively and understand what she said.

Many times when clients arrive for a massage session, they will be stressed or in pain. Take that into account when speaking with someone; you may have to work a little harder to get information out of her. Make the conversation all about the client, and ask questions that have specific answers, such as these:

- "How would you rate your pain on a scale from 1 to 10, with 1 being the lowest and 10 being the highest?"
- "Do you recall doing anything in particular that may have caused your back to start hurting?"
- "When did your injury occur?"

Words of Wisdom
Make a commitment to spend more time actively listening and less time talking.

REALITY CHECKPOINT

Let the client know up front that you aren't going to "fix" her in one session. In fact, never say you're going to "fix" anyone, in any amount of sessions. It's effective and appropriate to say something like this: "Mrs. Smith, you've been in pain for several weeks, so it may take several sessions for your pain to subside, but I'll do my best to bring you some relief today." You aren't promising anything, but reassuring the client that you're sympathetic and trying to help her.

You can't control the client's body language, but be aware of it—and don't forget to monitor your own. Sitting or standing with your arms crossed in front of you, for instance, looks like you are on the defensive—trying to block something—so try to remember to appear relaxed. When you give the appearance of being relaxed, it will help the client feel relaxed, and the communication between the two of you will be better.

The Informed Client

Be mindful that someone who is receiving a massage for the first time will not know what to expect. A new client who has had massage in the past must be informed about you and your business because you're going to be different from her previous therapist. There are brochures available from massage supply vendors that cover this subject: "Your First Massage." You might want to make up your own flyer with frequently asked questions and answers. Some possible questions are the following:

- How is getting a massage going to benefit me?
- Do I have to get undressed?
- Is it going to hurt?
- What if I feel uncomfortable during the session?
- How often should I get a massage?

Remember that the amount of clothing to be removed is always the client's choice. The best approach is to say that she can undress to her level of comfort and explain your rationale if you have to ask her to remove something in order to be able to work on an area. You might say something like, "I'll be able to work on your back much better if you will undress down to your underwear. You'll be covered with a drape during the massage, except for the body part I am working on." If you are practicing in a state with no draping law, or working on clients who have moved from a state where there are no regulations regarding draping, you should still insist on it.

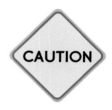

Let the client know that you'll be checking in with her regarding pressure or pain in certain areas during the massage, but that otherwise, it's her choice whether or not to converse during the session. Emphasize that you always want her to speak up if the pressure feels too deep or if she has any questions at any time—before, during, or after the massage.

It's just as important to talk with the client after the session. If you've done deep tissue massage, tell the client she might be sore for a day or two from the work you've done; otherwise, she may assume you've hurt her and not come back. Give aftercare instructions about drinking extra water, stretching, Epsom salts soaks, or whatever you recommend. Suggest rescheduling, but don't give a high-pressure sales pitch. Be sure the last thing you say to a departing client is "Thank you."

Written Communications for Clients

Every piece of paper with which your clients come in contact represents your business and is intended to communicate information. This includes everything from your intake form, to marketing materials like brochures and business cards, to billing notices and receipts. Promotion and advertising materials will be discussed in Chapters 13 and 14; here, we'll focus on the practical skills and forms needed for communicating effectively with clients.

Every written communication from your business should have your business name, address, phone number, e-mail, and website address at the top. Whether you order preprinted stationary or create a letterhead using your word processing program, choose a plain font that's easy to read, like Courier or Times New Roman.

If you choose a fancy font for your business name, use it for the name only and put the contact information and everything else in a plain font. People should not have to struggle to read your materials.

Using E-mail with Clients

E-mail is one of the most popular forms of communication, and little wonder. Technology has made it possible to contact people on the other side of the world instantly, without the expense of a long-distance phone call.

Your intake form should include a line for the client's e-mail address, with a qualifying statement such as, "Provide your e-mail address if you would like to receive appointment reminders, our newsletter, and notices of specials from our business. We do not share your e-mail address with anyone."

Always follow the basic rules of e-mail courtesy:

- Be careful not to irritate your clients by bombarding them with constant e-mails.
- Avoid abusing your client e-mail list to send out jokes, recipes, chain letters, or anything that doesn't directly concern your business with the client, no matter how cute or profound you think it is.
- Avoid using the abbreviations, such as BFF, OMG, ROFLOL, and other forms of techno-jargon; remember that this is a professional business communication.
- When e-mailing more than one person at a time, use the BCC (blind carbon copy) option. Putting your client list out for others to see is a HIPAA violation.
- Request an acknowledgement or response if the communication is an appointment reminder, or an invitation to an event that's time-sensitive.
- Always remember to include the subject line. Instead of just "Your appointment" use "Your appointment at Main Street Massage."
- Don't type in all capital letters. That's considered the e-mail equivalent of shouting.
- Use a standard signature line that includes the same contact information that's on your letterhead.
- Include an unsubscribe statement at the bottom of your e-mail, such as "You are receiving this communication because you personally provided us with your e-mail address. If you no longer wish to receive e-mail from Main Street Massage, please hit Reply and type Remove in the subject line. Main Street Massage does not share your e-mail address with anyone." If someone requests to be removed, act on it immediately.

The Client Newsletter

A client newsletter is one of the best communication tools you can use, and it's easy to implement. If you're not a writer, don't worry. There are a number of companies that cater to massage therapists by providing ready-made newsletters that can be customized with the name and contact information of your business.

If you belong to one of the professional associations, a client newsletter may be one of the benefits of membership. The template from ABMP includes numerous articles you can use for client education, and you can leave as much blank space as you like for inserting your own special promotions and office news. In addition to the educational articles, include any newsworthy items about your business, your staff, and yourself, such as conventions or continuing education classes or workshops.

Remember not to mention a client's name in your newsletter without her express permission; even something as mundane as announcing the winner of your monthly drawing for a free massage is a violation of confidentiality. On the other hand, it's also a nice touch to include client testimonials. Instead of putting a client on the spot by asking her directly, you might include an appeal in the newsletter requesting testimonials for future editions.

In the interest of saving trees and postage, an e-mail newsletter is the best way to go, especially if you have a lot of clients. It can be very expensive to mail printed copies. Take into account the rules of etiquette mentioned above regarding e-mail; they apply here as well. Figure 11-1 is an example of a client newsletter.

The Power of the Handwritten Note

A handwritten note might seem old-fashioned these days, but clients appreciate it when you take the time to send one. If you keep a box of blank note cards, you can use them for every purpose—writing a personal sympathy note when a client

The news from THERA-SSAGE

431 S. MAIN ST., STE. 2 • RUT HERFORDTON NC 28139 • WWW.THERA-SSAGE.COM • 828-288-3727

TMJ MASSAGE Dr. Donald Blanton, owner of Parkway Dentistry, will be the guest speaker at noon on Dec. 2. Everyone is welcome but space is limited , so please call to reserve your place. Fruit and sandwiches are provided. Dr. Blanton has referred many of his patients to us for TMJ Massage and will be speaking about TMJ dysfuntion and various treatment methods.

Contest Winner
Tom and Judy Jones won the Valentine's Day Couples' Massage contest and gave us their permission to say "Thanks! It was a great treat for a special day! We'll be back for more." They also enjoyed a limo ride to and from the massage provided by Elegant Rides. ♥

The Benefits of Massage

Did you know that massage can help relieve the pain and discomfort of many health conditions, including sciatica, carpal tunnel syndrome, and fibromyalgia? Postinjury, massage can help facilitate healing by increasing circulation, flexibility, and range of motion. Don't forget about stress relief! Massage can also induce profound relaxation. You'll feel your stress melting away.

The Best Time for a Massage: Anytime!

In the morning, in the evening...on Saturday... on your day off...after work, anytime. THERA-SSAGE is pleased to announce that we have expanded our hours and you can now book appointments up until 7 p.m. Monday through Saturday.

THERA-SSAGE STAFF NOTES

Mary Berry, one of our massage therapists, was married to Joseph Wheeler on February 15 in a beautiful service at St. John's Episcopal Church. They're spending their honeymoon skiing in Colorado. Mary will resume taking appointments in March.

Laura Allen, owner of THERA-SSAGE, has been chosen to serve on the Board of Directors of the Chamber of Commerce.

Jackie Kwan has just returned from Hawaii, where she attended a class in Lomi-Lomi, an indigenous Hawaiian massage that is often referred to as "the sacred dance." Jackie will now be offering Lomi-Lomi sessions at the reduced price of $75 for the first 20 people who book a session.

Chair Massage is available at your workplace for $60 an hour. Treat your staff and they'll be eternally grateful! Remember, a happy staff is a productive staff!

Community Education Schedule
Join us in our beautiful and spacious classroom for a class! Call 288-3727 for more details and pricing.

Monday 9-10 a.m. Eating Better with Raw Foods
Tuesay and Thursday 7-8 p.m. T'ai Chi Chuan
Wednesday and Friday 7-8 p.m. Yoga
Saturday 10 a.m. Yoga for Kids (12 and under)

Gift Certificates Are Available Online
You can now get a gift certificate directly from our website at www.thera-ssage.com

FIGURE 11-1 A client newsletter.

loses a loved one, a thank-you note for a referral someone sent, or a congratulatory note for a graduation from college or getting a promotion. It's the kind of gesture that only takes a couple of minutes, and it goes a long way. If an occasion calls for sending a personal note to a client and you're unsure of what to say, there are plenty of models available on the Internet and in etiquette books. Keep it short and sweet. Here are a couple of examples:

Dear Mrs. Cooper,
I read in the newspaper that your brother passed away, and I am so sorry for your loss. Please accept my deepest sympathy.

—Cathy Miller, your massage therapist

Dear Dr. Letty,
Congratulations on your retirement! It's incredible that you've been at the hospital for over forty years. I'm sure they'll miss you, but I hear you intend to do a lot of fishing and I hope you'll enjoy yourself.

Best wishes,
Patty Lynch, your massage therapist

Another occasion for a handwritten note is welcoming a new client. Massage supply vendors sell preprinted postcards bearing the phrase "Welcome to my practice." However, it only takes a minute to write one by hand, and it's much more personal.

ROADSIDE ASSISTANCE

I write my own "Welcome to my practice" cards on my blank note cards, and I write the body of the message ahead of time. My message says: "Thank you so much for choosing THERA-SSAGE. We truly appreciate your business." When I need to send one, I just write in "Dear Mrs. Smith," and it's done.

Form Communications for Clients

There are many times when a standard form can be used for client communications. The obvious ones are receipts, invoices, insurance-related paperwork, and other business needs. If you're using financial software, it will let you customize any finance-related forms you need for your business. There are also many software programs available that contain standard business letters for all kinds of occasions. Depending on your particular needs, you may prefer to write your own.

 For a sampling of blank form communications adaptable to your business, visit http://thePoint.lww.com/Allen-Business

You'll need to have standard form letters for other situations, such as the following:

- A client's check is returned to you by the bank for insufficient funds. Figure 11-2 is a sample letter.
- You are dismissing a client for some reason, such as arriving for an appointment under the influence of alcohol and behaving disruptively, or other inappropriate behavior (Fig. 11-3).
- You wish to thank a client for referring someone to your business (Fig. 11-4).

PORTSMOUTH SPORTS MASSAGE
2022 Trade Street
Portsmouth, NC 29091
828-919-4656
www.portsmouthsportsmassage.com

Marie Graves   March 2, 2010
901 Florence Way
Portsmouth, NC 29091

Dear Ms. Graves,

Check number _____ that you wrote to Portsmouth Sports Massage, dated _____, has been returned because of insufficient funds. We regret to inform you that we must also pass along the bank charge of $____, bringing the total amount you owe to $_____. Please stop by our office in the next _____ days and settle this matter. While we understand that everyone makes an occasional mistake, it is our policy after we have had two checks returned for insufficient funds to require payment by cash, debit card, or credit card. Thank you for your cooperation.

Regards,

Lydia Martin
Lydia Martin, LMBT

FIGURE 11-2 A returned-check letter.

Serenity Massage Therapy   **560 Happy Trails**
Colfax Gin, AZ 40404
219-098-5273

Janice Patton   November 29, 2010
21 Sapphire Parkway
Sedona, AZ 40408

Dear Ms. Patton,

I regret to inform you that you are being dismissed as a client of Serenity Massage Therapy. If you would like to have your client file to give to your new massage therapist, please sign the enclosed release form, return it in the SASE provided, and we will send it to you by registered mail.

Regards,

John Li
John Li, LMT

FIGURE 11-3 A client dismissal letter.

Jane Dungeness, LMT

775 Mainline
Ichabod, IL 20201
615-722-0101

Nancy Conner   April 10, 2010
1040 Coney Island Road
Ichabod, IL 20201

Dear Ms. Conner,

Thank you so much for your referral of David Alley to me for massage therapy. I truly appreciate your business and your confidence in my services.

                                      With much gratitude,

                                      Jane Dungeness
                                      Jane Dungeness

FIGURE 11-4   A referral thank-you letter.

ALTERNATE ROUTES

Employees

Your employer probably has forms for different types of written communications. Check with management before sending any written communications to a client.

Independent Contractors

Check with your employer before preparing any written materials for your clients. Even though you are self employed, you are representing someone else's business, and they may prefer that you use their forms for communications.

Business Partners

Agree on the form communications you're going to use prior to opening your business (e.g., letters and invoices). It will save time, and being consistent eliminates confusion.

STAFF COMMUNICATIONS

A business owner who knows how to communicate effectively with staff members is one who can speak the truth and be diplomatic about it at the same time. If you have only one employee, most staff communications can be handled verbally. An exception would be if you need to document an incident relating to the employee, or when giving a written warning, if you've already given a verbal warning. If a problem arises with a staff member, don't discuss it in front of everyone; discuss it privately with the person(s) involved.

It's up to you to set an example for staff communications. If you greet every client with a cheerful and welcoming attitude, that will rub off on your staff. If you make an effort to speak clearly and yet in a calm and quiet voice, that will rub off on your staff. Politeness breeds politeness. You want your employees to be polite to customers, polite to each other, and polite to you. Just remember to model that behavior, and everyone will follow your lead.

Going with the Flow

An enterprising therapist whom I know lives in a major city; he runs a massage therapy business that is strictly outcalls. He has a pool of about 25 independent contractors working for him, and all staff communications are handled by text messaging. When a request for massage comes in, he sends a text message to the whole staff, and the first person to respond gets the outcall. After he confirms with the therapist, he texts the other therapists to let them know the request has been filled. As a safety measure, the therapist texts when he arrives at the destination, and again when he is leaving the appointment.

Direct and Indirect Approaches

When you use a direct approach with a staff member, the main idea you want him to get is the first thing mentioned, followed by the evidence or supporting points you want to make. If you're delivering good news, or saying something that the employee is probably going to feel neutral or positive about, use the direct approach. You'll sound relaxed and confident when you're relaying the information; here's an example: "John, your package-deal offering on the Rolfing has been a great success. Your personal earnings are way up over the last couple of months, and the clientele is very pleased with the opportunity to save on your services."

ALTERNATE ROUTE AHEAD

Using the indirect approach is often a better way to communicate when you want to soften bad news, or to impart information you think might be received in a hostile or negative manner. You want to strike a balance between being truthful and still sounding sympathetic: "Karen, I'm afraid with the economy being as slow as it is right now, and with all the recent job layoffs around here, now just isn't the right time for me to increase the price of massage and give you a raise. I'll consider your request again in a few months." You gave the reasons first, and worked up to the fact that you couldn't give a raise right now, but left the door open for future consideration of the request. The employee may not be pleased, but if you had said, "Karen, you just can't have a raise now, the economy's not healthy," it would have sounded much worse and not sympathetic at all.

Not every issue for staff discussion is that serious. For instance, you might have to mention to a therapist that you can smell the garlic from last night's spaghetti on his breath—and don't hesitate to do that. Better for you to tell him than to have it come from the client he's breathing on. Remember that it's all about how you say things.

Staff Training

In addition to having a policies and procedures manual, and being sure your staff is familiar with it, you will need to conduct staff training. A new staff member should be given a tour of the office, shown where supplies are, and informed if there are any areas or equipment that are off limits.

Emphasize compliance with the code of ethics, Standards of Practice, and HIPAA requirements. Reinforce the fact that intake and exit interviews should be conducted in the privacy of the treatment room. A staff member who has been used to working alone could easily forget a detail like that, if she hasn't had to previously worry about anyone else being within earshot.

Train your staff to implement a **signature service**—something that sets your business apart, and that you want performed consistently by every therapist. Here are some examples of signature services:

- Putting a neck warmer or foot warmer on every client at the beginning of the massage.
- Offering chamomile teabags, cucumber slices (very refreshing!), or an herbal pillow for the eyes.
- Beginning or ending the massage a certain way, such as applying essential oils to the feet (with the client's permission, of course).
- Leaving a chocolate or cookie on the massage table for the client.
- Finishing the massage with a sinus massage and a hot towel over the face for a few minutes.
- Presenting the receipt on a silver tray accompanied by a bottle of water as the client is departing.

A signature service leaves a good impression on clients. Consistency creates a sense of familiarity and comfort, and having staff members trained to do things in a consistent way projects an aura of professionalism.

The Staff Meeting

Holding regular staff meetings is smart business. It's not only an opportunity to reinforce policies and procedures but also an opportunity to generate harmony and camaraderie among your staff members. Happy workers make a happy atmosphere. Staff meetings are the time to bring up issues that need correction, to discuss changes in policies and procedures, to brainstorm new ideas for services and marketing, and to recognize people for the good job they're doing.

ROADSIDE ASSISTANCE

I try to hold staff meetings at lunchtime and order in food as my treat for my employees. People are more relaxed when they're eating; it's a way for me to thank the staff for the work they do, and I try to temper any bad news or serious issues with praise.

Resolving Conflicts

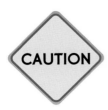

What if two staff members, both of whom you value, have a personality clash or some kind of serious issue with each other? Sitting down with the parties involved and acting as the calm voice of mediation is a good way to handle it. If it can't be resolved through open and honest communication, you may have to make a decision about which employee has to go. The key in this type of situation is to act swiftly. You simply can't let tension or dissension infiltrate your office; clients will pick up on it. Remember always that a massage setting is a place people come to de-stress, not to experience new stress. Handle problems immediately instead of giving them time to grow.

Written Communications for Staff

Written communications for staff are sometimes necessary. If you make a change in your policies and procedures, it should be communicated to staff members in writing. Here's an example of a simple memo: "Effective January 1, the Bella Spa policy concerning gift certificate redemption will change. The new policy is . . ." A copy should be given to everyone concerned.

If you use a bulletin board for communicating to staff members, you may want to request signatures at the bottom of each posting, acknowledging that they have read the notice. This is especially relevant when the subject is time-sensitive.

Most written communications for staff members are handled on forms (see below). However, just like the power of sending a handwritten note to a client, a handwritten note can be very effective when given to a staff member. An occasional "thank you for the good job you do" will make your employee feel appreciated.

Clear Expectations

For the most part, your expectations of staff members are spelled out in the policies and procedures manual, and in the employee or independent contractor agreements. However, the longer you are in business, the more you'll find that little things pop up that don't exactly warrant a policy and procedure—or at least you didn't think so, until the situation presented itself. You can think of those as opportunities to clarify your expectations, and to create new policies.

We discussed dressing professionally in the last chapter, but let's take that to the next level, as an extreme example of expectations being made perfectly clear. The policies of a worldwide recruiter that places massage therapy services on cruise ships go way beyond requiring staff members to wear a uniform. Here are a few of the rules that therapists must follow:

SUCCESS NEXT EXIT

- All underwear must be white so that no colors show through the uniform.
- Female therapists are not allowed to wear any nail polish.
- The only jewelry permitted is a pair of plain stud earrings; a wristwatch is not allowed, although a fob-style watch may be kept in a pocket.
- Full makeup is expected at all times.
- Women with short hair are expected to wear it "styled," and women with long hair are expected to wear it in a stylish "up-do"; no ponytails and no visible hair barrettes, pins, or other ornaments allowed.
- Male therapists are expected to be freshly shaved every day; no facial hair permitted.

You probably won't go to those lengths with your staff—or will you? It's your prerogative to do so, as long as you make your expectations clear and in writing at the outset. If your long-time therapist came in to work with a new nose piercing she got over the weekend, would you care?

If you expect staff members to participate in community service events for no pay, or require them to make their own reminder calls, or something as mundane as folding the sheets a certain way, the responsibility for communicating those things in writing is yours. When you let staff members know up front exactly what you expect, your business will run more smoothly. It's never fair to penalize anyone for failing to live up to an expectation that you haven't communicated clearly—and in writing.

BIG ADVENTURE AHEAD

COASTAL MASSAGE

800 Ocean Drive
City By the Bay, FL 83238
306-396-8787

Written Warning of Disciplinary Action

(Employee) or Independent Contractor: _Susan Alden_   Date _10/12/2011_

Details: _Susan has left work three times in the past thirty days without changing her linens and cleaning her room and was given a verbal warning after the second time._

The consequences of another infraction related to this will be:
____ days suspension without pay.
_X_ immediate termination from Coastal Massage.
____ reported to the proper authorities, including the police department and the Florida Board of Massage Therapy.

This disciplinary action was issued by _James Samuel, LMT_

I acknowledge receipt of this warning and understand the terms.
Susan Alden, LMT

FIGURE 11-5   A written warning of disciplinary action.

Form Communications for Staff

If something is serious enough to document, such as an injury on the job or an incident involving a staff member, a written record should be placed in the staff member's file and a copy given to the staff member. An incident report (see Fig. 9-3) should be filled out by management and signed by the employee. If the staff member refuses to sign the incident report, that should be noted as an addendum to the report.

There may be a need for a written warning of disciplinary action (Fig. 11-5). The purpose of this document would be to protect you from a lawsuit in the event an employee claims she was unfairly terminated; having one on file proves that you have made a previous attempt to address the problem with the employee.

REFERRAL RELATIONSHIP COMMUNICATIONS

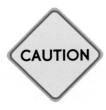

Your ability to communicate clearly, and your commitment to do so in a timely manner with fellow health care professionals and other sources for **referral**, will drive (or hinder) your success with referral relationships. The key to getting referrals from other health care practitioners is to let them know not only who you are and what you do, but also how professional you are in conducting your business.

Your written communications must be letter-perfect. All word-processing programs have a spell-checker function, but even that will ignore words that are used incorrectly, such as using "their" when you meant to say "there" or "hear" when you meant to say "here." Ask someone to proofread your written communications. A fresh pair of eyes will often detect something you overlook.

Cultivating Referrals

We briefly discussed the importance of following up on referrals in Chapter 10. In the health care field, it is expected that you as a professional will acknowledge and thank the source of any client referral and send in progress notes when appropriate. Referrals can be your biggest source of business, and it's certainly the case in my own practice. In addition to word-of-mouth referrals from your clients, which is the best advertising you can hope to get, there are many other sources you can seek out for cultivating mutual referral situations. Here are a few:

- Physicians
- Physical therapists
- Chiropractors
- Naturopaths
- Nurse practitioners
- Dentists
- Doulas
- Energy workers

OPPORTUNITIES AHEAD

Business Network International (BNI) is the largest professional referral organization in the world. If there's a chapter in your area, it would be a good idea to join. BNI is unique for several reasons:

- Only one person from each professional specialty is allowed to join in each chapter.
- Attendance is mandatory at regular meetings, for the success of the group; it's not optional.
- Admission to BNI is by application, and character and business references are checked.
- Any reports of unethical or inferior work reported to a member who has made a referral to you will result in an investigation; if found at fault, you can be dismissed from the group.

If the BNI chapter in your area already has a professional massage therapist as a member, you can apply to start another group. More about BNI and how it works can be found on the organization's website.

Be sure the people from whom you hope to cultivate referrals have your business cards and brochures. If other professionals are letting you display your literature in their offices, don't forget to provide your own business card or brochure holder. (Business cards and brochures, along with using the Internet for networking, are discussed in Chapter 14.)

ROADSIDE ASSISTANCE

When appropriate, I refer to other massage therapists and practitioners who specialize in certain modalities. For instance, when I think a client would benefit from a particular technique that requires specific training or expertise I don't have, such as craniosacral therapy, I'm happy to refer her to someone who does. In terms of scheduling, I also practice cross-referrals. Because my office is on Main Street, we often get walk-ins we can't accommodate right away. If I'm not able to schedule someone for a convenient time, I'll call another therapist in the client's presence and try to get her an appointment if she needs attention sooner than I can provide it. That service—and the referral itself—will come back to you; you can count on it.

Words of Wisdom
When you act interested in people and what they do, they'll be interested in you and what you do.

Maintaining a Referral Database

Creating and maintaining a referral database for your office is a great way to start. Systematically go through the telephone book and enter in your database program the contact information for every chiropractor, physician, and dentist listed in your area. Then you can do a mail-merge to send them all a letter at one time, or you can contact a select group of your choosing. Don't limit yourself to a certain type of doctor because sickness and stress go hand-in-hand; for instance, even though a urologist doesn't usually concern himself with muscle problems, he probably has patients suffering from stress he could refer to you.

You need to keep your database updated. Whenever a new physician opens a practice, it's usually reported in the local newspaper, along with the address of the location. Add the listing to your database. When the updated telephone directory comes out annually, check the physician listings against your database in order to keep your contacts current.

In the case of mutual referrals outside the health care world, keep a separate card file with the business cards you've collected, filed alphabetically by occupation. When a client asks, "Do you know a good plumber?"—the name is right at your fingertips. Remind your client to let the plumber (in this example) know you recommended him by writing it directly on the card: "Susie at Massage on Main sent me."

Meet and Greet

SUCCESS NEXT EXIT

For cultivating referrals, take advantage of opportunities to meet as many medical professionals in person as possible. Hospitals regularly offer free educational programs and short talks by doctors on a variety of subjects. These are advertised in the newspaper, or you could call the education coordinator at the local hospital and ask to be added to the mailing list. When you see that Dr. Barker is giving a 1-hour talk on fibromyalgia, make it a point to attend and to introduce yourself to him after the meeting—armed, of course, with your business cards. Someone is more inclined to refer clients to you when he can put a face with a name and has an impression of you as a professional member of the health care community.

One of the great things about the Chamber of Commerce, as mentioned in Chapter 1, is the opportunity to network. Think of how many other businesspeople are potential resources of referrals—almost everybody! Realtors are constantly meeting people who are just moving into town, as are contractors and others who are in the building trades. Hairdressers and manicurists are good sources of mutual referrals. Caterers and bridal shops, photographers, bed and breakfast owners—the list is endless. Don't limit yourself to referring only with other health care practitioners.

Your memberships in the Chamber, the merchant's association, civic clubs, and professional associations aren't worth the money unless you participate. You have to get involved—get out and go to the meetings, meet all the people you can, and spread the word about your business. Establish mutual referral relationships with as many people as you can, and reciprocate whenever you get the opportunity. Ask people for their business cards. Don't overlook your own clients—surely some of them are merchants or tradespeople and you could send business their way. It's a win-win situation.

EXPLORATIONS

If you are still a massage student, it's not too early to attend the free seminars offered by the physicians at your local hospital and to start networking with them. For instance, introduce yourself to the speaker, stating that you'll soon be graduating and going into practice, and that you'd like to focus on medical massage. Let the doctor know that you need bodies to practice on, and let him know that some of his patients (or he) could be receiving free massage from you while you're still a student. You may even work yourself into a job at the hospital or in the physician's office, if you haven't yet decided to go into business for yourself.

Written Communications for Referral Relationships

Bear in mind that every written communication is a chance to make a good impression. Any communications that you have with referral sources should be neatly typed, grammatically correct, and free of typographical errors. You'll need to write a letter of introduction to potential referral sources and cover letters to accompany the progress notes to physicians or other health care professionals who have referred to you. These can be form communications (discussed shortly).

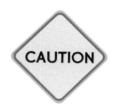

The Personal Touch

Unless you're the only massage therapist in your town, chances are there's stiff competition for referrals. Adding an element of a personal touch into your professional written communications can help keep you in the forefront, when another health care practitioner is considering making a referral. While your cover letter for progress notes may be a form communication, it's a personal touch to send a handwritten thank-you note for the referral itself—for every referral.

Taking a day to visit the offices of professionals who can potentially refer to you is a good idea. Introduce yourself to the receptionist, leave some cards and brochures behind, and invite her to your office to check out your facility; throw in a free 15-minute chair massage. A personal contact has more impact than a letter from an unknown face—and you can and should always send a letter within a few days after the meeting.

Form Communications for Referral Relationships

If not done in person, your first contact for a referral might be through a professional referral letter—a written introduction to inform other professionals who you are and what kind of services you provide. The letter can also be sent as a follow-up after you have met a potential source of referrals; be sure to mention where and when you met the person. A sample professional referral letter to physicians appears in Figure 11-6.

After you have received a referral from a physician, you should respond immediately with a thank-you note, including a promise to send updated progress notes. An example appears in Figure 11-7.

The progress notes should include a cover letter and a copy of the SOAP notes that have been recorded pertaining to the client (Fig. 11-8). An example of SOAP notes appears in Chapter 6. If the physician prescribed a certain number of sessions within a specific timeframe, or if the doctor failed to specify a number and you and the client decided upon a certain number as a care plan, include the SOAP notes from all those sessions.

Medical Massage Inc.

400 Hospital Drive ~ New Bethel, CT 70959 ~ 256-043-8787

Dr. Ramya Patel   January 12, 2010
Sunshine Family Medicine
200 Meridian Street
Sunshine, CT 70946

Dear Dr. Patel,
We met briefly last night when I attended your presentation on Chronic
Fatigue Syndrome at New Bethel Hospital. I am the owner of Medical
Massage, Inc., located in the Medical Park adjacent to the hospital. I
would like to introduce you to the services offered here, in the hope that
you will consider referring clients to our business.

Our staff members are all licensed by the state massage therapy board
and certified in medical massage. As you are aware, many of your clients
are probably suffering from stress-related illnesses. Massage therapy can
address that stress. In addition, we have therapists who specialize in
TMJ disorders, maternity massage, and orthopedic massage.

Massage can help relieve muscular pain, increase circulation, improve
flexibility, and aid in the restoration of range of motion post-trauma
and/or post-surgery. I am enclosing a brochure, *The Benefits of Massage*,
with more details about how massage can benefit your patients.
We accept major medical insurance from those companies who will pay
for massage. We also offer a discount to senior citizens.

We want to assure you that when you refer to us, you will receive an
acknowledgement and timely progress notes.

We are hosting an open house on January 31 from 9 a.m. until 5 p.m., and
we invite you to come and see our facility and talk with our staff members. If you are unable to make it that day, please feel free to call us and
set up an alternate time to visit Medical Massage, Inc. We look forward
to meeting you.

Regards,

Sherwin Bean

Sherwin Bean, LMT

FIGURE 11-6   **A professional referral letter.**

Medical Massage Inc.

400 Hospital Drive ~ New Bethel, CT 70959 ~ 256-043-8787

Dr. Ramya Patel   February 11, 2010
Sunshine Family Medicine
200 Meridian Street
Sunshine, CT 70946

Dear Dr. Patel,

Thank you so much for your referral of Michael Wells to our practice for massage therapy. We have suggested to Mr. Wells that he will benefit from 6-8 sessions performed over the next couple of weeks, and we will send you updated progress notes after his last session.

We appreciate your confidence in us.

Regards,

Sherwin Bean

Sherwin Bean, LMT

FIGURE 11-7   A professional referral thank-you letter.

ROADSIDE ASSISTANCE

I recently got a call from a therapist who had attended my insurance billing class. She left the class excited about the potential for new business opportunities, and as soon as she got home made a list of 30 doctors to whom she wanted to send introduction letters. Unfortunately, spelling was not her forte, and she failed to use her computer's spell-checker. She called me in tears to report that she had received letters back from five doctors chastising her about the typos in the letters, remarking how unprofessional they were. A couple of them had actually marked the mistakes in the letters. My advice was to rewrite the form letter—making it perfect this time, acknowledging the mistakes in the first letter, and sending it again. Ignoring a mistake won't make it go away. It's better to acknowledge it and strive for perfection the next time; at least the people who saw your mistakes will know you have enough integrity to do better.

Medical Massage Inc.

400 Hospital Drive ~ New Bethel, CT 70959 ~ 256-043-8787

Dr. Ramya Patel   April 13, 2011
Sunshine Family Medicine
200 Meridian Street
Sunshine, CT 70946

Dear Dr. Patel,

Thank you again for your referral of Michael Wells to our practice for massage therapy. Although the pain from his knee injury has subsided, Mr. Wells has decided to continue a course of monthly massage therapy for his own health and well-being.

During his visits to our office, Mr. Wells was seen by Edna Beggins, a member of our staff who specializes in orthopedic massage. Attached are the progress notes Edna prepared from the six visits Mr. Wells has completed.

We are grateful for your confidence in our services and appreciate your referrals to us.

Regards,

Sherwin Bean

Sherwin Bean, LMT

FIGURE 11-8   A professional follow-up letter to accompany SOAP notes.

POSTCARDS from the HIGHWAY

Tamsin Stewart

After working at a couple of unsatisfying jobs, I wanted to do something meaningful with my life; so in 1974 when my friend Lisa suggested I try to get a job with her massage therapist, I did. "You've always got your hands on everybody anyway," Lisa said. At the time 74 years old, Nanny, Lisa's therapist, ran her quietly famous salon in Los Angeles, and a great many of the era's female stars and starlets passed through her unmarked doors. From early morning until late evening, Nanny worked constantly, her bright little eyes usually closed, cooing, and humming to her "little ladies" as her arthritic but powerful hands stripped and squeezed their flesh. Minutes after meeting me she agreed to hire and teach me and took me straight into the inner sanctum to offer me one leg—she took the other—of a popular TV and film star of the day; and that was the beginning of my career.

I trained by her side for a few months and remained for a couple of years before leaving to start my own business. Did I have a license or formal education? Not necessary in those dark ages, so I bought a portable massage table and through rapid

(continued)

POSTCARDS from the HIGHWAY

Tamsin Stewart *(Continued)*

word-of-mouth gained entrance to beautiful homes in Beverly Hills, Malibu, and all over Los Angeles, working first with one famous singer-songwriter, then another, and then just about everybody in show business.

My circle of friends at the time included a stuntman. Along with his professional colleagues he had recently discovered Thomas Griner, an extraordinary muscle therapist who put stuntmen back together after they leapt out of tall buildings and rolled motorcycles off cliffs.

Griner had been in research engineering at NASA's Jet Propulsion Lab when he became so fascinated with how skeletal muscle becomes hypertonic, he left engineering and entered chiropractic college. Although Griner at first refused to teach me his work because I had no medical background, he soon relented because he realized I wouldn't go away until he taught me! I finally did go to massage school because I had to learn anatomy and physiology. My pride in being his student is matched by my amazement and awe of his abilities and my continuing gratitude. Because of him, my career was elevated to new heights, and I have remained in the field for more than 35 years.

I continued to work in Los Angeles, both in private homes and on movie sets; I traveled to the South of France and to New York and Philadelphia to work with theatrical clients, went on the road with rock stars, and to Washington D.C. with politicians. I had a large contingent of Saudi Arabian clients escaping the summer heat in Riyadh, and I was asked to work with the Saudi Ambassador to the United States, when he came to Los Angeles for the 1984 Olympics. When he asked me to move to Washington D.C. to become his private therapist, I accepted. I remained in his employ for 20 years, working with him, his wife and children, and his friends—including three U.S. Presidents. Traveling on his private plane as part of his entourage, I saw the world and stayed in the finest palaces and hotels. My career took me to many places I wouldn't have gone otherwise.

My advice to any new therapist is this: Don't believe everything you hear, read, or are taught; do believe you can make a real difference for good; do believe in the ability of muscle tissue to heal if properly treated; do believe your career can give you whatever you desire if you put into it what is required. And above all, of course: Believe in yourself and in your dreams.

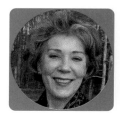

Today Tamsin Stewart focuses on teaching NeuroSoma, Thomas Griner's work. With his help, she developed a 104-hour graduate course over several years' time. She no longer travels, and consequently attracts only a few dedicated students who are willing to come to central Virginia to learn in the apprentice tradition. Tamsin is an Approved Provider of Continuing Education. You can read more about Tamsin Lee and the work she does at www.neurosoma.com.

SUGGESTED READINGS

Douglass, K. *Facilitating a Quality Culture Through Effective Staff Training and Competency Assessment.* http://www.pppmag.com/documents/V4N10_CC_Supp/p1_2_3_4.pdf. Accessed 01/06/2010.

Institute for Management Excellence. *Improving Verbal Skills.* http://www.itstime.com/aug97.htm. Accessed 01/06/2010.

Kelly Scientific Resources. *Running an Effective Staff Meeting.* http://www.kellyscientific.com.au/web/au/ksr/en/pages/business_services_running_an_effective_staff_meeting.html. Accessed 01/06/2010.

Steiner Leisure. *Dress Code for Beauty/Massage/Nail Technicians.* http://www.str.co.uk/gallerys/uniforms/femuni/femuni.asp. Accessed 01/06/2010.

My Personal Journey

In this chapter, we've discussed the various types of business communications. Using the examples that are provided, create your own standardized forms and letters for use in your business. If you don't yet have a business address, you can add it later. Save the forms and letters in files labeled Client Forms, Staff Forms, and Referral Forms.

My goals _____

_____

_____

What's in my way? _____

_____

_____

What action can I take to remedy the situation? _____

_____

_____

One-year progress update _____

_____

_____

PART V

Highway Visibility

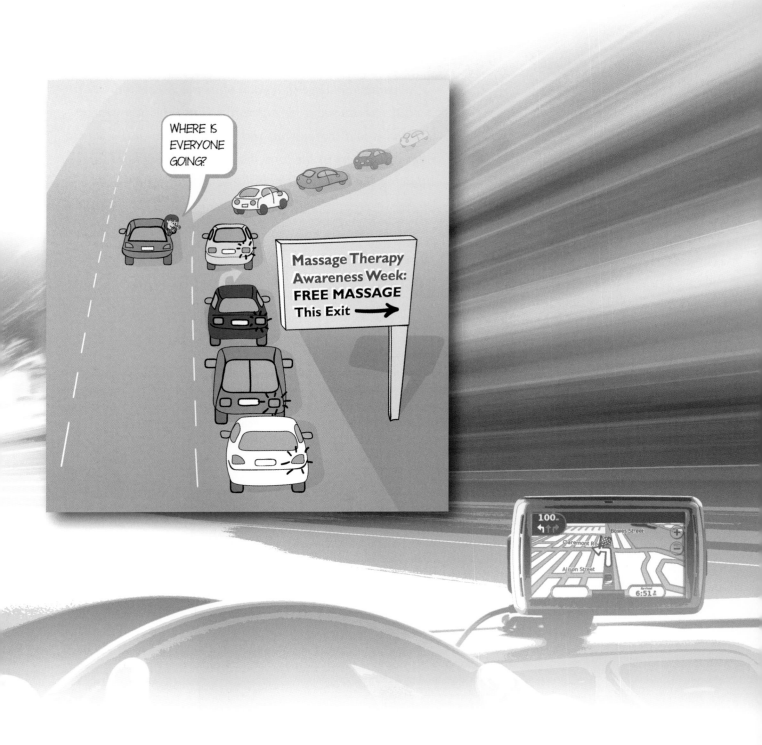

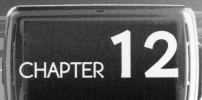

CHAPTER 12

The Marketing Mix: Product, Place, and Price

I've come to believe that each of us has a personal calling that's as unique as a fingerprint—and the best way to succeed is to discover what you love and then find a way to offer it to others in the form of service, working hard, and allowing the energy of the universe to lead you.

OPRAH WINFREY

KEY CONCEPTS

- The marketing mix includes the four P's: product, place, price, and promotion.
- In a service-based business, the person who provides the service is the real product, and self-confidence is indispensable.
- Maximizing your potential means taking advantage of every opportunity to promote and improve your business, with the goal of having every client become a regular customer.
- Client education is a form of product support that includes providing brochures and fact sheets listing the benefits of massage, and periodically hosting informational seminars or support groups for the community.
- The location of your business has a direct effect on the number and the type of clients you will attract.
- Creating a competitive advantage for your market position depends on analyzing the strengths and weaknesses of your business, and those of the competition, and acting on them.
- Tracking clients lets you gauge where your marketing efforts are the most effective and will help you update your market study periodically.
- Obtaining client testimonials, conducting and reporting case studies, and offering customer loyalty incentives are effective ways of increasing business.
- Setting prices involves a consideration of your own financial requirements, the value of your training and experience, the environment of your business, and research on what the market will bear.
- Three additional P's—people, punctuality, and physical evidence—are vital components of a massage therapy business.

- Everyone the client comes in contact with at your business setting has the potential to make an impression, including other customers.
- Punctuality is one of the most important qualities of a professional massage therapist.
- Clients will believe in the efficacy of massage therapy whenever physical evidence demonstrates the benefits.

The basic principles of marketing are often referred to as the marketing mix, or the four P's: product, place, price, and promotion. Three of the four P's will be discussed in this chapter; promotion will be covered in Chapter 13. An additional three P's—people, punctuality, and physical evidence—will also be discussed as components that are vital to a service-based business. Massage therapists, especially those who are just starting out in business, will find that cultivating the right marketing mix requires research, attention to detail, the use of good judgment, and the process of trial and error. Developing the most beneficial balance for your unique situation is an essential strategy for building customer relationships and running a profitable business. Finding out what marketing approach works for your particular business, and what doesn't, is part of the learning experience.

YOU ARE THE PRODUCT

You're probably thinking that massage is the product, but it isn't. *You*—the provider of the service—are the product. As with all service-based businesses, the objective is to make a positive impression on every client, with a goal of cultivating repeat customers.

Consider the fact that your potential clients are a diverse group of people who have different levels of experience with massage therapy. A client who is receiving his very first massage is going to recall that event whenever he has massage in the future, while a client who has had massage before will be comparing his first session with you to his previous sessions with other therapists.

If you're a new therapist just beginning your career, your technical expertise and experience are not yet the same as someone who's been practicing for 20 years. You can make up the difference by exuding professionalism, giving the best service you can give, and adding personal touches to your business. People want to be made to feel special for choosing to spend their time and money with you.

You want every client to leave with the impression that she has found exactly what she was looking for in a therapist. That's the real beginning of all the word-of-mouth referrals you hope to have coming your way. And it's the key to marketing yourself as the core product of your business.

A Sense of Self-Worth

A good salesperson has to have a belief in the value of his product in order to successfully sell it. Think about that in the context of *you* being the product, and selling yourself to the public as a massage therapist and a businessperson.

Your sense of self-worth is something that must be nurtured from within. By going into business, you're taking a leap of faith, so you have to have a certain amount of confidence in your ability to succeed; that's self-confidence, and it's about *what you can do*. Self-worth, on the other hand, is about *who you are*. It has nothing to do with how much money you have, whom you know, or where you live. Having self-worth means you realize what a valuable human being you are.

Those who choose massage therapy as a career are usually people who feel a deep satisfaction from helping others. And when it comes to business, we've all heard the old adage that "the customer comes first." However, we need to take care of *ourselves* first. Whether you are a lone practitioner or employ others, you are the most important product and representative of your company.

Consider the advice you give to clients every day:

- Eat sensibly, and drink plenty of water to keep your muscles hydrated.
- Get enough rest.
- Stretch several times every day.
- Get enough exercise.
- Take warm soaking baths.
- Schedule appointments for regular massage.

Do you follow that advice yourself? A self-employed person often works much longer hours than he would if he were employed by someone else. Massage therapy can be a physically demanding job, depending on a lot of factors, such as what modality you practice, how ergonomically efficient your workspace is, what kind of body mechanics you practice, even what kind of shoes you wear to work. You simply have to take care of yourself if you want to take care of others.

Value yourself in other ways, too. Sometimes difficult clients come along whom you just can't connect with and just can't please. It isn't about you, so don't take it personally and don't let them destroy your self-esteem. And as any business owner can tell you, sometimes the path to success is a rocky road. Whatever difficulties you experience, whether financial hardships, staffing problems, or other challenges, experiencing a rough time or an outright failure doesn't make you any less valuable as a person. You are still precious, so believe in yourself and take care of yourself.

Words of Wisdom
Your career isn't who you are; it's what you do.

Maximizing Your Potential

The phrase "maximizing your potential" should be a mantra you follow, in every business situation and each therapist/client relationship. For instance, meeting all the people you can, telling everybody you meet about your business, networking at every opportunity, and using smart promotion and advertising strategies (see Chapters 13 and 14)—all of these will maximize your potential to get people to think of *you* when seeking massage therapy. Once you get them in the door, you'll give them such a great experience that they wouldn't consider going anywhere else.

You want every client to become a regular customer. Regular clients will contribute to the financial stability of your business, and they will refer people to you. In addition to winning them over with your attentiveness to their needs, your professional demeanor, and your technical skill as a massage therapist, there are other inexpensive ways of maximizing your potential to turn every visitor into a returning customer.

Etienne Gibbs, author and motivational speaker, suggests that in order to maximize your potential, you should take an inventory of the skills that you have, and then look for creative ways to utilize them. For instance, you already know you possess the skill to perform massage. You don't have to be in luxurious surroundings to add extra touches to that skill, in order to impress clients.

Signature services were mentioned in Chapter 11, but don't stop there. A warm bathrobe and slippers for clients to slip into if they have to go to the bathroom is a good investment. A waffle pad or dense memory foam pad on the table and face cradle, a table warmer, a down comforter, and nice flannel sheets on your massage table make the client feel like she's in a cozy nest. A feather pillow is a good investment; some people aren't comfortable flat on their back, even with a bolster under their knees, and with a feather pillow, you can still get your hands under the head or neck if you need to. When the client is lying on the table, you want her to have that warm and nurtured feeling of being totally taken care of. Your technical skills will improve with experience, but providing those little extras will make you and your services stand out from the crowd from your first day in business.

Words of Wisdom
Successful people aren't necessarily any more talented than the majority. They simply find ways to maximize their potential and to use their talents and skills effectively.

Product Support

Product support can include any resource that gives the client information about you and your business. Product support includes client communications and client education.

Felicia Brown, an expert consultant in the spa industry, states that product support is anything that results in TOMA—Top of Mind Awareness. When it comes to being in business for yourself, TOMA is critical to your success. For example, when I was beginning in massage therapy, I wanted people to think of me as "The" massage therapist in town. I introduced myself to everyone, attended lots of networking meetings, gave my business cards out to everyone I met, and looked for as many opportunities as I could to get quoted in the paper or on the TV or radio news.

One of the best things about product support is that it usually doesn't cost any money. However, it does require effort on your part to be conscientious about taking advantage of as many circumstances as possible, in order to maintain Top of Mind Awareness. You want that customer state of mind to last as long as you're in business. Don't rest on your laurels once you're a success. Staying on top requires some effort.

Maintaining Contact

Product support—and Top of Mind Awareness—means maintaining contact with clients. Communication is absolutely necessary, if you want your clients to think of you—and the fact that they need to schedule a massage. The old saying "Out of sight, out of mind" is true.

Maintaining client contact starts with following up after the first session. Sending a "Welcome to my practice card" is an example (see Chapter 11). If a client was in a lot of pain when he came in, make a phone call a day or two later to find out how he's feeling. If a new client leaves your office without scheduling another appointment, making that call can get him back in. Along with the welcome card, you may want to include a discount offer for the next appointment, for those who didn't rebook before leaving the office. Instead of giving a discount to clients who have already made the decision to come again, you can target the ones who need an incentive, and this is a smart business move.

If a regular client suddenly disappears, call her to show concern. The conversation should be direct and to the point: "Mrs. Clay, this is Laura Allen, your massage therapist. I haven't seen you in a couple of months and was just wondering if you're doing okay? It's not like you to go so long between appointments, and I wanted to check in with you." When I've made that kind of call, I have found out that the client had been laid off from her job, or was taking care of her husband at home after a stroke, or some other catastrophe. If you don't call and ask, you'll never know, and the client may assume you don't care. If you don't feel comfortable calling, send a card instead. Take some kind of action to let the client know you are thinking of her and want to maintain contact.

Newsletters are one of the best tools for keeping in touch with clients (see Chapter 11). Direct mailings and other forms of maintaining client contact will be discussed in Chapter 14.

Client Education

People generally want to know how something will benefit them, and you can educate them about the benefits of massage! Providing brochures or fact sheets about massage is helpful to your clients. Client education is not only an obligation of your job; it empowers the client.

In many towns, there are support groups for people with all kinds of medical conditions: cancer, fibromyalgia, chronic fatigue syndrome, and so forth. Creating a list of contact information for these groups requires a few hours of effort on your part, but clients will appreciate the effort you've made in finding something that will help them cope with their situation. Educating clients and going out of your way to assist them is the best kind of product support. It makes a lasting impression when you go the extra mile to provide a more personal service.

If you have the space in your massage setting, consider hosting such a group meeting at your office. Consider inviting a physician to come and give an educational talk about a specific health condition or medical situation. At a minimum, you'll get appreciation for hosting the meeting, and you'll probably get a few new clients out of it, too.

ROADSIDE ASSISTANCE

In my office, I have a resource shelf, consisting of reference books and back issues of trade journals. If a client mentions she is suffering from a certain condition, I might pull out my pathology book for a quick consult, to help educate both myself and the client. Professional publications, such as *Massage Magazine, Massage & Bodywork*, and the AMTA's *Massage Therapy Journal*, publish articles every month on the efficacy of massage for different conditions. Copy articles of interest and share them with clients. They really appreciate it!

YOUR PLACE IN THE MARKET

Where to set up shop was discussed briefly in Chapter 2 as part of developing your business plan. Let's delve a little deeper because there are many factors to consider in choosing your location, as well as claiming your niche in the marketplace. Unless you've already decided to be a mobile massage therapist, the physical location of your business is a major determinant of your **market position**—a competitive comparison of your business relative to other businesses of the same type in your area. When looking for an appropriate business space, remember that you get what you pay for, but cost shouldn't be the only consideration. You must analyze the benefits of locating in a particular place. Here are some of the things to consider about cost vs. benefits when choosing a place:

- A high-visibility location, like Main Street, usually commands higher rent (or purchase price), but it will have more traffic than an office of the same size on a back street—even just one block back.
- A space in a large mall with a well-known anchor store will have higher rent, and more foot traffic, than one the same size in a strip mall.

- An office in an upscale neighborhood convenient to professional offices, exclusive boutiques, and fine restaurants will have a higher rent and will attract more affluent clients than an office in an industrial area.
- An office in a medical park will have high rent but will also be a prime spot for a medical massage business and the cultivation of doctor referrals.

A therapist practicing in a salon, a gym, the YMCA, or a similar place will have a certain amount of ready-made business. Chances are good that a percentage of the people already patronizing those businesses would use an on-site massage therapist and would help spread the word. On the other hand, if you're inside a salon or the Y, the chances are also pretty good that you won't get a lot of business coming in from outside sources, unless you really spend a lot of time, effort, and money to advertise yourself to other audiences. In a big city, the Y, a gym, or a salon may have a customer base of hundreds of people, and that would probably be enough to support you without your having to solicit outside business. In a small town or rural area, that may not be the case.

In a salon, gym, or even a chiropractor's office, massage is often viewed as a secondary service, and the employees in the primary business may have no idea of how to be supportive of massage therapy services. Educate them! If you're renting space in such a venue, give the staff members a free or discounted massage, tell them about the benefits of massage, and be sure they know what to say when one of their customers asks them about your practice.

Besides affordability and visibility, you should also consider the following:

- The amount of nearby competition.
- The ease of traffic getting in and out.
- Parking availability and accessibility for the handicapped.
- Whether the physical space meets your needs for an office.

While there's nothing wrong with improving your circumstances by moving to a better location, ideally you should establish an office where you intend to remain for a long time.

Wherever you decide to start your business, whether at home or at a prestigious address with a price tag to match, the function of the location is to provide a venue for the product—you—and your services. Don't get in over your head by getting a place that is going to strain your finances. You not only want it to be comfortable for your clientele, you also want it to be somewhere you'll look forward to going to and spending your workday.

Going with the Flow

Consider having an office inside a major corporation, either as a renter or as an employee. According to Forbes Magazine, SC Johnson, Cisco Systems, Allstate, FedEx, and Gannett, the major newspaper chain, all offer in-house massage as an employee benefit.

The Competition

I'm all for healthy competition; there are enough aching bodies and stressed-out people to go around. However, if there is a long-established massage therapy business right across the street from the office you're considering renting, you may want to rethink your choice—unless, of course, your business will have something drastically different. For instance, if the business across the street is an upscale day spa and your intent is to have a medical massage practice, there wouldn't be a competitive disadvantage. But if you're offering the same thing as the closest competitor, bear in mind that her customers are likely to be loyal to her if she's been in business for a long time.

If you do decide on a location that's near another massage establishment, be sure that your business name is totally different. Otherwise, first-time clients may confuse your business with the other place, not to mention that the competitor may think you're trying to copy his business or deliberately cash in on his name and fame.

Competing with Integrity

Value yourself enough to conduct your business, including competing for your share of the market, with integrity. Don't try to unfairly put the competition out of business. If the therapist down the block is charging $100 for a massage and you advertise that your new business charges only $50, you'll be perceived as someone who undercuts prices in order to steal business. (These prices are just examples; prices vary widely according to location.) Undercutting is unprofessional and simply not a good idea. You want to stand out from the competition—but not because your services are half the price. Competing fairly also relates back to the previous discussion of self-worth.

The Competitive Advantage

Competing fairly is not meant to imply that you shouldn't compete at all. Major corporations often use what is referred to as a SWOT analysis. SWOT stands for internal Strengths and Weaknesses and external Opportunities and Threats.

The **SWOT analysis** is a simple way of sizing up the competition, and determining ways to maximize your strengths, minimize your weaknesses, seize opportunities, and identify any potential threats to your business—in other words, get a competitive advantage. Bear in mind that in order to know anything about your competitors, you need to either visit them or depend on the word of someone you trust who has visited them, and obtain their business cards and brochures. You can't compete if you're ignorant of what they're offering and how they're presenting it.

Consider, for example, that a mile from your office there's a day spa offering massage. Let's say you make a visit in the interest of performing your SWOT analysis. Table 12-1 shows what your analysis might look like.

There are plenty of possibilities to give you a competitive advantage. Perhaps you have extended hours of operation, or a medical practice that's receiving doctor referrals; maybe you have equipment, such as a sauna, that the competition is lacking. When you do a comparison in the format of a SWOT analysis, right away you can see the pros and cons of your massage setting's location. You have to weigh those and decide the probability of a favorable outcome.

Clients Here, There, and Everywhere

Your place in the market is not only about your physical address. It's also about who your potential customers are, based on the location you've chosen, and the other factors in your marketing mix.

I know who my potential market is—everybody! I want all people to feel welcome in my business. The prices in my clinic are reasonable enough for most people to be able to afford to come here, and we accept health insurance. I live in a small town, so it's feasible, in my circumstances, that my market literally does encompass everyone. If you're seeking a niche market, such as pregnant women, or if you intend on doing sports massage and working only with athletes, you're

TABLE 12-1	A SWOT Analysis	
SWOT	**My Business**	**Competitor's Business**
Strengths	Better location due to traffic pattern	Signage much bigger than mine
	Handicapped-accessible	Steps in front, no wheelchair ramp visible
	Therapists trained in several modalities	Only offers Swedish massage
Weaknesses	Landscaping in front of office doesn't look appealing	Grounds in front are beautifully landscaped with plants and fountain
Opportunities	Opportunity to expand into suite next door	Lot is small, no room to expand
Threat	Rumor going around about a chain of spas coming to town	Chain of spas would potentially affect competition, too

making a choice to limit yourself to a specific clientele. Otherwise, why shouldn't you act as if everyone is a potential client? Just look at all the possibilities:

- People you have worked with in the past.
- People from your neighborhood.
- People who attend your church.
- People with whom you attended school or college.
- People you know from your child's school.
- People who work at businesses you patronize.
- People who are in your civic groups or clubs.

You have brief encounters with other people all the time, such as standing in line at the supermarket, sitting in the waiting room at a doctor's office, or even waiting for a bus. Each of these is an opportunity to make small talk with someone. Always have your business cards handy. (For a discussion of business cards, see Chapter 14.)

OPPORTUNITIES AHEAD

Tracking Clients

You want to keep track of how your clients hear about your business. The goal, of course, is to gain as many clients as possible through word-of-mouth referrals, and through your own efforts of talking to others about your business as mentioned above, because those don't cost anything.

Ask every new client who comes in how he learned about your business. Keep a simple tracking form on your desk, and record what each client tells you. Doing so will help you decide where your marketing efforts are being effective, and where they are being wasted. A sample client tracking form is shown in Figure 12-1.

Updating the Market Study

Doing a market study was part of the business plan in Chapter 2. However, that was not a one-time task. External forces can affect your business, and your market study should be updated every year or so, especially if your business is not

Client	Referred by	Yellow Pages	Newspaper Ad	Flyers	Radio Ad	Television Ad
J. Dunkle	R. Dunkle					
K. Robb		✗				
M. Pack	L. Flack					
D. Barre		✗				
C. Staly	F. Jones					
L. M. Cole	B. Cole					
P. Sayer	D. Harris					
A. Menno			✗			
G. Allan	L. Flack					

FIGURE 12-1   A client tracking form.

meeting your income projections. Instead of being discouraged, rely on market research and logical reasoning to modify your plan.

When you update your market study, note if there have been any drastic changes in the neighborhood since your business opened. Did the nearby mall lose their big anchor department store? Has the local economy suffered a decline for some reason? Do the other businesses around yours seem to be thriving, or barely surviving?

If there is a major change in the local economy, service-oriented businesses often suffer first; people who have to cut back financially will give up those things they don't consider to be necessities. Conversely, there could be an upswing in the local economy due to a new industry moving to town. Other businesses might be opening nearby, with new construction taking place, new people moving into town, more money circulating, and the many other things that happen when the economy is healthy. An economic boom could be the perfect opportunity to expand your business. (For times of economic downturn, see Chapter 13.)

It's wise to keep abreast of the changes that are going on in your community. If the newspaper announces that the five-year plan for a new highway will bring the road right through the front door of your business, don't wait until the bulldozer is in the yard to look for another place.

Customer Relations

The relationships you build with your customers will be key elements to your success. It costs less to keep an existing customer than it does to advertise in order to get a new one (see Chapter 14). Furthermore, if every person who visits your office has a favorable experience, and tells a friend, that begins to have a domino effect. No advertising is less costly, or more valuable, than your satisfied clients spreading the word. Be sure to thank a client whenever she sends someone your way. A handwritten note, or 15 extra minutes added to her massage at no charge, expresses your appreciation in a tangible way.

Sure, a customer will come back if she has an ideal experience the first time. The key to customer satisfaction is consistency. You want each person who patronizes your business to have that same ideal experience every time—the treatment room is cozy and clean, the appointment starts on time, the therapist is attentive to her needs, and so forth. A satisfied customer will be a repeat customer.

Testimonials

One effective method of getting new customers is to ask existing customers for testimonials. Of course, a word-of-mouth referral is a testimonial in itself, but a written testimonial can be used for advertising purposes, included in your brochure, or even framed and displayed in your office. Be sure to ask permission before using a client's name. If you use radio or television for advertising, you might ask a client to give an on-air testimonial.

Testimonials can also be helpful in getting you referrals from other health care professionals. For instance, if you want to approach a certain doctor about referring patients to you, and your long-standing client has mentioned that she is a patient of his, you could ask her if she would write a testimonial about how receiving massage from you has lowered her stress level or helped her fibromyalgia symptoms. Just say, "Ms. Jones, would you mind writing a short recommendation for me? I've got an appointment with Dr. Smith to talk with him about referring clients to me, and it would be helpful if I had a testimonial from one of his patients."

If you feel nervous about asking someone in person, you might solicit testimonials from your clients through your newsletter or e-mail updates. Here's an example:

> Therapy Plus is seeking client testimonials that we can use for advertising purposes. If you would be willing to write a few sentences about how our massage therapists have helped you, please send your testimonial to our e-mail address at info@therapyplus.

Once you have gathered some testimonials, don't procrastinate. Put them to good use!

Case Studies

A **case study** is a method of conducting research that relies on an in-depth investigation of an event or condition. Rather than a strictly conducted scientific experiment, a case study relies on gathering data and analyzing and reporting the results. In keeping with the rule of confidentiality, you should not use the client's real name if you publish or otherwise share the case study.

Case studies can serve a number of purposes, including

- Increasing your knowledge about the subject.
- Gaining clients for your business.
- Publicity for you if you publish your findings.
- Helping the subject(s) of the study through the benefits of bodywork.

You can easily set up a case study by choosing a health or medical condition that interests you, perhaps the condition you've seen most often among your clients, or some unusual pathology that you're curious about. Announce to your e-mail list or in your newsletter that you are seeking clients who are suffering from _____, who will receive massage at no charge or at a discount in exchange for being a research subject. Of course, you can't take more than one or two at a time unless you have plenty of spare time and enough money to support yourself.

The Massage Therapy Foundation holds annual contests for the best case studies and publishes the findings, and also awards research grants. There are particular ethical considerations to be observed when conducting a case study,

SUCCESS NEXT EXIT

OPPORTUNITIES AHEAD

including obtaining informed consent from the client to participate in a research project. You can find guidelines for conducting a case study, and read about past research projects, on the Massage Therapy Foundation website.

ROADSIDE ASSISTANCE

I've used case studies to attract clients for research purposes and performed the work with someone at no cost in order to explore the efficacy of massage on a certain health condition. In every instance, I have gained much more than a research paper. When I was researching Tourette's syndrome, the mother of a 15-year-old girl who had the condition was so grateful for the work I did with her daughter, she mobilized her entire family to buy gift certificates from my business for Christmas. That amounted to over $1000 of sales in itself, and I also ended up gaining three regular (paying) clients.

PRICING YOUR SERVICES

Setting fees was discussed in Chapter 4, and again in Chapter 7 in the context of figuring your break-even point. We'll revisit this important topic here, as a part of the marketing mix. The most important thing to consider when pricing your services is your budget, and how much money it realistically takes you to meet your obligations. You need to know how many massages you have to perform every month in order to pay your bills, and how much money you'd like to have over and above that, to save or use for other important purposes, like taking a vacation.

Some therapists charge by the minute, some by the hour; some charge a flat rate "per session," and the length of a session may vary. There are a number of things to think about when setting your prices. For instance, if you practice a special modality, such as Rolfing, that required more education than basic massage, or a modality that requires ongoing training, such as Trager or one of the Upledger techniques, you might feel comfortable charging a little more than the going rate for your work. Another consideration is the length of your experience; if you've been in practice for years, you may feel justified in charging more than a therapist who's fresh out of school.

Your work environment is another factor; if you have a luxurious office at a prestigious address, people will expect to pay a premium price for the surroundings. A massage on a cruise ship isn't really worth any more than a massage in your living room, if all you take into consideration is the value of your time performing the massage, but that's the point—a massage on a cruise ship is something special because it's taking place in the middle of the big blue ocean, during a vacation, when people have that "pamper me" mindset. Someone who might not bat an eye at paying $150 for a 50-minute massage while on a cruise might think that's an exorbitant price for an hour at your home massage office. She has the idea that she's paying not just for the massage but for the surroundings, and she's right.

Pricing Strategies

Along with your budget, your education, your level of experience, and the surroundings you are in, there are other things to consider when figuring out how to price your services. What the market will bear in your locale varies widely across all areas of the country. The attractiveness of your packaging, and whether or not you offer any discounted services, should all have an influence on your pricing strategies.

Think about retail establishments for a moment. On the high end is Macy's, on the low end is the Dollar Discount store, and 90% of other retail companies probably fall somewhere in between. Service businesses are much the same. Unless you're serving the poor by offering sliding-scale massage, or you have enough resources to open a luxurious spa, your business will probably be somewhere in the middle of that range.

What the Market Will Bear

"What the market will bear" refers to the going rate in your area. In order to determine what the market will bear, you have to find out what the other therapists in your area are charging, and be relatively in line with that, if your establishment and your offerings are similar. As discussed in Chapter 7 (see Table 7-1), there is a lot of variance from place to place in the usual and customary rate for massage. Even within the same town, a massage at the Y usually costs much less than a massage at an upscale day spa.

Undercutting the prices of other therapists was discussed earlier. Conversely, if the other therapists in your vicinity are charging $60 and you charge $100, you're taking a big risk—unless you have a clearly stated reason, like all sessions are an hour and a half long instead of the standard hour. There's nothing wrong with a variance of $5 or $10 more or less than what others in your proximity are charging, but if it's much more than that, there should be a clear justification.

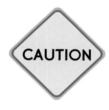

EXPLORATIONS

Call (or visit) the massage therapy businesses within a 10-mile radius of your proposed location to find out the fees for the services they offer. Figure out the average price of massage in your area. If one therapist is way out of line from the rest in terms of price, find out what is it about her service that warrants the price difference. It's a fair strategy to be informed about your competitors.

Attractive Packaging

Enhancing your menu of services was described briefly in Chapter 5, but let's look beyond that at the *packaging* of your services. Some therapists think the word "massage" is enough to describe what they do. However, having a descriptive menu adds a professional touch to your business. It can help educate clients about the different types of massage therapy available, thus increasing the possibility of selling them future services. Even if you provide only one modality, the intent is to describe what you're offering in an attractive way. The packaging of your services can enhance the client's perception—and add to your profits.

Many massage therapy schools today operate on the "smorgasbord" curriculum system, teaching a little of this and a little of that; perhaps you've had training in a number of modalities. Some schools focus only on neuromuscular therapy, or Eastern techniques, for example. The key is to take whatever it is you know, and make it sound as appealing as possible. Let's assume your education is in Swedish massage. Here are three different ways you could describe that on your menu of services:

Swedish Massage: $50 per hour.
Swedish Massage (light relaxation massage): $50 per hour.
Swedish Massage—A lighter massage for those seeking relief from stress and
    tension, guaranteed to make you float off into a cloud of relaxed bliss: $60
    per hour.

Notice that the third selection cost is $10 higher. The description makes it sound like more of a value. If I were seeking massage, I'd want the one that's going to make me float off into a cloud of relaxed bliss, wouldn't you?

Continuing with the assumption that your training has only included Swedish massage, let's look at other variations you could take from that to put on your menu. People who are pressed for time and/or money would appreciate the option of a half-hour focused on the neck and shoulders, or a half-hour foot rub. Look at these descriptions:

Neck and Shoulder Massage: $30 per half-hour.

The Stressbuster Massage—30 minutes of massage on your neck and shoulders, with a lavender pillow over your eyes and your feet elevated, will make you feel like a new person. Relax and feel the tension just melting away: $40 per half-hour.

Foot Rub: $30 per half-hour.

Tired Tootsie Revitalization—Your tired, aching feet will be massaged with pure organic peppermint oil. You'll love the hot towel wrap at the end, and the rest of your body will thank you for it: $40 per half-hour.

If you're given two identical gifts, one presented in an old paper sack, the other presented in a beautifully wrapped box, which one do you enjoy receiving more? It's all about the packaging.

Discounting Services

Discounting services can be done as a means of community service—you want to help someone who can't afford the regular price, so you offer a discount. Discounting services can also be an important part of your marketing strategy.

Consider offering an ongoing discount to certain populations. At my clinic, we give clients over 60 a $10 discount. Some therapists discount services to public servants, such as members of the police and fire departments. Here are some of the many other ways to gain and retain clients through discounting:

- Offer a discount on the client's birthday.
- Offer a discount for couples massage on anniversaries.
- Offer a discount to clients who pay in advance for x number of sessions.
- Offer a discount to families.
- Offer a discount to veterans and/or active military personnel.
- Offer a discount to other massage therapists and bodyworkers.
- Offer a discount to bridal parties.

ALTERNATE ROUTES

Employees and Independent Contractors

Be sure that the terms of your employment are clear regarding discounts. If the owner advertises a $20 discount, is she expecting you to take $20 less in pay? Is she absorbing the discount, or does she expect you to split the amount with her?

Business Partners

Use your financial software or otherwise document the discounts you give. Discounts are tax deductions.

Customer Loyalty Programs

Ideally, we will all cultivate clients who are loyal to us without having any kinds of customer loyalty programs. However, having such a program is an added incentive, and for some consumers, it's the icing on the cake when deciding where to take their business. Many of the massage franchises use such programs.

A **customer loyalty program** rewards the client for repeat business. A typical plan states that "Every tenth visit is free," or whatever number the therapist decides. You can monitor the visits by marking each session number in your appointment book, or you can provide the client with a card to be punched or marked off at each visit.

If you offer multiple services in your business, such as aesthetics or spa treatments, or you have modalities other than what the client usually receives, another good strategy is to give the customer a reward of some other service or product. This can introduce the client to the other options that are available and could result in purchases of multiple services during future visits.

A **referral reward** is usually offered in the form of discounts on future appointments. Examples are giving a client $10 off on massage for every new person she refers to you and/or giving a free massage for a stated number of referrals the client sends you.

Referral rewards are not appropriate between health care practitioners. The Code of Ethics of the NCBTMB states:

> The certificant shall refuse any gifts or benefits that are intended to influence a referral, decision or treatment or that are purely for personal gain and not for the good of the client.

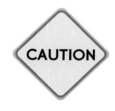

As health care professionals, we should avoid not only conflicts of interest but any *appearance* of a conflict of interest. We want physicians to refer people to us because of our ability to contribute to the health and well-being of their patients, not because we're paying them for every referral.

Referral rewards for clients may not be legal in all states, so check with your state's massage board before offering them. If allowed, they can be a real incentive for your frequent customers to send new clients your way.

Raising Your Prices

The rising cost of doing business is a fact of life, and there will come a time when you need to raise your prices. Set your prices high enough initially so that you won't have to raise them during the first year. Starting out with a lowball price and then raising it a month or two later will be perceived by clients as a "bait and switch" strategy.

If you find you aren't bringing in enough money to pay your bills in the beginning, the best thing to do is cut as many expenses as possible and make a concerted effort to attract more clients, instead of raising the fees on the ones you already have. The best time to raise prices is when your services are in demand. When you get booked ahead to the point where people have to wait a substantial amount of time to obtain an appointment, say 2 or 3 weeks, that's the time to raise your prices. It's a good practice to notify clients in advance of a price increase. You can accomplish that by sending a newsletter or other kind of direct mailing, sending it to your e-mail contacts, posting a notice on your website (see Chapter 14), and posting a sign in the waiting room.

Increasing your fee by $5 or $10 is not apt to cause you to lose a lot of business, but a $20 price increase would probably do you more harm than good, unless most of your clients are affluent. It's better to implement a modest increase periodically than a huge one sporadically. Use it as an opportunity to sell package deals.

Marketers call this the bad news/good news approach—letting a client know there's bad news, and then ending that notice on a positive note.

ROADSIDE ASSISTANCE

My price increase notice states: "Effective January 1, the fee for an hour of massage therapy will increase to $70. Please note that by purchasing a paid-in-advance package of six sessions, the discount will keep the cost to you at only $60 per session." Handling the price increase this way gives people time to prepare and generally results in more package sales.

EXPANDING THE MARKETING MIX

In addition to product, place, and price, when it comes to service-based businesses, three more P's should be included in your marketing mix: people, punctuality, and physical evidence.

People

People, in this case, refers not to clients, but to everyone in your business with whom clients interact—from staff members to other clients waiting in the lobby. Keep in mind that word-of-mouth is the best marketing tool you can have. Every person the client meets during her visit to your massage setting has the potential to influence her level of satisfaction—and to give her something to talk about.

For instance, another client in the waiting area can have a positive impact on the impression someone gets of your business, if she's standing there praising the massage and saying how much better she feels. But what if that person says something negative about the massage she just received, complains that the room was too hot or too cold, though she didn't mention it during the session, or otherwise acts disappointed?

In spite of your best efforts, there will always be the occasional person who enjoys complaining, and you'd like to keep that person away from your other clients, but sometimes you just can't do that. If such a situation occurs, the best thing to do is assure the unsatisfied client that you do hear, and care about, whatever he is complaining about, and if the situation calls for it, apologize and/or offer to do something to rectify the situation. At least the other clients who witness this exchange will perceive you as taking the high road instead of arguing with another customer.

Punctuality

Punctuality is one of the most important components of a service-based business. The wisest strategy is to organize your work schedule so that it's optimal for your body's clock. If you're not a morning person, and you know that, book your massage clients in the afternoons and evenings. That's better than scheduling appointments in the mornings and being chronically late and grumpy!

Many times clients are on their lunch break, or they've taken time off from their job, arranged a babysitter, or otherwise modified their schedule in order to have a massage. Haven't you ever had an appointment with someone and been totally impatient by the time he or she gets to you—an hour or more after you were told to be there? Client satisfaction is reinforced when the appointment starts on time.

Just like the interaction with the complaining client mentioned above, if you or another therapist in your office is late, and the waiting client is sitting there tapping her fingers impatiently, checking her watch, and looking upset about the delay, that could give a negative impression to a new client standing by. A happy and satisfied client is one who will schedule return appointments, talk favorably about your business, and send you referrals.

Words of Wisdom
Be on time!

Always leave enough time in between clients (a half-hour is ideal) so that you can go a few minutes over with the session if you need to, thus giving the client her full amount of appointment time. If you do find yourself running late for some reason, make it up to the client. If it's just a few minutes, I offer the client a free hand paraffin treatment as a thank-you for waiting. If you're more than 15 minutes late, it's a wise move to discount, or give the client the session for free. That could mean the difference in whether she returns or not. We all want our clients to be on time, and it's doubly important that we be on time for them.

Physical Evidence

Physical evidence is the goal for every massage session. Whether a client visits you for relaxation and stress relief, to relieve pain, or to increase mobility, the physical evidence is the result produced by the massage therapist. It doesn't mean you are going to "fix" or heal anyone. It means that the client will achieve relaxation, if that's what she is seeking, or will notice a difference in her pain level at the conclusion of the massage. When physical evidence is present, the client will know that massage therapy is good for her.

POSTCARDS from the HIGHWAY   **Christine Courtney**

I became an aromatherapist and a massage therapist by accident. I needed to make changes in my life, and I felt having a hobby would help me bring some balance into my life. I enrolled in a massage and aromatherapy course. I immediately fell in love with the essential oils and the whole concept of being able to maintain the health and well-being of my body mind and spirit through the use of massage and essential oils.

In 1999, I left my corporate job of 20 years to become self-employed. I have never regretted my decision because I love my work. Every day finds me awake and alert and ready to go! In the beginning, I had no idea what days or times would be the best hours to work, so I worked any day and any time (except Christmas day) that clients booked. On days when I had no clients but had scheduled it to be a working day, I walked around to the businesses in the area handing out business cards and special offer flyers. On weekends and evenings, I went to local ladies' club meetings, offering free talks on the benefits of massage and aromatherapy. If I didn't have a client to work on, I was working on getting a client!

Whenever I got nervous that my new career would not work, I would talk to one of the great supportive people I am lucky to have in my life. My husband is the leader of that "supportive group" and when needed he would encourage me, advise me, and help me to once again see the potential in myself. I would dust myself off, pick up my business cards and leaflets, and off I would go in search of that new client. I now teach aromatherapy and massage and following is the advice I give to students who want to "take the plunge" and change their career to work as a therapist:

(continued)

Christine Courtney (*Continued*)

Look after yourself physically. There is no point in telling clients that they need regular massage and how important it is that they look after themselves if you are not doing the same. Your physical body is one of your tools, and if you do not care for it, it will not hold up to the pace.

Stay current and up to date with your subject. Network; learn how to promote yourself and your business, and keep proper records. You cannot neglect the business of being in business, or you will not be in business for long.

The next thing is—and for me it is probably the most important—have inspiring and encouraging people around you. There will be days when your belief in yourself will wane. Make sure you have someone who will remind you of all the reasons you chose to become a therapist, who will help to lift your spirits and encourage you to keep going.

I am reminded almost every day why I chose this career. It is a privilege and a joy to work with people at the level I work. It is so satisfying to see someone come in to my clinic in distress and for her to leave a little better for having allowed me to work with her. It is wonderful to feel someone's day or health is that little bit better because of the work I do.

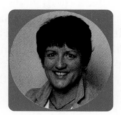

Christine Courtney is the owner and principal of OBUS School of Healing Therapies, located in Dublin, Ireland, with satellite branches in several other cities. She has trained as a Master Aromatherapist in France under Dr. Daniel Penoel and is a founding member of the Aromatherapy Council of Ireland. She is on the faculty at massage schools in the United Kingdom, Malta, and at THERA-SSAGE, Laura Allen's facility in North Carolina. Christine has also developed her own line of essential oils and skin care products. You can visit her website at www.aromatherapytraining.com.

SUGGESTED READINGS

Allen L. *One Year to a Successful Massage Therapy Practice.* Baltimore, MD: Lippincott Williams & Wilkins, 2008.

Brown F. *Do You Give Good TOMA?* http://.blog.spalutions.com/2009/01/17/do-you-give-good-toma.aspx. Accessed 01/20/09.

Dhillon A. *Self Help for Self Mastery: Building High Self-Esteem.* http://www.ananddhillon.com/blog/2008/07/building-high-self-esteem/. Accessed 01/20/10.

Gibbs E. *Maximizing Your Potential.* http://ezinearticles.com/?expert=Etienne_Gibbs. Accessed 01/21/10.

Harper C. *Fifty Habits of Highly Successful People.* http://www.lifehack.org/articles/lifestyle/fifty-habits-of-highly-successful-people.html. Accessed 01/21/10.

Kawasaki G. *Reality Check: The Irreverent Guide to Outsmarting, Outmanaging, and Outmarketing Your Competition.* New York, NY: Penguin Group, 2008.

Massage Therapy Foundation. www.massagetherapyfoundation.org. Accessed 01/21/10.

My Personal Journey

In this chapter, we've discussed the various components of the marketing mix, including how to package your services so that they are as attractive as possible. Start developing your menu of services by listing the modalities you are going to offer, and write descriptions that will make your offerings seem appealing to clients. Try writing several different descriptions for each service, and ask several friends or family members which one they find the most appealing.

My goals _____

_____

_____

What's in my way? _____

_____

_____

What action can I take to remedy the situation? _____

_____

_____

One-year progress update _____

_____

_____

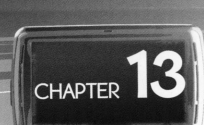

Promoting Your Business

There are people who make things happen, there are people who watch things happen, and there are people who wonder what happened.

JAMES LOVELL

KEY CONCEPTS

- Promoting a service business is selling an experience, rather than a product.
- A marketing budget is a necessity, because advertising is an unfixed expense that can easily spin out of control.
- The marketing budget should be revisited annually to reflect tracking results and the state of the economy.
- Carefully analyze the possible return on your financial investment, as well as your emotional investment, when choosing advertising venues.
- Treating a recession as a marketing opportunity is a strategy that can keep your business thriving during an economic downturn.
- The press release is one of the most useful no-cost promotional tools.
- Community service and philanthropy must be tempered by good judgment and by maintaining boundaries.
- The marketing budget and the marketing calendar should be created to work together; they depend on each other.
- Scheduling time every day to work on promoting your business will produce positive results.

Promoting your business is one of the most necessary tasks of being an entrepreneur and also one of the most fun and rewarding aspects of ownership. There are so many avenues to successful promotion; many are no-cost and low-cost, requiring only an investment of your time and your willingness to talk about yourself and your services. Marketing your business serves three main purposes: to draw interest, to educate potential clients, and to create the desire for your services. Your opportunities are only as limited as your imagination!

THE FOURTH P: PROMOTION

The word "promotion" encompasses all the efforts that go toward advancing your massage therapy business. *Promotion* can include those methods of marketing that don't require money. Everything—from the message on your answering machine to the simple act of talking to others about your services, handing out business cards and other printed materials to the advertising you buy—is a form of promotion. *Advertising* includes all the promotional materials and activities you have to pay for (see Chapter 14).

Promoting a service is different from promoting a specific product. For one thing, service is intangible; it's an *experience* that is inseparable from the place it's performed, whether in your office or the client's home or some other location. Every experience you provide in your service business is unique; no two massages you give will be exactly the same. The objective, of course, is for the experience to be great every time, and that's what you'll promote.

Like the other aspects of business, successful promotion is much easier to achieve if it's planned, in an organized way. Haphazard, disorderly promotion doesn't work. The goal of effective marketing is reaching your intended audience with a positive message about who you are and what you do, sparking enough interest that people will want to experience your service for themselves.

In addition to being effective, your promotional efforts also have to be affordable for you. Marketing is not a fixed expense such as rent, and the potential is there for it to be a very low percentage of your overhead—or for it to break the bank and send you into a financial tailspin. Next stop on the highway to success: your marketing budget.

HELP JUST AHEAD

Your Marketing Budget

Some costs are essential when you're creating a budget for marketing your business, unless you're working strictly from word-of-mouth referrals. These four essentials are the Yellow Pages, your own Internet presence, signage, and business cards. Once you've figured out these costs, you'll have a better idea of what you can afford to spend on other forms of promotion and advertising. These topics are discussed in detail in Chapter 14; they are mentioned here because they're a vital part of the overall budget.

You must have the money to pay for necessities—rent, utilities, telephone, and so forth—or advertising isn't going to do you much good. Calculate your break-even point without any advertising factored in (see Chapter 7). Then, once you have a realistic picture of the basic expenses of keeping the doors of your business open, you'll be able to budget a comfortable amount for marketing. I recommend sticking to that amount religiously for the first year. Marketing textbooks call this the **residual approach**—spending what you can afford only after you have covered your necessary expenses. They also say this is the least desirable method for setting a budget, and while that may be true for large corporations, they play by rules that are different from those for small businesses. Even if their balance sheet shows a huge loss, somehow they still manage to keep those television commercials coming. That probably won't be the case for you or me.

Most marketing books say that the first year or two you're in business, you should expect to spend 30% of your gross income on promotion and advertising. For example, if you've projected your first year's income to be $20,000, that would mean almost $7000 would be your advertising budget—a very substantial amount of money. While this might be okay in theory, wouldn't you prefer to keep some of that money for yourself? It can be done. You have to carefully weigh your options and make informed choices about where to spend your money. The cost of advertising varies greatly from place to place, and just like other expenses, it will cost more in a big city than in a small town.

Creating your marketing budget is not a one-time task. As time goes by, you'll find out, through careful tracking, where your marketing dollars are having the most beneficial effect and where you should save your money (see Chapter 12). Your budget should be revised every year; you cannot assume the budget you had for last year will work for next year. The economy—and your business— could go up or down, or your circumstances could change in some other way. And the longer you are in business, word-of-mouth referrals will gradually replace the need for extensive promotion and costly advertising, thereby cutting down on the amount of personal time you have to spend compared to when you were starting your business.

The Cost-Per-Person Formula

Marketers frequently use the term **ROI**, for **return on investment**: the amount of money brought in as a result of money spent. How much does it cost, who is the audience, and how many people is it going to reach—those are the questions you need to ask before committing to spending your hard-earned money on promoting your business.

You can calculate your ROI using the cost-per-person formula. Unless your bank account is endless, you have to figure out where you can get the biggest bang for your buck; your objective is to reach the most amount of people for the least amount of money. There's a big difference between paying $500 for an ad in the Sunday paper that will be seen by 40,000 subscribers and paying $500 for a plastic phone book cover that's only going to 1000 people. To demonstrate that difference, use simple math:

$500.00/40,000 = 0.0125 cent per person
$500.00/1000 = 5 cents per person

It's not hard to see which one is the better deal.

You can take this a step further and calculate your ROI based on how many people actually come in in response to a promotion, if you're doing the smart thing and tracking your results. If you spend $500 and get five new clients from that effort, it appears on the surface that you've invested $100 per person—but that's not realistic. One or more of the new visitors might have more than one appointment or turn into a long-term client. Gift certificate sales and word-of-mouth referrals could follow. It's feasible that you may even recoup the entire amount or make more—a great return on investment.

REALITY CHECKPOINT

Steering Clear of Ineffective Advertising

Business owners are bombarded with promotional offers and advertising opportunities, and even if you're so inclined, you just can't take advantage of every one of them. In order to stick to your budget, you have to learn to say, "Thank you, but I'll have to pass this time; my advertising budget is already used up for this year."

There are numerous "opportunities" that you should avoid, with a few caveats. For example, if your child asks you to buy an ad on the Little League calendar, or your mother asks you to buy an ad in the church cookbook, I'm not suggesting you turn down the request, as long as you can afford the cost of the ad. However, if it's not a family member prevailing on your guilt or good nature, think about those types of ads very carefully. They usually have a very limited audience. Chances are the Little League calendar is only going to be seen by other parents who have kids on the league. The church cookbook will spend most of its time sitting on the shelf, and when someone looks in it, she's searching for a recipe, not looking for your ad.

Let's examine a few other examples of advertisements that have either a limited potential audience and/or limited exposure over time:

- Ads on school calendars and programs
- Ads on theater and play programs
- Ads on promotional items that wind up in the junk drawer
- Ads in school yearbooks
- Ads on maps
- Ads in civic organization cookbooks
- Ads in coupon booklets
- Ads in periodicals that have a limited target audience, unless you share that same target audience

Does this mean you should never advertise in any of these places? Of course not; there are exceptions to every rule. You may want to show support for the local theater group, if it's a pet cause of yours, in spite of the fact that the printed programs will probably go in the trash as the patrons leave the building.

Consider the promotional items. There are "smart" promo items, and some that aren't so smart. Everyone uses pens; that's a smart item. Sticky notes are great giveaways to office workers. A tape measure might be a nice-looking promotional item, but how often is it used? It's probably going to go straight to the junk drawer.

Look at a few of the other things mentioned above. Coupon booklets are another thing that often get tossed in a drawer and forgotten about until they're long expired. School yearbooks are passed around for a week or two and relegated to the bookshelf. Maps are usually used by people passing through, not locals who would be repeat customers. Periodicals that are geared to a very narrow audience, such as the *Fraternal Order of the Police Journal*, are only going to be seen by people who are members of that organization.

Where to advertise is a personal choice, and people sometimes have their own reasons, other than money, for choosing a certain marketing venue. If you have the money to spare, certainly you should advertise anywhere you want to, even if it's not "productive," as long as it makes you feel good. However, don't forget the main objective, which is for your promotion to be seen by as many people as possible. Just remember when you make your choices, the cost is coming out of your budget, and the more you spend in one place, the less you have to spend somewhere else—maybe somewhere that would be more productive in terms of results.

ROADSIDE ASSISTANCE

I advertise my massage business on the prescription drug bags at a local pharmacy. Although it's not a venue I normally would choose, it's a family-owned company, not a chain, and the owners are regular customers of my business. They also purchase a lot of gift certificates for their employees' birthdays and other occasions. I estimate that they spend about $6000 a year in my business. I get ad space on 25,000 of their drug bags for less than $300. It's a reciprocal relationship; I'm supporting another local merchant who supports me.

No-Debt Marketing

When you first open your business, it's tempting to advertise anywhere and everywhere in an effort to become well known in as short a time as possible. Unless you have plenty of extra money, you must avoid that urge, or you'll find yourself in a financial strain. If you take out a start-up loan or use credit for capital expenditures such as a building, equipment, or an office furniture, you have something tangible to show for it—an asset. But don't get into the trap of using borrowed money or credit cards for advertising expenses.

After you have some cash equity built up in your business, you can raise your regular monthly advertising budget if you're ready to commit to contract advertising or more aggressive paid marketing. But you don't want to still be paying for an ad in last Sunday's paper a year from now, and if you put it on a credit card, that's what you'll be doing.

REALITY CHECKPOINT

Remember the important questions we asked above: What is the cost, who is the audience, and how many people is it going to reach? Add one more question: Do I have the expendable cash available to do this? Following those principles will help you choose the best forms of promotion and advertising that you can realistically afford.

Thriving in an Economic Downturn

OPPORTUNITY AHEAD

When the economy is in a downward spiral, consumers are more careful about spending money. There's a segment of the population that views massage as a luxury item, instead of a vital part of health care, and during a recession, luxury items are one of the first things to go. When people are ready to spend the fewer dollars they have, you want them spent with you, not the competition. Giving the best level of service possible has been discussed in several chapters, and it is definitely what will keep people coming back—even when they have less money.

During a time of economic uncertainty, the *perceived value* to a consumer becomes a bigger factor when he's confronted with a choice of where to spend money. When people are tightening their belts, here are some strategies for surviving and thriving:

1. *Help people save money.* Other than offering an occasional discount or special, avoid discounting your basic services. Instead, strengthen your efforts to sell more package deals, or try offering shorter sessions at a lower rate.
2. *Take care of your existing customers.* The people who remain loyal to your business deserve little extras as tokens of your appreciation, such as an extra 15 minutes on their massage session occasionally, or a special discount on their birthday. It's cheaper to keep existing customers than it is to advertise to get new ones.
3. *Maintain contact.* Keep in touch with your customers, and renew contact with those who haven't been in recently. An e-mail newsletter or blast offering a special, a handwritten note, or a personal phone call may be just the thing to get them back in the door.
4. *Develop a complementary service.* A service related to what you already do, such as offering hand paraffin treatments as an add-on to a massage, will bring in extra income. I've calculated that it costs $0.18 per person to give a hand treatment to a client; if I sell it as an add-on for a mere $5, I'm still making $4.82 profit on it.
5. *Take credit cards.* If you are not already accepting credit cards, during an economic downturn is the time to begin. Using a credit card gives the client the option of paying over time, but you still receive your money immediately.
6. *Create strategic partnerships with other complementary businesses.* If, for instance, there's a beauty salon nearby, partner with them to offer "Queen for a Day." The client can get her hair and nails done, and get a massage, for one agreed-upon price, and you'll be splitting the profits.
7. *Maximize promotional opportunities.* Keep in mind that many businesses are forced to lower their prices during a recession, and that includes media outlets, such as newspapers and radio or television stations. You may be able to get better advertising rates and can thus enjoy the opportunity to enhance your promotional efforts while staying within your budget.
8. *Cut expenses only where service won't suffer.* While a customer would notice you shortening a massage by 20 minutes, she's not apt to notice that you're buying cheaper paper towels for the bathroom or buying office supplies at garage sales.

9. *Develop multiple streams of income.* If you have a website, for example, there are numerous opportunities for affiliate programs that will bring you steady money, and a little here and there can really add up over time. Everyone from Google to Massage Warehouse is a prospect. Stick with reputable companies, and avoid anything questionable or potentially offensive.

10. *Be creative in your efforts to earn money.* If one day of the week is really slow for appointments, you might publicize like this: "Every Tuesday between 9 a.m. and 12 p.m., Therapy Plus is offering seated massage. Walk-ins welcome. Come in and get a great chair massage for $1 per minute." Then use the downtime to catch up on other marketing efforts, and on business and housekeeping chores. Chances are you won't have time, you'll be so busy doing chair massage.

11. *Accept health insurance.* As discussed in Chapter 5, accepting insurance is a buffer against recession. People who can't afford to pay the full price for massage therapy will still come for massage if they can manage the price of a co-payment.

12. *Keep a good attitude, and realize that this, too, shall pass.* Over the past 100 years, there have been numerous recessions in the United States, at least two per decade, with the average one lasting 11 months.

ALTERNATE ROUTES

Employees

You may not have input into the promotional efforts of your employer, but you can still *promote yourself*. Make it a point to tell a couple of new people every day where you work as a massage therapist, give them a card, and tell them to be sure to ask for you.

Independent Contractors

You can promote yourself, or collaborate with the owner, to split the cost and effort of mutual promotions, depending on the circumstances of your work contract. Discuss it with the employer.

Business Partners

Agree on who will handle promotional details, so that important responsibility doesn't fall through the cracks. One person may be responsible for keeping the calendar updated, while the other orders promotional items. Keep each other accountable for your efforts.

Using a Recession as a Marketing Tool

If the economy is in a recession, it always seems to be the main topic of the daily news: woeful statistics about plant closings and layoffs, businesses folding, and foreclosures. It's a stressful time for many people. What do stressed-out people need? Exactly—massage!

When you can't hide your head in the sand about the fact that the economy is weak, use it as a focus for marketing. While putting the suggestions in the list above into practice, build your promotional advertising around the recession. For example, here's a catchy blurb for the slow-day chair massage:

Short on money? Don't let the recession get you down! Come into Therapy Plus for a 15-minute Stress-Buster Massage for $15. It won't break the bank!

You might send coupons for $10 off with something catchy on them, such as "Recession Relief," to clients who haven't been in recently. Mention the recession in your newsletter, along with a few lines about how stressful times are for people and how stress-relieving massage is. Offer a discount on the first visit to anyone who brings in her unemployment check stub or layoff slip. When times are bad, people like to feel as if others are commiserating with them, so don't ignore a recession—capitalize on it!

Going with the Flow

Massage Magazine, reporting on a survey conducted by Readex Research for Associated Bodywork and Massage Professionals during the beginning of the recession in 2008, stated that 42% of massage therapists expect their businesses to continue having an increase in revenues, despite an economic downturn, with only 5% of therapists expecting a decrease in business. The Bureau of Labor Statistics predicts that the demand for massage therapists will grow by 19% during the decade of 2008 to 2018.

Free Publicity

Nothing serves your business better than free publicity, and of course, word-of-mouth referrals are the best free advertising you can get. You want to create a "buzz" around your business, having as many people talking about it in a positive way as you can and being in the media spotlight as often as possible.

Most massage therapists don't have the luxury of an unlimited marketing budget, but they need exposure in order to generate awareness about their business. Getting your name out there at no cost to you can be accomplished if you take advantage of the numerous opportunities to do so. The key is to make free publicity a top priority and to be diligent about working at it consistently. You'll be surprised at the amount of free publicity you can actually get, if you're willing to make the effort.

The Power of the Press Release

When it comes to promoting yourself, you have to toot your own horn, and don't be shy about it. One thing massage therapists often overlook as a free marketing tool is a press release. A **press release** is a no-cost short announcement about something you've accomplished, an event you've participated in or will be participating in, or other pertinent news. Check your local newspapers, free tabloids, and websites or blogs that specialize in community news to get the names of the business editors, and address all press releases to them. There are numerous occasions that could warrant a press release, starting with your graduation from massage school—you don't even have to wait until your business is open! Box 13-1 is an example.

Other opportunities for sending out a press release include the following:

- Opening your business
- Attending continuing education, to learn a new skill
- Attending a professional conference or convention
- Participating in, or hosting, a community service event
- Hosting a free seminar or other event
- Having an article or a book published
- Teaching a class
- Speaking at a public event
- A new therapist, or other employee or contractor, joining your practice
- Getting a new job or joining someone else's massage practice
- Being appointed to a public board
- Moving your business to a new location
- Being honored with an award

BOX 13-1   Sample Press Release No. 1

MacAllistar Completes Equine Massage Training

Susan MacAllistar of the Ellenboro community has completed training at the Center for Equine Massage in Boulder, Colorado. MacAllistar has had a lifelong love of horses, and for the past 5 years has been employed as the administrator at The Whole You School of Massage & Bodywork. After witnessing the profound changes that massage facilitates in the human body, she decided to attend the equine school and learn massage techniques for horses. She plans to offer her services to horse owners all over western North Carolina.

- Making a media appearance, such as being interviewed on radio or television
- Passing a milestone in your business, such as reaching an anniversary or giving your five-thousandth massage

Box 13-2 is another example of an informative press release.

No one will know what you're up to if you don't tell them! Publicize your accomplishments; clients are impressed when they read about them. Even if you are a brand-new therapist and you're working for someone else, use the power of the press. Box 13-3 is an example.

ROADSIDE ASSISTANCE

Did you notice that the name of my business is in all capital letters? I did that on purpose, and it's that way on our sign and all our printed materials—and on all advertising. Having it all in caps makes it stand out. You can do the same with your business name.

Community Service

Participating in community service is worthy of a press release. No one participates in community service just for the purpose of getting free publicity, but it is an opportunity, and you should take advantage of it. Performing community service gives you a heartwarming feeling, but unless you have the money to place philanthropy above the need to earn a living, choose carefully when you decide where and how to be involved in community service. This is an area where you have to balance your desire to give with protecting your financial stability. For example, if you donate ten massages to a charity benefit and they are all redeemed in a month, that would substantially cut into your income.

A community service event that's too far away from your office is not apt to bring you much business. Weigh the situation carefully before you jump in. Don't fall into the trap of automatically saying yes every time someone calls on you.

REALITY CHECKPOINT

BOX 13-2   Sample Press Release No. 2

Allen Attends National AMTA Convention

Laura Allen, owner of THERA-SSAGE in Rutherfordton, has just returned from attending the national convention of the American Massage Therapy Association (AMTA) in Atlanta, Georgia. The AMTA convention is an annual event that attracts more than a thousand massage therapists from all over the country. While at the convention, Allen attended a continuing education class in the dissection of the shoulder taught by internationally known instructor, David Kent, and learned valuable information about rotator cuff injuries.

BOX 13-3   Sample Press Release No. 3

Byers in Practice at THERA-SSAGE

Will Byers, a recent graduate of The Whole You School of Massage & Bodywork in Gilkey, North Carolina, has joined THERA-SSAGE in Rutherfordton in the practice of massage therapy. Byers specializes in rehabilitative massage and particularly enjoys working with athletes to aid in injury recovery and help enhance their performance. Byers is from the Green Hill community and looks forward to welcoming clients into his new practice at THERA-SSAGE.

Newspapers and local tabloids will usually publicize community service events at no charge, in the "Community Happenings" section or whatever similar feature they have. Box 13-4 is an example.

Community service can take many forms. You could donate massage services to hospice workers, give foot massage to the residents in a nursing home, or open a sliding fee clinic. It can also mean simply helping someone in need because you're inclined to do so.

Responsible Giving

Even when it means free publicity, there's a limit to how much of your time and resources you can give away without causing yourself any undue stress. Create a policy for responsible giving (see Chapter 9), and adhere to it. For instance, you may decide that you can afford to donate two massages per month to worthy causes or attend two community service events every month. Think of your policy as one of your boundaries, serving the purpose of keeping you from overextending yourself, time wise and financially.

Donating gift certificates for services is a good alternative if attending an event is impractical or wouldn't bring in much business. For example, you're not likely to get enough business from a Cub Scout meeting to make it worth the time you'd have to spend out of the office, but you could provide gift certificates for massage for their fundraiser. Even though a certain amount of the gift certificates won't ever be redeemed, you've garnered good will by giving the donation, and gathered potential paying clients from those who do redeem the certificates. It's also a good strategy to donate a half-hour massage that can be upgraded to an hour for $20 or some similar deal. Many people will go for the upgrade.

Don't forget to keep records of what you give away. A donation can be a tax deduction; discuss it with your tax preparer. Giveaways should be factored into your budget as well as your work schedule. If you aren't yet reaching your break-even point, the $50 session you just gave away might have paid your water bill. Or let's say you've set a goal of having a steady ten clients a week, and you've already got them. Where are you going to fit in those free massages you promised? Will you have to work late or come in on your day off? Consider these things in the context of responsible giving. Sometimes, in order to maintain your boundaries, you have to *just say no*.

BOX 13-4   Sample Press Release No. 4

Massage Therapy Event to Benefit Humane Society

Mary Martinez, a licensed massage therapist and owner of Mary's Mobile Massage, will be at the Sunshine Community Humane Society on Saturday, February 2, from 9 a.m. until 2 p.m. offering chair massage for $1 a minute. All proceeds go to the Humane Society to help spay and neuter animals.

ROADSIDE ASSISTANCE

I donate gift certificates to certain events every year: our local Habitat for Humanity fundraiser, the Breast Cancer Awareness Week fundraiser, the Chamber of Commerce Reverse Raffle, the Power of the Purse silent auction to benefit the abused women's shelter, and a few others. These organizations know they can count on me, and knowing when these annual events are going to be held allows me to plan ahead for giving. I always get good results; I don't think I've ever had a recipient who didn't end up making return visits, purchasing a gift certificate, or referring someone else.

Words of Wisdom

My desire to be in service exists in harmony with my need to be responsible for myself.

Public Speaking

Whenever you have the opportunity to do public speaking, seize it—and publicize it in a press release. Civic groups, merchants' associations, the Chamber of Commerce, church groups, and support groups are always looking for public speakers. Chances are that many of your clients belong to such groups, and you should belong to as many as you have the time for yourself. Let them know you are available to talk about the benefits of massage in general or specific topics such as "Massage Therapy and Fibromyalgia" or "Massage Therapy and Stress Relief." The host group will probably publicize the event as well, so coordinate with them. Box 13-5 is an example of a press release for speaking at a public event.

EXPLORATIONS

Make it a point to attend several presentations offered by other speakers as the opportunities arise, and take notes: who was stimulating, who held the attention of the audience and who didn't, and figure out why. Note the things that made it a good or bad speech; for example, a good speaker may have used a lot of humor, or included an engaging slide show or other visual aids, while a poor speaker may have spoken in a monotone or used a lot of filler words. Attending your local chapter of Toastmasters, an international organization aimed at improving public speaking, can also give you the tools to enhance your public speaking skills.

The Snowball Effect

The excitement of opening day will inevitably die down, especially if you don't immediately get all the clients you had hoped for. But don't be discouraged. Building a business is a process that takes time, and fortunately, you can probably count

---

BOX 13-5   Sample Press Release No. 5

Grant Speaking on Massage Therapy and Arthritis

Alan Grant, a licensed massage therapist and owner of Professional Massage Associates, will be speaking on the topic "Massage Therapy and Arthritis" at the monthly meeting of the Holly Springs Senior Citizens Club. The meeting will be held at noon, October 20, at Quincy's Cafeteria, where the members will enjoy a dutch-treat meal before Grant's presentation. Please call Alan at 989-4040 by October 19 to reserve your seat.

**BIG
ADVENTURE
AHEAD**

on the snowball effect. When a snowball rolls down hill, it collects more snow as it rolls along, getting bigger and bigger, and gaining more and more momentum. Business is like that, too.

You can't expect to be rolling in money your first year or two in business. Even if you get all the clients you want or need, you still have to recover your start-up costs before you'll be able to show a profit. But with each passing day, your reputation as an effective massage therapist, and your reputation as a businessperson with integrity, will be gaining momentum, just like that snowball. One person will tell another, and that person will tell someone else, and that person will pass the word, and so on.

Your experience and your expertise at running your business will gain momentum, too. Every day you'll be you making progress on the highway to success.

YOUR PROMOTIONAL CALENDAR

There are 365 days in a year, and at least as many ways for you to promote your massage therapy practice. The goal is for you to create a marketing calendar that can coexist in harmony with your marketing budget. Planning ahead is necessary, in order to maximize the best use of your time and your advertising dollars. Having a written plan for your business promotions will help you avoid spending impulsively on publicity—which can put your finances in the red zone.

Formulating your marketing strategy should be like competing in a chess game: If you want to win, you have to think three moves ahead. You should aim for your promotional calendar to be booked at least 3 months in advance; 6 months to a year is even better. Bear in mind that you can make adjustments if your marketing budget doesn't meet your projections or, better yet, exceeds them.

Your promotional calendar should include community events in which you want to participate, public speaking engagements, holiday promotions, and everyday promotions. An example of a promotional calendar appears in Figure 13-1.

Marketing on a Schedule

Marketing experts claim that consistency is the key when it comes to successfully promoting a business. Have you ever noticed how department stores cycle the things they put on sale? Examples are the January white sales and the August back-to-school sales. Establishing a cyclical pattern for yourself will simplify your marketing efforts.

While allowing for a certain amount of flexibility, creating a schedule that will function year after year will enable you to maintain better control over the budget. Keep your marketing budget in plain sight while working on the schedule. It will be a reminder of the spending threshold when planning your promotions. Think carefully about each event or promotion you're scheduling, and, as mentioned earlier, the possible return on investment. Include the venues and the events that will pay off for you—and leave out the ones that won't.

The first year or two you're in business is the time for all-out publicity efforts. Fill your promotional calendar, and set goals for your first-year marketing schedule. For example, during your first year in business, strive to schedule the following:

- Your grand opening and/or ribbon-cutting ceremony
- A public speaking engagement every quarter
- A chair massage event once a month
- Monthly participation in a Chamber of Commerce or merchants' association event
- An in-house promotion once a month
- Hosting or participating in a community service event every quarter

JANUARY	FEBRUARY	MARCH	APRIL
10 Red Cross blood drive at the office 15 Chair massage at Winter Festival	1 Start Valentine's Day gift certificates and couples massage contest ads 14 Draw for winner	5 Chamber Spring Fling 10 March Madness promo two-for-one	7 Booth at Bridal Fair 16 Speak to Kiwanis Club 20 Start Mother's Day ads
MAY	JUNE	JULY	AUGUST
1 Start month-long graduation special 20 Start Father's Day ads	2 Chair massage at College Career Day 18 Host Business After Hours	4 Chair massage at JulyFest 15-22 Christmas in July gift certificate special promo	1 Start ads for back-to-school special
SEPTEMBER	OCTOBER	NOVEMBER	DECEMBER
5 Anniversary special w/radio live remote	1 Chair massage at Octoberfest	15 Ad kickoff for Christmas gift certificates	8 Client appreciation open house 8-23 Blanket drive for women's shelter

FIGURE 13-1   A sample promotional calendar.

- A media appearance on radio or television at least twice during the year
- An open house at your business at least once during the year
- Sending out press releases for all of the above

When compiling your marketing calendar, utilize the slow periods too; they're great times for running special promotions. If you're just starting out, you won't have any history to tell you what your slow periods may be, but in talking to a lot of other therapists, I've found that many of them have noticed the same trends I have. Slow periods in service businesses normally occur at three times: right after New Year's, when people are recovering from holiday spending and other excesses; when school gets out for the summer and many people leave town for vacation; and a week or two in the fall after school starts, when people have spent a lot of money getting their children ready for the school year.

You should be able to forecast slow periods by the second year in business, assuming you keep a careful watch on your sales. It's not smart to discount services when you're busy; do it when you're in need of the business. Slow periods are also good times to spend more time out of the office, such as attending community service events or out-of-town conferences.

Community Events

Community events should be the first thing you put on the calendar; after all, you're trying to attract and educate the people in the community about your business. In most towns, the Chamber of Commerce or merchants' association will have a schedule made out many months, sometimes a year or more, in advance, of important events like community festivals. These are usually listed on the organization's website.

In my town, for instance, the Mayfest is the first Saturday in May and the Octoberfest is the first Saturday in October. I always participate in those events because they attract thousands of people, so they go on my calendar at the beginning of every year. There are a number of other annual events, such as the Classic Car Ride-In, the annual Founder's Day, and the All-School Reunion Day, that attract a lot of attention, and it serves my business to have a presence there—either a chair massage tent or an informational booth. Those also go on my calendar at the beginning of the year.

Even if a booth or a chair massage tent is not appropriate, certain types of community events can be opportunities for networking, passing out business cards, and meeting and greeting other members of the community. These include the Chamber of Commerce's annual picnic, business-after-hours events, and community or neighborhood suppers.

Be as diligent in scheduling attendance at community events as you are in scheduling clients when you're first starting out. The more exposure you get, the more quickly people will get to know your name and know about your business. The word will spread!

Holiday Promotions

Begin by putting the obvious holidays on the calendar—the ones that are potentially good for gift certificate sales: Valentine's Day, Mother's Day, Father's Day, and Christmas are all prime times for promotions. Other trends in gift certificate sales aren't quite as obvious; for instance, the week school gets out for the summer, gift certificate sales go up because parents buy them as thank you presents for their children's teachers. Though not as big as other holidays, it's still a time for a definite spike in sales. June is the traditional time for weddings and college graduations—two other big opportunities to promote gift certificates and packages. You might take advantage of some less common holidays, such as Grandparent's Day and Secretary's Day.

Other holidays can also be ripe opportunities for gift certificate sales—for instance, Thanksgiving. A sample ad for Thanksgiving might say, "Someone's slaving over a hot stove to make your Thanksgiving dinner. Show your hostess you appreciate her with a gift of massage." The same blurb could be used for Easter, Labor Day, or any other day when friends and families usually come together to celebrate.

When publicizing gift certificate sales that are targeted at holidays, it's wise to start campaigning 2 weeks ahead of time. Don't wait until the holiday is upon you to advertise it.

Everyday Promotions

Every single day is the right day for marketing your business. Pretty much daily, someone calls my office to ask if there are any specials on that day, and the same thing can happen at your massage practice. The public is looking for a special, just the same as if they were reading the grocery store handout to see what's on sale—so give them a deal!

Instead of trying to come up with something different every day, offer a monthly special (and don't forget to put it on your promotional calendar). If you've been trained in more than one modality, mix it up. For instance, if your clients tend to get the same Swedish massage every visit but you've learned how to do Lomi-Lomi in a continuing ed class, you might offer a discount on that for a month. Mention to every client that it's on special, and explain what

Lomi-Lomi is. During cold weather is a good time to offer a special on hot stone massage or hot paraffin treatments. Or try offering a lunchtime special of a half-hour massage.

You'd be amazed at all the silly "special days" that exist on the calendar. You can find hundreds of them on the Internet, along with important dates in history, and all manner of other observances that last a day, a week, or a month. For example, June is Professional Wellness Month. June 17–23 is National Headache Awareness Week. June 2 is Leave the Office Early Day. All three of those days lend themselves perfectly to a promotion! January is Red Cross Month. Host a blood drive at your office, and give a discount on massage to everyone who donates. November 11–17 is National Food Bank Week. Have a canned food drive, and give a $5 discount to everyone who brings in five cans of food. There is a promotional opportunity literally every day.

You may want to consider offering a special to first-time clients. A slow period is a great time to offer a twofer—two massages for the price of one—to your existing clients, with the stipulation that the other recipient must be a first-time visitor. It's a way to reward your regular clients and attract some new ones. Here are a few other ideas for everyday promotions:

- Make one day of the week Family Day, and offer a discount if more than one family member has an appointment on the same day.
- Pick your least busy day of the week, give it a catchy name (Manic Monday, Freaky Friday), and offer a special to people who come on that day.
- Instead of discounting, offer an added service with a full-price massage, like a free paraffin hand treatment.
- Send out an e-mail or text message stating that you have x number of appointments left for the week and that the first person who calls will get $10 off. You can, of course, give that deal to as many people as you like.

Remember, promotions are meant to advance your business. While you don't want to give away the store by continually discounting, you have to allow for a certain amount of discounts when you're just starting out as an incentive to get people in the door. It's worth a $10 discount, or even half-price like the twofer, in order to build your clientele to the saturation point.

Words of Wisdom
When you reach the saturation point and can't take any more clients, say "I'll be happy to put you on my waiting list." It makes a big impression on people when you're in demand!

The 30-Minute Marketer

Setting aside 30 minutes on your schedule every day for marketing tasks is one of the most important things you can do to promote your business. Put your half-hour of marketing time in your appointment book, and treat it with the same importance as you would an appointment with a client.

The daily time can be spent creating new forms of publicity, brainstorming for new promotional opportunities, scheduling participation in community service events, lining up media appearances, sending direct mailings, or writing press releases. It can be something different every day, but the point is you have to consistently devote that time to the advancement of your business. If you schedule your marketing time on a daily basis, you'll have plenty of leeway, for instance, when planning your holiday ad campaigns or writing those speeches you're going to make when you take advantage of public speaking opportunities.

Client Retention Marketing

Remember that it's less expensive to keep existing clients than it is to advertise for new ones. Your regular, established clients can be your best advertisement, in terms of giving testimonials and providing referrals for your business.

Client retention marketing can be summed up in one sentence: Keep in touch!

Send a regular newsletter (see Chapter 11) to your clients, either hard copy or e-mail (see Chapter 11). Send a birthday card. Send a handwritten note when you see your client's name in the paper for some accomplishment or a sympathy card when there's been a death in the family. Call those clients who haven't been in lately. Send a postcard that says something like "We haven't seen you lately, and we've missed you! Here's $5 off on your next massage." Let them know you haven't forgotten about them.

Target your existing clients with specific advertising geared at bringing in referrals, such as offering the twofers or family days mentioned above. Remember to offer package deals; they're the best form of client retention marketing. When you get people to pay in advance in exchange for getting a substantial discount or a free session for *x* number that they've purchased, you're guaranteed that they'll be in for at least that many sessions, and you've helped your immediate cash flow.

ROADSIDE ASSISTANCE

The best thing you can do to enhance client retention should be taking place in your office at every visit: asking if the client would like to schedule another appointment. When I gave my very first paid massage as a newly licensed therapist, I was worried about appearing too pushy if I asked the client to reschedule. She was almost out the door when she turned to me and said, "Aren't you going to ask me if I want to make another appointment?" I got over it right there on the spot, and it quickly became second nature to ask every client. It should be the second most important thing in your vocabulary, right after "thank you."

POSTCARDS from the HIGHWAY Nina McIntosh

Like many others, I came into a career in bodywork for a number of reasons—personal (needing desperately to quit living in my head), financial (I thought, wrongly, that it would be an easy way to make a living), altruistic (it seemed a satisfying way to help others feel better), and probably a bunch of other reasons, conscious and unconscious.

I was living in Denver, working at a stuffy psychiatric hospital as a social worker. For fun, I took a weekend massage class and that was the beginning. I seemed to have a knack for it, and I realized I wanted to get on with my life in a different way. I felt drawn to setting aside my current career and launching out into massage. I attended what was then the Boulder School of Massage, a little school in a small house at that time. To help me with the transition, I received the basic Rolfing series of ten, which was transformational for me.

I practiced massage with modest success for 3 years, making almost every boundary mistake I wrote about later in *The Educated Heart*. And then I realized I was always talking about Rolfing and was fascinated by it. My own Rolfer, Tom Wing, was (and is) a sensitive, intuitive, and kind man, who inspired me to go to the Rolf Institute. Long story short, I was a Certified Rolfer for the next 25 years or so—sometimes working at it only part-time because of health or family obligations; sometimes fairly successful, in terms of numbers of clients, and sometimes not.

(continued)

POSTCARDS from the HIGHWAY   Nina McIntosh *(Continued)*

To write this piece, I looked back over my career and was surprised at what I discovered. I had known that having a supportive bodywork community was important to me, but I had not suspected what a huge difference it had made. I see that I was happiest and busiest when I was actively engaged in the Rolfing community. That meant having frequent contact with other Rolfers I respected and who were excited about the work. It also meant going to workshops, having help from nearby teachers one-on-one, and getting lots of bodywork for myself. This wasn't particular to the Rolfing community; I saw that it was true for colleagues who were involved in other kinds of bodywork. Those who had an active, positive, supportive community, especially one they were involved with frequently, seemed to make their enthusiasm for their work last longer.

Let's face it: As massage therapists and bodyworkers, we're still swimming upstream all the time. The culture certainly recognizes us more than they did 30 years ago when I started, but we still need all the support we can get. When I teach massage school students, I urge them to stay in touch with each other when they graduate, especially if the class seems close. I think it would be great if more schools would set up ways for alumnae to get together regularly. Community may not be the answer for everyone, but it certainly was for me.

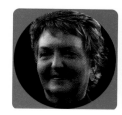

Nina McIntosh authored *The Educated Heart: Professional Boundaries for Massage Therapists, Bodyworkers and Movement Teachers*, 3rd ed. She was honored with the Aunty Margaret Machado Humanitarian Award at the World Massage Festival in 2010. After a brave battle with ALS (Lou Gehrig's disease), Nina passed away on July 18, 2010.

SUGGESTED READINGS

Allen L. *One Year to a Successful Massage Therapy Practice.* Baltimore, MD: Lippincott Williams & Wilkins, 2008.

Brown E. *How to Create a Massage Marketing Plan.* http://www.massagebusinesscenter.com/marketing-plan-article.htm. Accessed 02/01/09.

Bureau of Labor Statistics. *Occupational Outlook Handbook 2010–2011: Massage Therapists* http://www.bls.gov/oco/ocos295.htm. Accessed 01/31/10.

Johnson S. *The Enviable Lifestyle: Creating a Successful Massage Therapy Business.* Booksurge Publishing, 2008.

Massage Therapists Carry On, Despite National Economic Downturn. Massage Magazine. http://www.massagemag.com/News/print-this.php?id=2849. Accessed 02/03/09.

Piehl G. *Massage Marketing Tips That You Can Feel Good Using. Massage-Marketing-Tips.com.* Accessed 02/01/09.

Recession History in the United States. http://www.recessionhistory.com/. Accessed 02/03/09.

Roseberry M. *Marketing Massage: From First Job to Dream Practice.* Clifton Park, NY: Milady, 2006.

My Personal Journey

In this chapter, we've discussed the key elements of effective promotions. Using the suggestions from the chapter, create a potential marketing budget and calendar for your first year in business.

My goals _____

_____

_____

What's in my way? _____

_____

_____

What action can I take to remedy the situation? _____

_____

_____

One-year progress update _____

_____

_____

Effective
Advertising

CHAPTER 14

Many a small thing has been made large by the right kind of advertising.

MARK TWAIN

KEY CONCEPTS

- The business name, logo, and slogan, as well as consistency in advertising, will help build brand recognition for your business.
- Making good use of the tools you already have on hand, such as your signage, printed materials, and telephone, and having them serve more than one purpose are an effective use of marketing dollars.
- Effective advertising contains a clear message of who, where, what, when, how, and/ or why your business is the best source for people who are seeking the service you provide.
- Classified ads contain text only; the five main types of display ads can be used across all forms of print media.
- Print ads are those that appear in newspapers, the Yellow Pages, periodicals, flyers, and direct mail pieces.
- Direct mail has the advantage of being easy for tracking results and the disadvantage of being expensive.
- Radio advertising can include personal interviews, theme music, and your slogan.
- Television advertising may be traditional commercial advertising, or you could gain exposure through public access television.
- Internet marketing includes having your own website, online networking, banner ads, or pay-per-click advertising; using the database listings provided by the professional massage and bodywork associations; linking to other websites; and e-mail.

BRAND RECOGNITION

A **brand** is a combination of a concept, symbols, images, experiences, and associations that people attribute to a person, a product, or a business. A brand that gets widely known is said to have **brand recognition**. Massage Envy, for example, enjoys brand recognition, but you don't have to be a big chain to cultivate some of the characteristics of brand recognition. Following some of the same practices that major companies use will help your business stand out in the mind of the consumer.

Your name and your logo, if you have one, are a part of your brand, and you want people to recognize them. If you're not artistic, there are many software programs that can help you create a logo; your business name may actually be your logo, or you may have a separate symbol in addition to your name. Graphic designers tend to be expensive, but you could hire one, or barter your massage services, to get a professionally designed image for your company. Either way, the goal is for people to immediately recall you and your business when and wherever they see your name and/or logo.

Marketing experts say that advertising must be done *consistently* in order to be effective. Moreover, it takes six to nine exposures for an ad to register in a person's mind, regardless of the medium.

When it comes to any type of print advertising, for instance, you can help create your brand recognition by as simple an act as using the same font all the time. Notice the difference between the two advertisements in Figure 14-1. While both ads contain the same information, using both of them isn't going to create recall in the minds of the public. The better strategy is to choose the font you like best and use it consistently for all printed materials. Choose a font that's easy to read. If youv do choose an elaborate font for your business name, choose a simpler one for the body of your message on your marketing materials.

Having a slogan, or motto, that captures attention is another way to build your brand recognition. Think of some of the well-known slogans used by big corporations that are embedded in the public consciousness: "It's the real thing" (Coca-Cola) or "Just do it" (Nike). A catchy phrase gets attention, and when it's used consistently on all of your printed materials and advertising, people associate it with your business. My own slogan is, "It's time to take care of yourself." It appears on my business cards, brochures, and all advertisements directly underneath my business name. Others I've seen are "Rest. Relax. Revitalize" and "Have

---

| **M & M Massage & Bodywork**

Mary Scoggins, LMT & Mike Jones, LMT

invite you to celebrate our *Grand Opening* **July 6 at 9am**

340 S. Main St. Mayberry, NC

828-289-4444 www.mandmmassage.com | *M & M Massage & Bodywork*

Mary Scoggins, LMT & Mike Jones, LMT

invite you to celebrate our Grand Opening July 6 at 9am

340 S. Main St. Mayberry, NC

828-289-4444 www.mandmmassage.com |

FIGURE 14-1 Consistency in print advertising. Left: Newspaper ad with easy-to-read font. Right: The same ad but with a font that is too fancy and difficult to read.

you had your massage today?" Think of one to suit your business, and use it consistently on all your printed materials and other forms of advertising media. You can also use it when you answer the telephone, and have it as the recorded greeting on your voice mail; for example, "THERA-SSAGE, where it's time to take care of yourself. Can I help you?"

TOOLS ON HAND

There are many components of your business that can serve more than one purpose. Since they're already there, use them to your best advantage to publicize your massage practice. Your signage, your business cards and brochures, the telephone, fax, and e-mail—all of these are must-haves for establishing brand recognition and conducting business. They can function as promotional tools, too, and you should get all the mileage you can out of them.

Signage

How well a sign works to promote your business depends largely on how easy it is for people driving by to see it. Besides placement, the height and overall size, readability, and illumination are other important factors.

If you're renting a space instead of owning, get your landlord's permission before planning signage for your business. In addition, check with your town and county council and/or zoning board to make sure you know about any restrictions before you order your sign. It would be a shame to spend a lot of money for a customized sign, only to be told you can't put it up where people can see it. Your sign should be as visible as possible, preferably located where it can be seen from the street so passersby will be able to read it, react to it, and stop safely.

It's smart and sensible to use the same font for your signage that you use for all the materials that represent your business. Maintain your sign in good repair, because it's usually the first impression people get as they approach your business. If the sign is painted, be sure to refresh the paint every year or two so it doesn't appear faded. If it's an illuminated sign, replace any burned-out bulbs right away.

Printed Materials: Business Cards and Brochures

Professional-looking printed materials are a vital part of publicizing your business. The business card is often the first form of contact people have with your business. Someone may come into the office to pick up a brochure, with the thought of making a future appointment or gift certificate purchase; the impression she gets from the brochure could make the difference in whether she actually becomes a client or not. Figure 14-2 shows an example of a business card and brochure for the same massage therapy practice.

Your business cards and brochures have to be distributed; they won't be effective if they sit on the desk in your office. The Chamber of Commerce always has room for members to display their marketing materials. Numerous locales, from your county tourism office to the local Wal-Mart, have card racks or bulletin boards you can use.

Be sure to provide your cards and brochures to any other health care practitioner you have a referral relationship with. Provide your own holder.

Hotels and motels have racks for brochures of local businesses and attractions in their lobbies. Take your brochures around to local bed and breakfasts, gyms, salons, the police and fire departments, bridal shops, photographers,

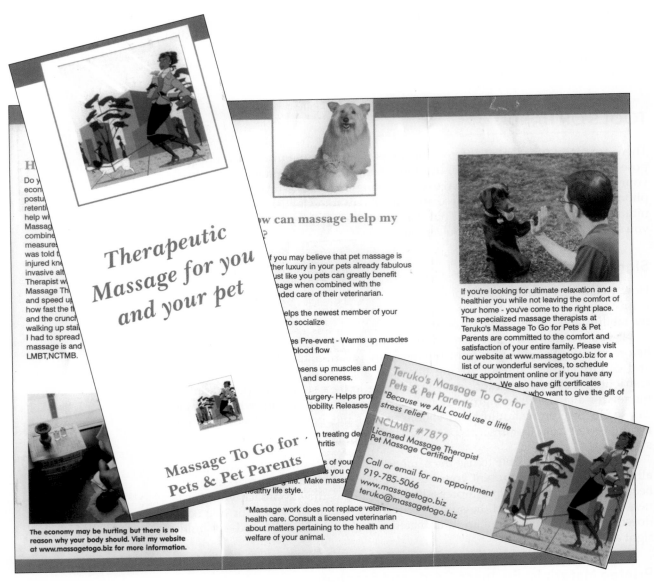

FIGURE 14-2   A matching brochure (A) and business card (B).

and real estate agents. Many business owners will reciprocate when it comes to distributing marketing literature. If you have an empty shelf or table you can use to display the cards and brochures of other entrepreneurs, make that offer whenever you're in the store or office of a small business owner. It's mutually beneficial.

Be sure your cards and brochures match, or at least look harmonious, in order to reinforce recognition of your brand. It doesn't make sense to have a smorgasbord of printed materials that don't harmonize with each other. Your business cards and other marketing aids have your contact information, so they should be easy to read and pleasing to the eye. If the name of your business does not convey what you do, the actual service must appear on the card directly under the business name. For example, *Inspire* is a pleasant-sounding name, but without the words "Skin and Body" underneath the name, it doesn't convey what the business is about.

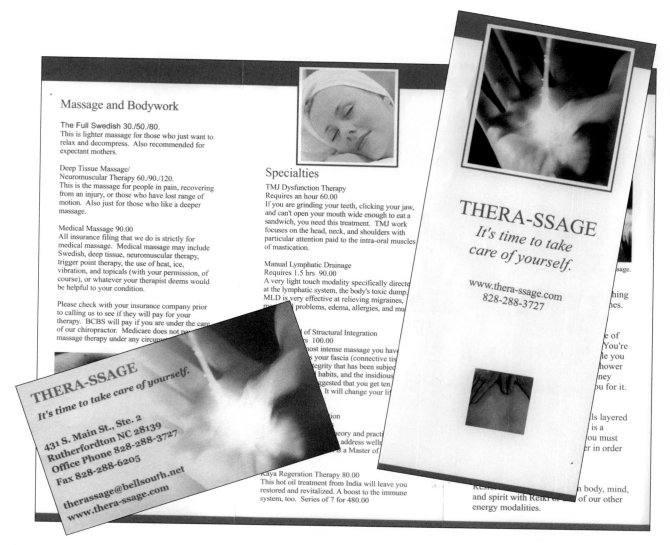

FIGURE 14-2 *(Continued).*

Printed materials can have multiple uses, as shown in Figure 14-3. The business owner has been careful to create pieces that are visually pleasing and has maximized the way they can be used in a coordinated way. For example, the back of the business card is a preprinted client referral reward. The oversized postcard doubles as a brochure, listing the staff members and their specialties of service, as well as a client upgrade incentive. Attractive blank note cards are used as "welcome to my practice" cards and any other purpose that calls for a personal note.

Your business card is one of the least expensive and most effective forms of advertising you have. Here are some places you might not have thought of to leave cards:

- On the table with the tip, every time you eat out.
- In payment envelopes when paying local bills.
- Between the pages of a library book as a bookmark to be found by the next borrower.
- In the student lounge at the local college campus.
- With the local Welcome Wagon.

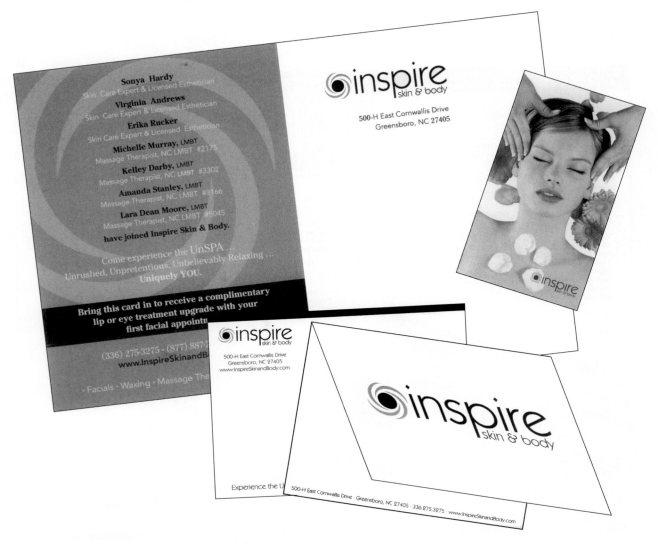

FIGURE 14-3 Multiuse printed materials.

ROADSIDE ASSISTANCE

Do you sometimes forget to refill your business card case, go to hand a card to someone, and you don't have one? My advice is every night on your way out of the office, make it a habit to put two cards in your wallet or purse. Put a few in the pocket of each of your coats and jackets and keep some in your car. If you stop anywhere on the way home, or whenever you're doing errands, make it a point to give at least one card to someone—the clerk at the store, or someone you've run into. Don't be shy! You'll become more comfortable with promoting your business as time goes by.

The Telephone

The telephone, a necessary part of office equipment, should be a marketing tool, as well. For example, when someone calls your office and you have to put her on hold, don't make her listen to dead air or canned music. Instead, have a recorded message about your business: "Thank you for holding. Your call is important to us. Massage Connection is having a special this month on hot stone massage for only $75, a savings of $20. Book yours today."

Be sure the message on your answering machine or voicemail is direct and not too long, or people will hang up before they hear the end of it. Another idea is to incorporate your slogan into your message; it will help reinforce brand recognition: "Thank you for calling THERA-SSAGE, where it's time to take care of yourself. We're open from 8 to 8 Monday through Friday and 8 to 1 on Saturday. Our special this month is couples massage for $100. Please leave your name and number and we'll return your call as soon as possible."

Your message must be clear and concise. Avoid having loud music playing in the background, don't giggle, and don't let your 4-year-old record your phone message, no matter how cute you think it is; the general public will not be amused, and it doesn't present a professional image.

REALITY
CHECKPOINT

Text Messaging

A text message is like an e-mail, except it's delivered to a mobile phone instead of a computer. It can be used like the Monday morning scheduling blast, to announce specials, or it can be a great way to fill an appointment that's been canceled on short notice. You could send out a text message, such as "THERA-SSAGE has had a cancellation at 4 p.m. this afternoon. If you would like to take that appointment, please respond immediately by text or phone to 288-3727. First come, first served."

You don't want to be intrusive, so ask your clients if they would like to be contacted by text messaging.

The Fax Machine

The Monday morning scheduling blast can work as well with faxing as it does with e-mailing or text messaging. In the interest of saving trees, use e-mail or text when you can, and fax when you can't. The same courtesy should be exercised when faxing as when sending e-mail; don't send repetitive unwelcome faxes. But if you belong to a merchant's association or the Chamber of Commerce, chances are either you can arrange for them to send a fax broadcast for you, or the organization will provide the membership with a listing of contact information of the other members, including your business.

Going with the Flow

The efficacy of massage therapy in treating various conditions has been backed up by many recent and ongoing peer-reviewed research projects. Highlighting some of these in your advertising will reinforce that massage can provide a lot of real health benefits. According to AMTA, research has shown massage therapy to be effective for decreasing pain and fatigue in cancer patients, reducing the frequency of headaches, helping alcohol withdrawal symptoms, relieving postsurgical pain, and lowering blood pressure, among other things. When you include facts such as these in your advertising, you're likely to get calls from people who have never considered massage as a possible help for their condition.

Your Elevator Speech

"Hi, I'm Laura Allen. I'm a licensed massage therapist and the owner of THERA-SSAGE on Main Street in Rutherfordton. We offer massage and bodywork, chiropractic, acupuncture, spa treatments, and aesthetic services. May I give you my card?" That's my elevator speech.

An elevator speech is a metaphor for a quick verbal blurb about your business. In addition to an introductory message, you'll need a short speech about massage

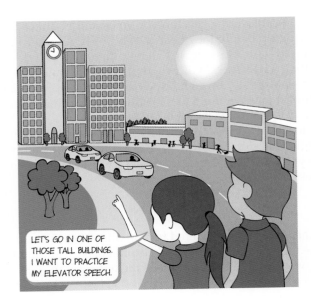

in general. You should be able to tell people in just a minute or two how your services can benefit their health.

Say you've just given your introduction to someone and he asks, "I've never had a massage before; what's it going to do for me?" Remember, people want to know how something will benefit them. Here's your answer: "Massage is really effective at relieving stress, helps relieve muscle pain, increases the circulation of blood and lymph, and brings oxygen to the muscles."

You can take the elevator speech a little further, if you like. While I never touch anyone without asking, over the years I've gotten a lot of clients by giving a short sample of massage while talking to them. For instance, at a meeting or an event I might notice that someone keeps rubbing her neck. I'll go right over and say, "I'm Laura Allen and I'm a massage therapist. I can't help noticing that you keep rubbing your neck. May I put my hands on you for a moment?" I can't recall ever having been turned down. During the few minutes I spend giving a brief massage, other people might line up—and I'll give them a card and ask them to call me. Obviously, a few minutes of massage won't correct any problem, but it can ease pain. Even 5 minutes of therapeutic touch can do a lot—including convincing the person that she needs to call you for an appointment. Mission accomplished!

BIG ADVENTURE AHEAD

ROADSIDE ASSISTANCE

I'm from the South, where we use the phrase "How are you doing?" as a greeting, instead of "hello." Although we might not actually want to hear details, a lot of people will tell you how they're doing, especially if they have a complaint. I'm sure it's common in other places, too; people are ready to tell you about a pain they have, their latest surgery, or their medication. Whenever I get that kind of response, my ready-made answer is, "Did you know that massage can really help the sciatica that's bothering you?" Then I give my "benefits of massage" message. I try to use it at least once a day.

BASIC ADVERTISING CRITERIA

As mentioned in Chapter 13, promotion refers to anything you do to market and advance your business, and many of those efforts are no-cost or low-cost.

Advertising refers to forms of marketing that are purchased. In order to be effective, the advertising you buy should meet certain criteria:

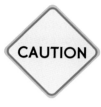

- The message of the advertisement is clear.
- The advertisement piques curiosity so the audience wants to know more.
- The advertisement conveys the value that you and your business provide.
- The advertisement tells who you are.
- The advertisement tells what you do.
- The advertisement tells where, when, and how and/or why you do it.
- The advertisement tells why you are the best source for the service your business offers.
- The advertisement reaches the audience you want to target.

TRADITIONAL MEDIA

Different advertising venues require different approaches. For instance, a TV commercial will contain different components than an advertisement in the Yellow Pages or the newspaper. However, the information that needs to be conveyed is the same.

Any traditional media outlet that you choose for advertising, such as a newspaper or radio station, will usually provide ad design or copy writing services for free when you purchase the space or air time. It's up to you, of course, to supply the specific information you want the public to know. The successful outcome of your advertising depends on providing the media with a clear and concise message about your business, so they, in turn, can give the public the same.

Newspapers

The newspaper can be an effective vehicle for advertising and building your brand recognition. Although this may not be representative of every locale, my county has a population of about 65,000 people, and the daily newspaper has about 40,000 subscribers, so I could reach almost two thirds of the populace by placing an ad in the paper. Remember, though, what the marketing experts say about advertising consistently. A random ad every once in awhile is not an effective way to bring in clients. Many newspapers are also available in a digital version on the Internet (including ads), but printed copies are still popular in most places. If you have an ad or a press release in a newspaper's print edition, it will appear on the Internet as well.

Classified ads are text ads, and while they're okay for selling a used car, display ads are more effective at drawing attention. There are five basic types of display ads:

- *Business card ad*: Contains your name and contact information, your logo, and nothing else. This is as good as a basic ad in a business directory or Yellow Pages listing.
- *Coupon ad*: Encourages new customers to try your services. It's easy to track the effectiveness of a coupon ad.
- *Informational ad*: Can be written like a story about your business, or written in an FAQ (frequently asked questions) format. It gives more details than other types of display ads.
- *Sales ad*: Invites people to take advantage of a discount during a specific period of time.
- *Spotlight ad*: Focuses attention on a specific aspect of your business, such as a certain service you offer, or it could be about you or other staff members.

The most effective ads are simple in layout, easy to read, short, and to the point. Avoid using large blocks of print and fancy fonts. The main component of a newspaper ad should be the headline, to draw the reader's attention, and a subhead, like your slogan mentioned above, followed by the body of the message, any terms or conditions, and graphics or illustrations. A good ad has ample white space; avoid trying to pack too much information into a small area.

Newspapers will usually give you a price break in the form of a package deal if you commit to a certain number of ads per year. When you're just starting out in business, check into those rates and figure out how many fit into your budget, and use that information to plan your advertising campaigns.

The Yellow Pages

REALITY CHECKPOINT

People have been turning to the Yellow Pages for business contacts almost as long as the telephone has been in existence. This reliable place is still where many people go to look up a telephone number, so it's smart to have a listing for your business.

Like any print advertising, the cost will depend on the amount of space you purchase, whether or not you include color or photographs in your ad, and other enhancements such as borders or fancy graphics. For a Yellow Pages listing or display ad, you can also expect to pay more in a big city than you would in a small town.

Particularly in metropolitan areas, the Yellow Pages often fail to differentiate between therapeutic massage and the massage that we'll just refer to as adult entertainment. In the Yellow Pages in my area, there are two headings, "Massage" and "Massage Therapy." Our state massage board has informed the telephone company repeatedly that legitimate massage therapists are obligated to have their license number printed with any advertisement and has asked many times to list the "other" type of massage in the Adult Entertainment section. The phone company is a huge bureaucracy, and unfortunately, trying to make such a change has been unsuccessful in my state. Be sure that your Yellow Pages ad clearly states that you perform therapeutic massage. If required by your state, include your designated initials and license number. If you are nationally certified and/or a member of a professional organization, including those affiliations in the ad will reinforce the message that you're not performing sexual massage.

Periodicals

Periodicals include magazines, inserts, and tabloid papers. They can be effective places to build brand recognition and attract business, depending on what audience they reach. For example, a weekly shopper's magazine that's distributed freely, or a newspaper insert or supplement, will reach a wide audience, compared to a subscription magazine that focuses on a certain segment of the population. If your business is focused on maternity massage, advertising in a woman's magazine would make sense. If your practice focuses on sports massage, advertise in a publication for athletes.

Metropolitan areas usually have a number of local and regional publications. You won't be able to recoup the cost of an ad in a national magazine, but you will in a local periodical. The complementary travel magazines that are usually found in hotels and airports could be good ad sources for you if you're located nearby such places. While they're primarily geared toward travelers, it's safe to assume that at least some of the people they reach are those who travel to your area repeatedly for business or to visit family; they could turn into repeat customers.

OPPORTUNITIES AHEAD

If your local Chamber of Commerce or Tourism Development Board publishes a magazine, it can be a good place to advertise, too. Such publications are always given to newcomers who stop in and are widely distributed at the businesses of Chamber members, at visitor centers, and at local tourist attractions.

The Humble Flyer

The humble flyer is a handy way to stretch your advertising budget. For just the cost of printing, and an investment of time on your part, you can put them all over the town. My flyers are probably on a minimum of 40 to 50 bulletin boards all over the county. If there is a college or university in your town, every floor will have a bulletin board. Town squares often have bulletin boards, or there may be one outside the town hall. They're in malls, convenience stores, restaurant lobbies, hospitals, libraries, and literally everywhere. Arm yourself with a stack of flyers on brightly colored paper and spend some time driving around. You'll be surprised at how many places you can find to put them up—for free.

Direct Mail

Direct mail has advantages and disadvantages. The great advantage is using it to easily contact your existing clients or to target all the people in a certain zip code. Direct mail companies can handle everything for you from the creation of the card or letter itself to the labeling and mailing to your target audience. Many offer targeted mailings based on consumer research; for instance, you can send a mailing only to people who have had massage before, or to people who have had or inquired about other holistic health services.

The disadvantage is that direct mail can be expensive, especially if you use the cost-per-person formula. In 2010, it costs $0.29 to send a postcard, and that's not counting the price of the card. If you're sending enough pieces to qualify for bulk mailing rates, your cost will be lower.

The results of direct mail campaigns can be very easy to track, and this lets you know if you're getting a good return on your investment. For instance, you could send out a mailing that says "Call 955-1212 to hear about our February spa specials. Give us the secret code from your postcard and we'll tell you if you're an instant winner of a free day at the spa." Based on the number of responses you receive, you'll find out if that was an effective use of your advertising dollars for future decisions about where to spend your money.

Radio

Radio can be a great advertising medium that's cost-effective. Radio advertising is usually offered in bundles of x number of ads, and the price depends on the station's total number of listeners, or **market share**, as well as the length of the ad, the frequency with which it appears, and the time of day that the ad runs. It's cheaper to run an ad at midnight than it is to run one during morning drive time when people are on the way to work.

Cultivating a relationship with the salespeople and disc jockeys at your local radio station can really help you. If you can't afford the station's advertising packages when you're just starting out in business, offer free gift certificates in exchange for ads, and of course, don't give away more than you can afford. Ask for an interview to talk about the benefits of massage therapy. They might welcome the opportunity, and if you don't ask, you'll never know. AMTA has a CD containing prerecorded ads about Massage Therapy Awareness Week, which is held annually in October, available to members for sharing with their local radio station.

Another strategy, when you can't afford a big advertising package, is to ask the station salesperson to let you know about any special events you could sponsor for a one-time fee. In the past, I've sponsored such things as Christmas Eve music, election results, basketball tournaments, car races, and other events. It's actually a great approach; instead of a random announcement, the airwaves are saturated with your ad for the duration of the event.

Your brand recognition can be reinforced through radio advertising, by including your slogan in your ad, and/or by choosing a theme song or jingle for your advertisements. The staff at the station will be able to take care of licensing issues related to the music you choose, or if your talents lie in that area, record something that you've written just for your business.

Bear in mind, as you do when choosing any advertising medium, what audience you'll reach with a particular station. For example, a conservative talk radio station has a different audience than a classic rock, gospel music, or college radio station. Any station you are considering advertising with should be able to tell you the demographics of their listeners. An FM station will usually have a bigger market share than an AM station, and you can expect to pay more at a big, popular commercial station than you would at a smaller station.

Television

Before you jump to the conclusion that you can't afford television advertising, do some investigating. For instance, I currently have an ad with our local cable company, and at the time of this writing, it only costs $90 per month. My ad appears on one of the weather channels, and it's in a rotation format; how many times it appears in a 24-hour period depends on how many other advertisers have ads on that channel at a given time. I've watched the channel to see how often my ad runs and found that it rotated at least once every hour or two. It isn't an action video, it's an informational ad for THERA-SSAGE, Massage & Bodywork, with our contact information, including our website. Of course, if you have the money, you can be as grand as you want to with your TV commercial.

One of the greatest opportunities for television exposure is public access television. In the early 1970s when cable TV was relatively new, the Federal Communications Commission decreed that stations in the 100 largest markets in the United States must provide three channels for state and local governments, education, and public noncommercial use. Don't let the word "noncommercial" be a deterrent; it doesn't mean you can't share information.

If you're not familiar with public television, tune in, and you'll see shows about everything from yoga to how to raise soybeans, in the interest of educating the public. Most cable stations will supply not only free air time for public access but also free use of their equipment and production personnel; the law obligates them to do so.

Even though you can't make an outright commercial for your business, you could do a show about the benefits of massage in general or a series about massage for different health conditions. If there is already a show about massage on one of your local public access channels, contact the host about the possibility of appearing as a guest. Visit your local cable company to find out what options are available to you. You could also approach a local commercial station and ask them to have you appear in a feature about massage; they're always looking for items of human interest.

If you will be appearing on television, be sure to send out a press release. It's a newsworthy event, and it will make a great impression on clients.

THE INTERNET

The Internet has made the world a very small place, and it is a hotbed of marketing opportunities that you shouldn't pass up. Even if you don't have a website, there are hundreds of places on the World Wide Web that will let you list your business at no charge or for a nominal fee.

If you're nationally certified, or a member of a professional association such as AMTA or ABMP, your affiliation automatically entitles you to be included in their searchable database of therapists. If you are a practitioner of a modality that has an association, such as the Guild for Structural Integration or the American Reflexology Association, you can be listed on their website at no charge if you desire. Membership in your Chamber of Commerce or local merchants' association usually includes the same benefit.

There are Internet applications that let you sell gift certificates and even book appointments online. The marketing opportunities are almost boundless.

Your Website

If you are the owner of a service business, most people will expect you to have a website. You can get one for little expense, and it's a big time-saver. When someone calls asking about services, prices, and so forth, you can, of course, chat if you have the time. But if you're busy, ask the caller if he has Internet access and refer him to your website. Tell him he can make appointments or purchase gift certificates online. It saves people the trouble of driving to your office, and out-of-town people who want to purchase a gift certificate for a local friend or relative will make a lot of use of this convenience.

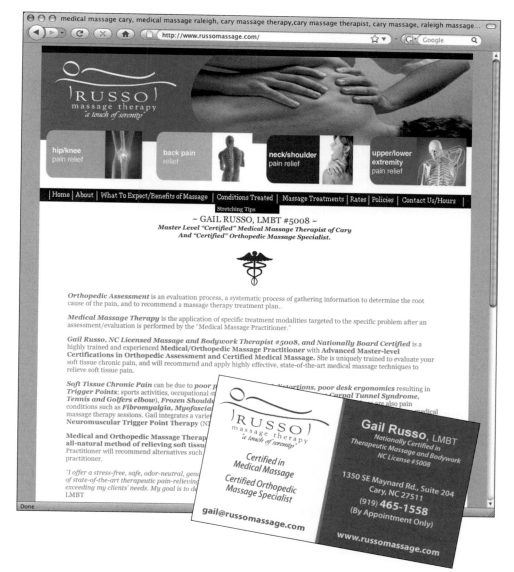

FIGURE 14-4   A matching website (A) and business card (B).

The professional massage associations have websites available to members that you can have up and running in the amount of time it takes you to type in your contact information. Numerous software programs can easily walk you through the steps of building your own website, or you can pay a professional to build one for you.

The most important features of a website are easy navigation and readability. If you choose to build your own, some basic rules will ensure that the visitors to your website will have a good experience:

- Avoid busy backgrounds. Text shows up the best on a solid background.
- For the text, use basic black or darker colors that will stand out and fonts that are large enough and easy to read.
- Break the text up into small sections.
- Leave enough "white space" on the page. Don't try to fill every inch.
- Add interest with pictures or graphics.
- Be sure you have the correct key words optimized on your website. Key words are what the search engines look for when they're searching the Internet, and "massage" and "bodywork" are examples of words that will get you listed in those categories.
- Use the spell-checker! Ask several people to proofread it before you make the website live.

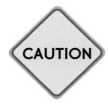

Certain Internet host providers will give you a website for free, but you should avoid those, because of the obscurity of the web address you'll be assigned. Your website address, or URL (uniform resource locator), should be the same exact name as your business, if at all possible. You could save yourself a modest amount of money by going with one of the free services, but you might wind up with a very long or obscure URL that doesn't even seem like your own.

It's worth the small amount of money you'll spend to get a web address that's easy for people to remember and that will fit on your business cards. When you purchase your web domain or website name, be sure to reserve it for multiple years. Always make the payments on time, because someone may be waiting in the wings to snatch your business name. Domain providers often have a waiting list of people who want to reserve a certain name.

Keep in mind that you're working toward brand recognition. Having your website match, or at least closely harmonize with, your business cards and other printed materials will reinforce that recognition. An example of a website and business card that complement each other appears in Figure 14-2.

Words of Wisdom
Jump on the technology bandwagon and get a website! If your competitors have one, and they probably do, they'll be getting business that might otherwise have come to you.

Going with the Flow

You can use affiliate marketing as an income stream. Many companies will pay you per click for advertisements placed on your website. Be selective in the companies you choose, and be sure you have final approval over which ads appear on your site.

Online Promotion: To Pay or Not to Pay

There are many ways to direct traffic to your website. Your website address should be included on your business cards, brochures, and other marketing materials. It should also appear in every piece of print advertising you have and mentioned in any radio or television ads.

Be prepared for the barrage of solicitations from search engine companies or third parties guaranteeing that they'll move you to the top of search engine listings; the same promise goes out to everyone, and there's only one spot at the top. Banner ads or pay-per-click links on other websites to yours can also run into a lot of money; Yahoo, Google, and other vendors charge a minimum amount per day for sending visitors to your website.

It's best, of course, to get as many people to visit your website as possible without spending money to attract them. Here are some effective strategies:

- Update your website regularly. If people visit a couple of times and see the same old thing, they're not apt to return.
- Make it available on your website for people to sign up for your mailing list, newsletter, or free e-zine.
- Remind visitors to bookmark your website.
- Post weekly or monthly specials on your website; people will return to see what they are.
- Have a blog on your website.
- Host a forum on your website so the public can interact.
- Make use of Internet networking, linking, and e-mail to publicize your website (see below).

If you're not Internet savvy, get someone who is comfortable online to help you. The Small Business Administration offers many classes in Internet marketing for a minimal fee of $5 or $10; community colleges have affordable classes, and there are plenty of free tutorials on the web.

Internet Networking

Internet networking doesn't cost a penny, so it's an obvious choice for advertising your business. There are many social and business networking websites available, and the more you participate, the more exposure you'll get. People frequently use the so-called social networks to talk about their business, publish links to their website, and otherwise promote themselves. Some of the most popular are

- Facebook www.facebook.com
- LinkedIn www.linkedin.com
- MySpace www.myspace.com
- Plaxo www.plaxo.com
- SelfGrowth www.selfgrowth.com
- Twitter www.twitter.com

Besides joining as many networks as you can, there are a lot of other steps you can take to get exposure on the Internet, such as visiting and commenting on other people's blogs about massage and/or small businesses. You might have to create a password and a profile in order to be able to comment, so be sure your profile prominently mentions your business.

Words of Wisdom
It's estimated that 70% of employers now search social networking sites before hiring an applicant. It's very possible that potential clients could do the same, so be sure your professionalism is on display.

There are many hundreds of massage and holistic-related communities on the Internet, with forums, link exchanges (see below), chat rooms, classified ads, and discussion boards. My personal favorite is www.massageprofessionals.com. At the time of this writing, there are more than 5000 members, 300+ different groups, and 300+ discussions taking place. People share research, ask each other for advice, and discuss common problems. Join the conversation, and mention your business, your credentials, your area of expertise, your publications, school affiliations, memberships, awards, and anything else that will help you establish yourself in the business world as well as the massage profession. The massage and bodywork community is truly a global community, and it's great to connect with others from all over the world. An investment of time is the only thing required to participate—and that's an investment in the health and longevity of your business.

Be aware that there is a lot of overlap on many of those networks, with both friends and business associates often belonging to the same network. You might want your friends to see the picture you've posted showing you dancing on the bar at your high school reunion, but you don't want your business associates or potential clients or employees to see any such thing. Use common sense and discretion when you're networking on the Internet.

ALTERNATE ROUTES

Employees and Independent Contractors

Even though you're not the business owner, you can still have a personal website to advertise the fact that you're a massage therapist, stating the location where you practice, the business phone number, and a link to that website.

Business Partners

Agree on a company to build and maintain your website. If you're going to do it yourself, determine which partner is responsible for regularly updating the site and taking care of technical problems. Keep a folder with contact information of the contracted administrator or webmaster, domain assignment company, and instructions for updating passwords accessible to all partners, in case circumstances require another partner to take over the website maintenance.

Productive Linking

The Internet is full of opportunities for free links, and you should take advantage of as many as you can. Numerous massage and holistic health websites will let you place a link to your website for free. If you retail products in your practice, many manufacturers will include a link to your website as a distributor, at no cost to you. You can also exchange links with other massage therapists and post your link on any of the social or business networks mentioned above.

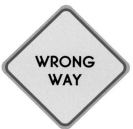

You must be very careful, however, about where your links are placed. As a massage therapist, you do not want connections to your website on any sites that have inappropriate associations, such as adult content, Internet gambling, and dating services. This requires extra diligence, because even if you avoid directly linking to such a site, if you connect to any other site that's linked to those types of sites, you become guilty by association, so to speak. Before placing a link, carefully peruse each site for questionable content and for links to other sites containing questionable content.

Don't forget to link all your own networking sites to your main website and to each other.

SUCCESS NEXT EXIT

EXPLORATIONS

Spend some time on the Internet searching for websites where you would like to place a link as soon as you have your own site. Save them in a specified folder in your bookmarks.

E-mail

E-mail is another good way to promote your business. It's fast and it's free, after the initial cost of your Internet access. As mentioned elsewhere, you can use e-mail to send out newsletters, publicize specials and events, introduce new services you're offering, make announcements about new staff members joining your practice, take customer satisfaction surveys, and even remind people of their appointments.

Words of Wisdom
Save a tree—use e-mail for promotion!

One of the most effective uses of e-mail marketing is the Monday morning e-mail blast. First thing Monday morning, check your schedule and then send out an e-mail similar to this:

Good morning from Mack at Main Street Massage! I have the following appointments available this week: Tuesday at 3 p.m., Thursday at 9 a.m., Friday at 11 a.m., and Friday at 2 p.m. Please call immediately or reply to this e-mail to set up your appointment before they're gone; first come, first served.

It's almost a given that the phone will ring, as people who might have been considering making an appointment are informed that you have only a few left.

E-mail is also a great way to send out a "press release," the same way you'd send one to a newspaper (see Chapter 13). If you belong to the Chamber of Commerce or a merchant's association, you have access to the organization's e-mail list of your fellow members as well; it's one of the benefits of belonging. If you attend a continuing education class and learn new skills, get an article published, make a media appearance, win an award, or have any other noteworthy news, send an e-mail. People will be impressed by your accomplishments—and that's part of business promotion.

Using an e-mail service such as Constant Contact or iContact to manage your bulk communications is convenient and inexpensive. List management, spam filtering, easy-to-use templates, and attractive stationary to make your e-mail more visually appealing and professional looking are just a few of the benefits. You can also schedule communications in advance, allowing you to plan ahead for keeping in touch with your clients.

One caveat: A number of companies sell targeted lists of e-mail addresses, such as people who have visited other massage therapy websites before. Contacting people through e-mail who have never initiated any contact with you, and whose address you've purchased from a third party, is not appropriate. Be sure to follow the rules of e-mail courtesy in Chapter 11.

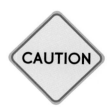

Angela Palmier

"Massage therapy? I like getting a massage, but to make a career out of that? I don't think so." That was the start of my massage therapy career—and that was my quote. Fifteen years ago massage therapy did not have the level of acceptance that it has today, and especially not in Southern Illinois. While I've had multiple roadblocks placed in my path, I never let them get in the way of realizing my goals. I challenge you to accept those "roadblocks" as opportunities to educate, form relationships, and inspire you throughout your career.

Each year, massage therapy schools in the United States graduate about 60,000 students, yet the average life span of a massage therapist is 6.3 years. While those numbers are very sobering for a new therapist, those of us who have not only survived but thrived in this industry have several common characteristics, and I'm honored to share some of the critical factors that have contributed to my success. First, I created a niche. I specialized in treatment of the knee. From a minor to moderate injury or one severe enough to require surgical intervention, I worked very diligently to attain an "expert" status, and referrals came quite easily. When you focus your practice in a specific area, not only does it lend credibility, but it also makes your marketing efforts much more simple and effective.

Second, I recognized the importance of diversification. While I did enjoy the hands-on work, I also knew that by opening myself to other opportunities I wouldn't be limited. Mom was right: Don't put all your eggs in one basket. I became an educator and later cofounded and co-owned a successful massage school. This provided an outlet for me to utilize skills other than the hands-on work.

Third, I owned and continue to own my career. Each and every day I spend time directing and driving my career growth. I research trends in the profession and monitor the activities of the industry stakeholders. Where I find areas of interest or concern, I advocate for or work to protect and enhance the profession I love so much.

A very valuable lesson I've learned is that you need to take care of yourself. Your body must be able to withstand the mental and physical stresses that are prevalent in our profession. Eat, sleep, exercise, always monitor your body mechanics, and get regular massage!

I believe one of the most important things you can do to maintain and promote your business is to give back. Invest in yourself by investing in the profession. Become a mentor, volunteer for professional associations, and support the research that is being done to validate what we as therapists already know. Volunteering for the associations that support the profession through advocacy, education, leadership development, and research is key to ensuring the viability of our profession and thereby assisting you in your career.

Finally, what I consider to be the most important factor in my personal success is finding the right mentor or mentors. Immediately after graduation, and to this very day, I seek out those people who embody the traits that I find to be most important. As my professional goals change, I immediately start searching for a mentor who can help me develop the skills needed to reach those goals. I've even resorted to "mentor stalking." When we cross paths, please ask me all about it! I hope I've inspired you in some way by sharing my story, and I look forward to hearing yours!

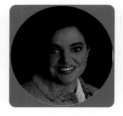

Angela Palmier, along with her business partner, Christopher Alvarado, is the principal of Resource ETC, providing consulting services for schools, instructor training, leadership and volunteer development, as well as facilitating strategic planning sessions for nonprofit and for-profit organizations. Angela is a past President of the American Massage Therapy Association, Illinois Chapter, as well as a donor and volunteer for the Massage Therapy Foundation. To learn more about Angela's work, visit www.resourceetc.com.

SUGGESTED READINGS

American Massage Therapy Association. *Massage Therapy Research.* 2009 Massage Therapy Industry Fact Sheet. http://www.amtamassage.org/news/MTIndustryFactSheet. html. Accessed 02/015/10.

American Research Group, Inc. 10 Rules for More Effective Advertising. http://american-researchgroup.com/adrules/ Accessed 02/05/10.

Cullins J. How to Drive People to Your Site. http://www.sitepronews.com/archives/2002/mar/1.html. Accessed 02/05/10.

Intelesure. Winning Tips and Strategies for Top Performance Advertisi. http://www.intelesure.com/webapp/articles/a6.htmlng. Accessed 02/11/2009.

Waters S. Effective Newspaper Advertisement Types: The Display Ad. http://retail.about.com/od/marketingsalespromotion/a/effective_ads.htm. Accessed 02/05/10.

Webopedia. Text Messaging Abbreviations. http://www.webopedia.com/quick_ref/text-messageabbreviations.asp. Accessed 02/05/10.

My Personal Journey

In this chapter, we've discussed the elements of effective advertising. Using the definitions of the different types of display ads as a guide, create one display ad for each of the five types.

My goals _____

_____

_____

What's in my way? _____

_____

_____

What action can I take to remedy the situation? _____

_____

_____

One-year progress update _____

_____

_____

APPENDIX

Business Forms for Every Need: a Listing of Sample Business Forms and Letters in This Book		
Chapter		**Title of Form**
1	Figure 1-1	A sample self-inventory
1	Figure 1-2	Chronological resume
1	Figure 1-3	Functional resume
1	Figure 1-4	Combination resume
4	Box 4-1	Opening day checklist
4	Box 4-2	Opening day checklist for home practitioners
5	Figure 5-1	Health insurance claim form
5	Figure 5-2	Practitioner's lien
5	Figure 5-3	Intake form
5	Figure 5-4	Statement of informed consent
5	Figure 5-5	Assignment of benefits form
5	Figure 5-6	Authorization to release personal information
6	Figure 6-1	Professional SOAP notes
7	Figure 7-1	Balance sheet
7	Figure 7-2	Profit and loss sheet
7	Figure 7-3	Cash flow statement
7	Figure 7-4	Daily ledger
8	Figure 8-1	Employment agreement for massage therapist (employee)
8	Figure 8-2	Job description for massage therapist (independent contractor)
8	Figure 8-3	Noncompete agreement
9	Figure 9-1	Policy and procedure manual
9	Figure 9-2	Billing for a missed appointment
9	Figure 9-3	Incident report
11	Figure 11-2	Returned check letter
11	Figure 11-3	Client dismissal letter
11	Figure 11-4	Thank you for your referral
11	Figure 11-5	Written warning of disciplinary action
11	Figure 11-6	Professional referral letter
11	Figure 11-7	Professional referral thank you letter
11	Figure 11-8	Professional referral follow-up letter to accompany progress notes
12	Figure 12-1	Client tracking form
13	Figure 13-1	Sample promotional calendar

GLOSSARY

Accounts Payable All money that is owed by a business. *See also* liability.

Accounts Receivable All money that is owed to a business. *See also* asset.

Asset One of any number of tangible items, such as property, equipment, and furnishings, that are owned by a business itself or the owner.

Assignment of Benefits Form A form a client signs that authorizes an insurance company to pay the therapist directly.

Authorization to Release Personal Information A form that authorizes the therapist to share a client's personal and medical information with a third party, such as an insurance company or attorney.

Balance Sheet A document that tracks the financial state of a business, including assets, liabilities, and equity of the owner.

Brand A combination of a concept, symbols, images, experiences, and associations that people attribute to a person, a product, or a business.

Brand Recognition A measurement of the extent to which consumers recall, or recognize, the attributes of a particular brand.

Break-Even Point The point at which business income exceeds expenses.

Budget A statement of the financial position of a business for a definite period of time, based on projected income and expenses.

Business Plan A written summary of the purpose, goals, and strategies for starting a business, including a detailed plan for how the objectives of the business will be accomplished, with projected income and expenses.

Capital Investment The money an owner invests in a business.

Case Study A method of conducting research that relies on an in-depth investigation of an event or condition; rather than a strictly conducted scientific experiment, a case study relies on gathering data and analyzing and reporting the results.

Cash Flow Statement A document that tracks the revenues coming in and expenditures going out of a business during a given time period.

C Corporation A business structure that offers protection of personal assets; partners receive stock in the corporation in exchange for investing money, work, or both; it may be owned by another business entity.

Certified Financial Planner (CFP) A financial planner who has achieved certification through education, examination, experience, and agreeing to abide by ethical business practices.

Code of Ethics A set of rules governing professional moral behavior that practitioners agree to observe while performing their duties as health care providers.

Confidentiality The safeguarding of personal information; keeping private whatever a client shares with a therapist.

Co-Payment The amount of money a client is responsible for paying out-of-pocket at time of service; it may be a set amount or a percentage of the total cost of service.

Corporation A body formed and authorized by law to act as a single person although constituted by one or more persons and legally endowed with various rights and duties, including the capacity of succession and usually protection of personal assets of the owner(s).

Cover Letter A brief introduction to prospective employers that clearly states the job you wish to apply for and highlights the key points of your resume.

Customer Loyalty Program An incentive program that rewards clients with free services after a stated number of visits have been completed.

Daily Ledger A daily record of income and expenses.

DBA (Doing Business As) A method of identifying a business, often used by sole proprietors.

Deductible The amount of money a client is responsible for paying out-of-pocket on an annual basis before insurance will pay; a set amount chosen by the policy holder to suit his particular financial circumstances.

Demographics Data regarding the characteristics of a certain population, such as average income, average age, and average amount of education.

Depreciation Deducting a portion of the original cost of a business asset from taxable income over several years as the value of the asset decreases.

Draw Money taken out by the owner until such time as the amount invested in the business has been returned.

Dual Relationship An association between two people that goes beyond the professional relationship, for example, when a therapist has more than one relationship with a client, such as a familial, friendship, romantic, sexual, or other business connection.

Employee A worker who is paid hourly wages or a set salary, whose schedule and work activities are under the employer's control, and who is subject to withholding tax.

Employer Identification Number (EIN) A number issued by the IRS to identify a business entity, such as a partnership or corporation, for federal tax purposes; also referred to as a federal tax identification number.

Equity The monetary value of a property or business beyond any amounts owed on it.

Executive Summary   An introduction to the business plan that pulls all the key points of the plan together; it appears at the beginning but isn't written until the rest of the plan is complete.

Fee Schedule   An explanation provided by a health insurance company or provider network stating the amount of money that will be paid for services.

Gross Income   The total amount of money a business takes in, before taxes and expenses are paid.

Hard Copy   Paper, as opposed to electronic, documentation or records.

Hardware   The computer, printer, and any accompanying devices.

Health Insurance Claim Form (HICF)   The standardized form used to file an insurance claim; it may be paper or electronic.

Independent Contractor   A worker who is self-employed but conducts business in another's place of employment; is usually paid hourly, by the job or on commission; and is not subject to withholding tax.

Informed Consent   A client's agreement to receive treatment after having been informed of what the treatment will entail.

Intake Form   A form used to collect a client's personal and medical information; can include the statement of informed consent.

Intangible Assets   Business assets that are difficult to put a monetary value on, such as a well-known business name and customer goodwill.

Key Words   Words used as reference points for finding information on the Internet.

Liability   Money owed by the business itself or by the owner on behalf of the business.

Limited Liability Company (LLC)   A relatively new type of business structure that has members instead of shareholders and combines features from other structures.

Major Medical Insurance   An insurance plan that covers the cost of most health care visits, prescription drugs, hospitalization, and other medical equipment and services.

Market Position   A competitive comparison of your business relative to other businesses of the same type in your area.

Market Share   The percentage of the total available market that is being serviced by a business.

Marketing   Any method of promoting a business.

Market Study   The gathering and evaluation of data regarding consumers' preferences for products and services.

Market Survey Analysis   The data collected from a market study compiled into a reader-friendly, summarizing report.

Mission Statement   A concise statement of the goals and purposes of a business.

Mentor   An experienced therapist, businessperson, or other person who can serve as a sounding board, teacher, or trusted counselor.

Net Income   The total amount of money leftover after all taxes and expenses are paid (profit).

Networking   Creating and sustaining mutually beneficial relationships between business owners for support, education, and sharing of ideas and possible referrals.

Overhead   The expenses of operating a business.

Partnership   A legal business relationship between two or more individuals.

PDA (Personal Digital Assistant)   A handheld computer that can be used to send e-mails, keep track of appointments, keep client files, and many of the other tasks a full-size computer can do.

Personal Injury Case   A lawsuit filed by or on behalf of an injured party who believes the injury to be caused by the fault or negligence of another party.

Power Differential   A concept used to describe a relationship between two people who are not peers and thus hold different amounts of power within that relationship.

Practitioner's Lien   A form signed by a client acknowledging he is personally responsible for all payment owed to the therapist, if his insurance doesn't pay all or part of the charges.

Press Release   A no-cost short announcement about something you've accomplished, an event you've participated in or will be participating in, or other pertinent news.

Profit and Loss Sheet   A document that shows whether a business is operating at a profit or a loss; also called income statement.

Provider Network   A list maintained by an insurance company of health care practitioners who have agreed to provide services to their policyholders, usually at a reduced fee, and to abide by all their policies and procedures.

Referral   Recommending a client to another practitioner or specialist.

Referral Reward   An incentive usually offered in the form of discounts on future appointments, to thank clients who have referred you to others.

Residual Approach   Spending only what you can afford after necessary expenses have been covered.

Resume   A document to introduce a job seeker to employers, which details contact information and qualifications such as work experience and education.

ROI (Return on Investment)   The amount of money coming in as a direct result of the money being spent.

Roles and Boundaries   The defined parameters of a therapeutic relationship and each person's part in it.

Scope of Practice   The legal delineation of a professional person's practice, including limits on the breadth of functions that may be performed.

Self-Employment Tax   Social Security and Medicare tax paid by people who work for themselves.

Shareholder   A person who owns stock in a corporation.

Signature Service   An action beyond regular expected service, performed consistently with the intent of impressing the client and setting your business apart from others.

SOAP Notes   A form of documenting client progress during massage sessions. S = Subjective; O = Objective; A = Assessment; P = Plan. Also called progress notes, SOAP notes are used by many health care practitioners.

Software   Computer programs for applications such as word processing, graphic design, and database creation and maintenance.

Sole Proprietorship   A business structure having one owner.

Subchapter S Corporation   A corporation that is taxed different than a C corporation but still offers protection of personal assets; it must be owned by individuals and not by another business entity.

SWOT Analysis   A strategic planning method for evaluating the internal strengths (S) and weaknesses (W) of and external opportunities (O) and threats (T) to a company or business, in order to gain a competitive advantage.

Tangible Assets   Assets of a business, such as equipment, furnishings, and cash on hand.

Therapeutic Relationship   The relationship between a practitioner and a client; includes the observation of confidentiality, reliability, and the mutually agreed upon roles and boundaries of each party in the professional relationship.

Worker's Compensation   Insurance provided by an employer for a worker who is injured on the job.

INDEX

Note: Page numbers followed by "t" indicate table.

RRS1011